CHICAGO STUDIES IN PRACTICES OF MEANING

Edited by Jean Comaroff, Andreas Glaeser, William Sewell, and Lisa Wedeen

Inclusion

The Politics of Difference in Medical Research

STEVEN EPSTEIN

THE UNIVERSITY OF CHICAGO PRESS

Chicago and London

The University of Chicago Press, Chicago 60637
The University of Chicago Press, Ltd., London
© 2007 by Stephen Epstein
All rights reserved. Published 2007.
Printed in the United States of America

21 20 19 18 17 16 15 14 13 12   3 4 5 6 7

ISBN-13: 978-0-226-21310-1 (paper)
ISBN-10: 0-226-21310-2 (paper)

Library of Congress Cataloging-in-Publication Data

Epstein, Steven, 1961–
    Inclusion : the politics of difference in medical research / Steven
Epstein.
        p. ; cm.
    Includes bibliographical references and index.
    ISBN-13: 978-0-226-21309-5 (cloth : alk. paper)
    ISBN-10: 0-226-21309-9 (cloth : alk. paper)
    1. Medicine—Research—Social aspects—United States. 2. Human
experimentation in medicine—Social aspects—United States. 3. Clinical
trials—Social aspects—United States. 4. Minorities—Medical care—
United States. 5. Health and race—United States. 6. Social medicine—
United States. I. Title. [DNLM: 1. Research Subjects—United States.
2. Classification—methods—United States. 3. Cultural Diversity—
United States. 4. Politics—United States. 5. Population Groups—
United States. W 20.5 E64i 2007]
    R853.S64E67 2007
    610.72—dc22

                                                        2006039689

CONTENTS

ACKNOWLEDGMENTS

With a project that has become so enmeshed in my personal and professional life over a period of many years, it is hard to know how to single out for thanks any particular individuals out of all those who have helped me to grow into the person who, along the way, I have become. But it is a great pleasure to be in a position to acknowledge at least some of those debts here. I apologize quite sincerely for the inevitable omissions.

My first and most abundant thanks go to the individuals who agreed to be interviewed for this book. I have never failed to be amazed by the willingness of very busy people to make time for the intrusions of researchers. In addition, several of them, including Pat Dunn, Gary Ellis, Terry McGovern, Curt Meinert, Judy Norsigian, Marty Rouse, Jeanne Stellman, and Eiji Uchida, helpfully provided me with access to research materials.

This project would not have been possible without financial and institutional support from various sources. I am especially grateful to the Robert Wood Johnson Foundation (and to Al Tarlov, David Mechanic, David Colby, Barbara Krimgold, and Lynn Rogut), which provided me not only with an Investigator Award in Health Policy Research but also, as a consequence, with membership in an interdisciplinary community of health policy researchers. Additional crucial funding came from the National Science Foundation's Ethics and Values Studies program (administered by Rachelle Hollander), grant no. SRB-9710423. Any opinions, findings, and conclusions or recommendations expressed in this material are those of the author and do not necessarily reflect the views of the National Science Foundation or the Robert Wood Johnson Foundation. The University of California, San Diego, supported this work in various ways, including through the provision of sabbatical leave, but also through a Hellman Faculty Fellowship in the Arts and Humanities and Social Sciences. I am grateful to the Center for AIDS Prevention Studies at the University of California, San Francisco (and to Tom Coates, Ron Stall, and the administrative staff), for hosting me as a visitor. In addition, I had the benefit of participating in a residential research fellowship at the University of California's Humanities Research Institute at UC-Irvine. I am grateful to David Theo Goldberg and the HRI staff for their assistance, and to the members of the group—organizers Leigh Star and Martha Lampland, along with Geof Bowker, Rogers Hall, Jean Lave, Martin Lengwiler, Janice Neri, Ted Porter, Mimi Saunders, and Judith Treas—for comradeship, productive intellectual exchange, and detailed comments on my work.

The University of California, San Diego, has been a wonderful home to me as I carried out this project. I am grateful to my colleagues in the Department of Sociology and in the Science Studies Program for their encouragement and intellectual feedback. I owe a special debt to UCSD's graduate students for all that I have learned from them. Several of them— Nielan Barnes, Paul Chamba, Christine DeMaria, Josh Dunsby, Mark Jones, David Ribes, and Marisa Smith—served as research assistants for this project. I also am grateful to the Sociology Department staff for their assistance—especially Barbara Stewart (1946–2005), who never failed to express her unqualified support for me and my work.

Many individuals at or associated with the University of Chicago Press have helped to bring this body of work into materialized form. The wise, warm, and witty Doug Mitchell has been a tremendous editor as well as an eloquent conversationalist. Matt Avery, Peter Cavagnaro, Susan Cohen, Liz Demeter, Tim McGovern, Clair James, Catherine Rice, and Maia Rigas all contributed in important ways.

I owe an enormous debt to Tom Gieryn, Kelly Moore, Rayna Rapp, and Stefan Timmermans, each of whom read the entire manuscript in draft form and gave me excellent suggestions on how to improve it. In addition, many colleagues over the years have given me extensive commentary on individual chapters or on associated journal articles. These include the audiences at many colloquia and conferences where I have presented this work. They also include Madeline Akrich, Judy Auerbach, Marc Berg, Chloe Bird, Mary Blair-Loy, Charles Briggs, Héctor Carrillo, Adele Clarke, Peter Conrad, Steve Cornell, Josh Dunsby, Richard Elovich, Kristin Esterberg, John Evans, Anne Figert, Jill Fisher, Scott Frickel, David Theo Goldberg, Jack Goldstone, Sandra Harding, Val Jenness, Mark Jones, David Kirp, Andy Lakoff, Catherine Lee, Paul Lichterman, Margaret Lock, Natalia Molina, Michael Montoya, Ingunn Moser, Dorothy

Nelkin, Nelly Oudshoorn, Trevor Pinch, Ken Plummer, Jonathan Rabinovitz, Jenny Reardon, Chandan Reddy, Annelise Riles, David Rothman, Leslie Salzinger, Andy Scull, Nayan Shah, Steve Shapin, Janet Shim, Susan Silby, John Skrentny, Marisa Smith, Colin Talley, France Twine, Jonathan Warren, Carol Weisman, Meira Weiss, Sarah Wilcox, Howard Winant, Daniel Wolfe, and Mayer Zald.

In addition, many other individuals have given me advice about the project, and I have benefited from intellectual interchange with them. These include Dennis Altman, Olga Amsterdamska, Robert Aronowitz, Ron Bayer, Sam Bozzette, Troy Duster, Jeffrey Escoffier, Wendy Espeland, Andy Feenberg, Shereen El-Feki, Eric Feldman, Cori Hayden, Carol Heimer, Lori Heise, Sheila Jasanoff, Jonathan Kahn, Jerry Karabel, Rick Kronick, Les Levidow, Kristin Luker, Harry Marks, Cal Morrill, Mary-Rose Mueller, Alondra Nelson, Brian Powers, Barbara Hernnstein Smith, David Snow, John Torpey, Paula Treichler, and Jeff Weintraub.

A portion of the material in chapter 12 appeared previously in different form as "Sexualizing Governance and Medicalizing Identities: The Emergence of 'State-Centered' LGBT Health Politics in the United States," *Sexualities* 6, no. 2 (May 2003): 131–71, and is used by permission of Sage Publications Ltd. Isolated paragraphs from other previously published articles can be found scattered throughout this text; those articles include: "Inclusion, Diversity, and Biomedical Knowledge Making: The Multiple Politics of Representation," in *How Users Matter: The Co-Construction of Users and Technology*, ed. Nelly Oudshoorn and Trevor Pinch, 173–90 (Cambridge, MA: MIT Press, 2003); "Bodily Differences and Collective Identities: The Politics of Gender and Race in Biomedical Research in the United States," *Body and Society* 10, nos. 2–3 (2004): 183–203; and "Institutionalizing the New Politics of Difference in U.S. Biomedical Research: Thinking across the Science/State/Society Divides," in *The New Political Sociology of Science: Institutions, Networks, and Power*, ed. Scott Frickel and Kelly Moore, 327–50 (Madison: University of Wisconsin Press, 2006).

I am thankful for all the support I have received from friends over the course of my work on this book, including Sarita Groisser, who scoured the page proofs for typos. My parents, Burt and Bede Epstein, and my sister, Audrey Epstein, have provided unflagging encouragement. My life partner and intellectual companion Héctor Carrillo has played too many roles to enumerate, but I am grateful each day for all of them.

ABBREVIATIONS

ADAMHA	Alcohol, Drug Abuse, and Mental Health Administration
AHRQ	Agency for Healthcare Research and Quality
CDC	Centers for Disease Control and Prevention
CBER	Center for Biologicals Evaluation and Research (FDA)
CCWI	Congressional Caucus for Women's Issues
CDER	Center for Drug Evaluation and Research (FDA)
CRO	contract research organization
DHHS	Department of Health and Human Services
FDA	Food and Drug Administration
GAO	General Accounting Office (U.S. Congress)
ICH	International Conference on Harmonisation of Technical Requirements for Registration of Pharmaceuticals for Human Use
IRB	Institutional review board
JAMA	*Journal of the American Medical Association*
LGBT	Lesbian, gay, bisexual, and transgender
NCI	National Cancer Institute (NIH)
NDA	new drug application
NICHD	National Institute of Child Health and Human Development (NIH)
NIH	National Institutes of Health
NIMH	National Institute of Mental Health (NIH)
OMB	Office of Management and Budget (White House)
OPRR	Office of Protection from Research Risks (NIH) (later replaced by the DHHS's Office for Human Research Protections).
ORWH	Office of Research on Women's Health (NIH)
PhRMA	Pharmaceutical Research and Manufacturer's of America
PHS	Public Health Service (NIH)
SAWHR or SWHR	Society for the Advancement of Women's Health Research (later renamed the Society for Women's Health Research)
WHI	Women's Health Initiative

Health Research and the Remaking of Common Sense

*The orthodoxy of sameness and the orthodoxy of the mean, which has domi-
nated much of the thinking in medical science . . . often impaired our attitude
toward clinical research in those days—we tended to want to reduce the human
to that 60 kilogram white male, 35 years of age, and make that the normative
standard—and have everything extrapolated from that tidy, neat mean, "the
average American male."*

Dr. Bernadine Healy, former director of the
National Institutes of Health

Since the mid-1980s, specific ideas about what it means for humans to
differ have refashioned medical research and practice in the United States.
Two decades of reform—reflected in policies about who gets studied and
how they are studied—have placed group identity and group difference
squarely in view within the biomedical arena.[1] Socially significant categories and characteristics such as sex and gender, race and ethnicity, and
age,[2] used routinely when people assert their belonging or are classified
by others, have taken on a new salience within modern medicine.

That these socially meaningful aspects of personhood divide humanity
into medically distinguishable populations has become a commonplace
assertion, even a cliché:

- "Men and Women Are Different," declared the title of an editorial in
a medical journal in 2004. "Sex differences have been noted in most
major cardiovascular diseases," the author observed, and "medicine is
not exempt from the basic biological fact that men and women are
indeed different, and may need to be treated therapeutically as such."

According to the *New York Times*, researchers "have found that men and women sometimes report different symptoms of the same disease, and that certain drugs are more effective in one sex than the other, or produce more severe side effects in one sex."[3]

- Television news broadcaster Peter Jennings reported in 2002 that hundreds of children die each year from reactions to medications. Because the drugs have not been tested in pediatric populations, these children have become the victims of "guesswork" in the determination of proper dosages.[4]
- In an article about how medical researchers were seeking members of racial minority groups to participate in clinical trials, the *Charleston Post and Courier* quoted a registered nurse and oncology research coordinator in 2005: "When you do a randomized trial with an all-white population, you can only extrapolate to the white population. . . . You don't know if it actually works in African-American or Hispanic populations."[5]
- In 2005, the U.S. Food and Drug Administration (FDA) licensed a pharmaceutical drug called BiDil for treatment of heart failure in African American patients only. Having failed to demonstrate the drug's efficacy in the overall population, BiDil's manufacturers reinvented it as an "ethnic drug" and tested it only on African Americans.[6]

Characteristic of this way of thinking is the assumption that social identities correspond to relatively distinct kinds of bodies—female bodies, Asian bodies, elderly Hispanic male bodies, and so on—and that these various embodied states are medically incommensurable. Knowledge doesn't travel across categories of identity—at least, we can't presume that it does. We are obliged always to consider the possibility that the validity of a medical knowledge claim stops dead when it runs up against the brick wall of difference. While some experts, policymakers, and health advocates have embraced this way of thinking about bodies, groups, and health as obviously valuable, and others have dismissed it as pernicious or silly, my goal is to do neither of the above. I seek to understand, first, how a particular way of thinking about medical difference in the United States helped give rise to an important strategy to improve medical research by making it more inclusive. Second, I intend to show how this strategy gained supporters, took institutional form, and became converted into common sense. Third, I want to shed light on its various consequences for government agencies, biomedical researchers, and pharmaceutical companies, as well as for the social groups targeted by new policies. And finally, by comparing this approach to other ways of thinking about the meanings of identities, differences, and inequalities in biomedical contexts, I aim to understand the extent to which the new common sense might lead to better health and a more just society, as well as the extent to which it either falls short or takes a wrong turn.

An evaluation of the merits of this emphasis on bodily difference might begin by considering a second set of recent claims:

- According to the U.S. National Center for Health Statistics, out of every 1,000 babies born to U.S. mothers whose race was identified as "White" or "Asian or Pacific Islander" or whose ethnicity was "Hispanic or Latino," fewer than 6 died within the first year of life. By contrast, the infant mortality rate (the number of deaths per 1,000 live births) was 8.6 for "American Indian or Alaska Native" mothers, and 13.8 for "Black or African American" mothers.[7]
- According to the same source, a white woman born in the United States in the early twenty-first century could expect, on average, to live 11.5 years longer than an African American man.[8]
- On the basis of a public opinion poll, researchers from Harvard University reported in 2003 that two-thirds of black people in the United States believe that the health care they receive is inferior to that of whites. One in five white respondents agreed with them. Eight out of ten blacks in the study attributed the substandard care to bias, intended or otherwise, on the part of physicians. Only one in five white respondents thought this was the case.[9]

Reports of health disparities—inequalities with regard to health status, access to health care, or experiences within the health care system, measured according to factors such as race, class, gender, geographic location, and sexual identity—have become ubiquitous in recent years.[10] While there is a general sentiment that they constitute a significant social problem, the precise meaning of these disparities has been a matter of some debate.[11] Concern over these disparities also coincides with growing frustration about other problems: the plight of the more than 40 million Americans who lack health insurance (a problem unique to the United States among countries within the so-called developed world), the high price of pharmaceutical drugs, and the quality and character of health care as organized and rationed under the system known as managed care.[12]

Will the new focus on embodied difference lead to the elimination of health disparities? To some extent, the new emphasis that takes categories of human difference as basic units of analysis in medical research and medical treatment has coincided and cooperated with research on these disparities. But in other respects, this way of attending to difference—equating group identities with medically distinct bodily subtypes—has precluded direct attention to reducing inequalities in the domain of health, while encouraging the misleading notion that better health for all can best be pursued through study of the biology of race and sex.[13]

ONE SIZE FITS ALL?

Today's pronouncements about medical differences are often accompanied by self-conscious reflection on social change within biomedical institutions—indeed, by strenuous criticism of past deficiencies. For years, a range of health activists from outside the establishment have issued stinging critiques of neglect by researchers of women, racial and ethnic minorities, and others who have fallen beneath the radar screen.

Well-established biomedical insiders also have had their say. Bernadine Healy, who served as the first (and so far only) female director of the National Institutes of Health (NIH) from 1991 to 1993, commented in 2003 on the worldview that prevailed until relatively recently among medical researchers. When Healy denounced "the orthodoxy of sameness and the orthodoxy of the mean" (see the epigraph at the start of this chapter),[14] she targeted a double whammy of biomedical insensitivity: not only were groups such as women, children, the elderly, and racial and ethnic minorities routinely under-studied in clinical research,[15] but it was assumed that the absence of these groups didn't matter much, because the findings from studying the "normative standard"—middle-aged white men—could simply be generalized to the entire population. Yet the more that researchers have included distinct groups among research subjects, critics have argued, the more it has become apparent that differences do matter and that we cannot just extrapolate medical conclusions from white people to people of color, from men to women, or from middle-aged adults to children or the elderly.

These are not isolated sentiments. Since the mid-1980s, an eclectic assortment of reformers has argued that expert knowledge about human health is dangerously flawed—and health research practices are fundamentally unjust—because of inadequate representation of groups within research populations in studies of a wide range of diseases. The critics have included prominent elected officials, like former member of Congress Patricia Schroeder, who, as cochair of the Congressional Caucus for Women's Issues, asked "Why would NIH ignore half the nation's taxpayers?"[16] Voices calling for change also have come from the ranks of grassroots advocacy groups, clinicians, scientists, professional organizations, and government health officials.

Collectively, reformers have pointed to numerous culprits in the general failure to attend to biomedical difference, but in their bid to change them, they primarily have targeted the state. Reformers have trained their attention on the U.S. cabinet-level Department of Health and Human Services (DHHS) and especially two of its component agencies: the NIH, the world's largest funder of biomedical research, currently providing about $27 billion annually in research grants;[17] and the Food and Drug Administration (FDA), the gatekeeper for the licensing of new therapies for sale.[18] Under pressure from within and without, these federal agencies have ratified a new consensus that biomedical research—now a $94 billion industry in the United States[19]—must become routinely sensitive to human differences, especially sex and gender, race and ethnicity, and age. Academic researchers receiving federal funds, and pharmaceutical manufacturers hoping to win regulatory approval for their company's products, are now enjoined to include women, racial and ethnic minorities, children, and the elderly as research subjects in many forms of clinical research; measure whether research findings apply equally well to research subjects regardless of their categorical identities; and question the presumption that findings derived from the study of any single group, such as middle-aged white men, might be generalized to other populations.

These expectations are codified in a series of federal laws, policies, and guidelines issued between 1986 and the present that require or encourage research inclusiveness and the measurement of difference. The new mandate is reflected, as well, in the establishment, from the early 1980s forward, of a series of new offices within the federal health bureaucracy; these include offices of women's health and offices of minority health that support research initiatives focused on specific populations. Versions of the inclusionary policies also have been adopted by the "institutional review boards" (IRBs) located at universities and hospitals across the United States—the committees that review the ethics of proposals to conduct research on human subjects. As a result, these policies affect not just those researchers seeking federal support or those companies seeking to market pharmaceuticals; they may apply, in some fashion or another, to nearly every researcher in the natural or social sciences performing research involving human beings.

In other words, if indeed we are witnessing a repudiation of so-called one-size-fits-all medicine in favor of group specificity, then the shift is apparent not just in the realm of free-floating ideas. It is anchored to institutional changes—new policies, guidelines, laws, procedures, bureaucratic offices, and mechanisms of surveillance and enforcement—that are the products of collective action. These changes matter for those who carry out medical research on humans: researchers are obliged to alter their work practices to comply with new requirements if they want to get funding, and so must pharmaceutical companies, if they seek to get their products on the market. But the changes also matter downstream: they may affect any person who, now or in the future, becomes obliged to claim the status of "patient." More diffusely, but importantly, they also matter insofar as they alter social understandings of what qualities such as race and gender are taken fundamentally to be.

Yet this redefinition of U.S. biomedical research practice has been little remarked upon by social scientists. Several scholars have provided excellent accounts or analyses of recent attempts to include greater numbers of women in biomedical research.[20] In addition, an important and growing body of literature by science studies scholars, while not precisely focused on questions of research inclusion, is analyzing how concepts of race are used in biomedicine—especially, new scientific attempts to take findings from the genetic study of populations and use them to make claims about the medical meaning of race.[21] However, there has been almost no scholarly attention to the broad-scale attempt to dethrone the "standard human" and mandate a group-specific approach to biomedical knowledge production—an identity-centered redefinition of U.S. biomedical research practice that encompasses multiple social categories.[22]

I call this set of changes in research policies, ideologies, and practices, and the accompanying creation of bureaucratic offices, procedures, and monitoring systems, the "inclusion-and-difference paradigm."[23] The name reflects two substantive goals: the inclusion of members of various groups generally considered to have been underrepresented previously as subjects in clinical studies; and the measurement, within those studies, of differences across groups with regard to treatment effects, disease progression, or biological processes.

This way of thinking and doing is by no means the only, or the most important, way in which biomedical research has changed in recent decades. During those same years, as the sociologist Adele Clarke and her coauthors have noted, medicine itself has been remade "from the inside out"—through innovations in molecular biology, genomics, bioinformatics, and new medical technologies; through vast increases in public and private funding for biomedical research; through the ascendance of evidence-based medicine; through the rapid expansion of a global pharmaceutical industry constantly searching for new markets and engaging in new ways with consumers; and through the resurgence of dreams of human enhancement or perfectibility by means of biotechnologies.[24] The point, then, is not to understand how the inclusion-and-difference paradigm has changed "medicine," as if the latter were a fixed target, but rather to consider how this particular emphasis has intersected with the other transformations that have taken place in the domain of biomedical research and the health care sector generally.

The Time and Place of Difference

Although a shift away from the inclusion-and-difference paradigm could certainly occur, at present this model is reasonably well institutionalized within DHHS agencies. Unlike policies that depend for their survival on the support of a particular politician, bureaucrat, or political party in power, the inclusion-and-difference paradigm has sunk roots and seems to have developed its own staying power. It grew up in the Republican administrations of the 1980s and early 1990s, flourished under the Democratic administration of President Bill Clinton, and mostly has survived—despite some explicit attempts to roll it back and halt its expansion—under Republican President George W. Bush.

Interestingly, formal policies concerning inclusion and difference in biomedicine are mostly restricted to the United States—at least so far. Biomedical research and pharmaceutical drug development are increasingly global industries that crisscross national borders, and it is not unreasonable to imagine that policies promoted by a dominant player will diffuse gradually to other countries or that those countries, on their own, will adopt similar institutional responses. To date this has happened to a limited extent, and not without resistance. This peculiarity explains why I focus on the United States, a narrowing of gaze that otherwise might seem surprising when tracking a global industry. I argue that the nation-state, as well as national political struggles, remain powerful contributors to the definitions of medical and social policies, categories, and identities.[25] Many of the policies that I consider are, if not specific to the United States, then applicable only to those persons or firms seeking U.S. federal funding or regulatory approval. However, given the prominence of the United States in this arena—organizations headquartered in the United States account for about 70 percent of the global drug development pipeline[26]—the consequences of U.S. policies for the rest of the world are not insubstantial. And the general questions concerning the medical management of difference have implications for every country that engages in social and technological practices of differentiation and difference-making across human subgroups—that is to say, all of them.

The nation-specific character of this response to difference also has important implications for the framing of the analysis. To the extent that these concerns appear at present to have a special resonance in the United States, then it would not make sense to attribute their emergence into public debate to any inexorable law of scientific or social progress. Instead, the approach will be to look closely at U.S. culture, politics, and history and the particularities of U.S. biomedical and political institutions to explain why debates about identity and difference have left such a distinctive and indelible mark on biomedicine in this country in the late twentieth and early twenty-first centuries. Rather than treating the inclusion-and-difference paradigm as an obvious scientific development, this analysis examines why new understandings about research and human differences have emerged in the United States and supplanted the common sense that prevailed previously.

Of course, it is not hard to imagine why appeals to include women, minorities, and other groups in biomedical research might acquire traction in the United States in recent years. In the wake of what has been called the "minority rights revolution,"[27] U.S. political culture now typically promotes equality of opportunity and diversity as worthy social goals, though remedies such as affirmative action have been under increasing attack. And the idea of the United States as a multicultural society has become much more taken for granted, even in the face of resistance.[28] Compared to other countries, the United States is also typically seen as a place where "identity politics"—the assertion of political claims in relation to social identities such as "woman," "Latino," or "Native American"— looms large.[29] Even though the phenomenon that the sociologist John Lie has called "modern peoplehood"—the formation of "an inclusionary and involuntary group identity with a putatively shared history and a distinct way of life"—is everywhere present, certain countries, such as the United States, are more likely to establish policies with respect to these categories, while others seek instead to subsume difference under a broader conception of national citizenship.[30] Finally, given the particular prominence and cultural authority of the biosciences in the United States, it seems not unlikely that this country would witness the emergence of what might be called "bio-multiculturalism."[31]

Yet this program for the medical recognition of difference has gone against the grain of powerful trends toward standardization within biomedicine during the same recent decades in the United States—universalizing tendencies reflected in the movement to develop uniform, evidence-based guidelines for patient care, as well as efforts by both the FDA and the pharmaceutical industry to standardize the drug approval process across national borders.[32] And conversely, the focus on broad social categories, such as women, also has contrasted with the alternative ideology of personalized medicine, the plan to target therapies at the individual.[33] Thus, when viewed against the backdrop of dominant tendencies within biomedicine—emphases on the universal and the individual—the group-based inclusion-and-difference paradigm would seem to lie betwixt and between.

Moreover, the implementation of new inclusionary policies and practices encountered concrete resistance on multiple fronts. Some critics rejected the empirical claim that groups such as women in fact had been under-studied. Defenders of scientific autonomy opposed the politicizing of research and argued that it should be up to scientists, not policymakers, to determine the best ways to conduct medical experiments. Conservatives decried the intrusion of "affirmative action," "quotas," and "political correctness" into medical research. Ethicists and health activists expressed concern about the risks of subjecting certain groups, such as children, to the risks of medical experimentation in large numbers. Statisticians and experts on the methodology of the randomized clinical trial argued that requiring comparisons of population subgroups was not only scientifically unsound but also fiscally unmanageable and that it might bankrupt the research enterprise. And many proponents of medical universalism argued that biological differences are less medically relevant than fundamental human similarities: when it comes right down to it, they insisted, people are people. Claims about racial differences, in particular, seemed to sit poorly alongside well-publicized findings by geneticists that, on average, genetic differences within the groups commonly called races are actually greater than the genetic differences between those groups.[34] If racial classifications are biologically dubious, why were legislators and health policymakers calling for labeling research participants by race and testing for racial difference in clinical studies? Some critics went further, charging that the new medical understandings of race and sex differences were eerie echoes of social prejudices from the past, when scientific reports of bodily differences had provided a veneer of respectability to claims that both women and people of color were not just socially, but biologically, inferior.

Given these varied arguments against the new policies and the logic behind them, we should not take for granted the rise of inclusion and the measurement of difference—still less the particular forms these have taken. The birth and maturation of this paradigm require explanation. Indeed, the more we examine the new inclusionary policies, the less obvious they appear—and hence the more we can learn by studying them in depth.

For example, the whole premise of the reforms is to reverse a past history of exclusion and inequality—but, as is so often the case, "history" here is a contestable matter. To what degree can it be established that medical research used to focus on middle-aged, white men and took them to be the norm or standard? And how much have research practices really changed in response to the new policies? Has there been a revolution in medical knowledge-making? Another set of questions concerns the unexamined choices embedded within the inclusionary remedy: Out of all the ways by which people differ from one another, why should it be assumed that sex and gender, race and ethnicity, and age are the attributes of identity that are most *medically* meaningful? Why these markers of identity and not others? And are there differences among these types of difference, such that the same policy remedies may not be appropriate for each case? In the most general sense, how can we know when to assume that any particular way of differing might have medical consequences? And when is it proper to invoke the unity of the human species—to assert that a body is a body is a body?

Pros and Cons

At least in part, this wave of reform offers an important and valuable corrective to past medical shortsightedness. It exemplifies the more general point, made by feminist theorists and theorists of multicultural citizenship, that sometimes the pursuit of genuine social equality requires policies that *do not* treat everyone the same—policies that affirm group rights and establish new practices of group representation.[35] These reforms also are broadly consistent with the important perception, expressed variously by feminist theorists and science studies scholars, that the formal knowledge of experts sometimes may be improved through the contributions or redirections introduced by those who have been made marginal to the knowledge production enterprise.[36]

But an emphasis on difference-making also rightly invokes concern when difference essentially is taken to be a biological attribute of a group. These, too, are very contemporary preoccupations: in 2005, Lawrence Summers, the president of Harvard University, ignited a fiery debate when he wondered aloud whether the underrepresentation of women in science and engineering professions might actually reflect innate differences between the sexes.[37] Attempts to treat racial differences as biologically based—as in, for example, the claim that I.Q. tests or other standardized tests track natural differences in mental ability between racial groups—likewise have proven resilient, though they, too, have been the subject of much criticism.[38] To the degree that the inclusion-and-difference paradigm also suggests—albeit in a nonpejorative way—that biology is fundamental in distinguishing races and genders, its logic appears consistent with these other rhetorical moves.

How then, should the inclusion-and-difference paradigm be evaluated? If it were a simple matter of declaring these changes "good" or "bad," the case would be far less interesting than it turns out to be. My strategy will be to link an investigation of the causes and consequences of these new policies and practices with a detailed analysis of their associated cultural and political logic, including ways of standardizing and classifying human beings, beliefs about the meaning of difference, and possibilities for establishing "biopolitical citizenship." On the basis of that analysis, I will argue that although reformers' characterizations of the biomedical *status quo ante* were not entirely accurate, they nonetheless did bring attention to a real and important problem. And the solutions that have fallen into place, while imperfectly designed, have in some respects been positive and praiseworthy from the standpoint of both improved health and social justice—even if a formalistic emphasis on compliance with rules sometimes has obscured or interfered with the substantive goals that originally animated the reforms.[39]

However, I also will argue that these reforms have unintended consequences that merit especially close study. By approaching health from the vantage point of categorical identity, they ignore other ways in which health risks are distributed in society. By valorizing certain categories of identity, they conceal others from view. By focusing on groups, they obscure individual-level differences, raising the risk of improper "racial profiling" or "sex profiling" in health care. By treating each of the recognized categories in a consistent fashion, they often ignore important differences across them. And by emphasizing the biology of difference, they encourage the belief that qualities such as race and gender are biological in their essence, as well as the mistaken conclusion that social inequalities are best remedied by attending to those biological particularities. While the inclusion-and-difference paradigm is certainly preferable to any narrow biomedical practice of exclusion, and while it may generate useful knowledge for specific purposes, the net effect of these unintended consequences is to make it a problematic tool for eliminating health disparities. Rather than tackle the problem of health disparities head on, we have adopted an oblique strategy that brings with it a new set of difficulties.

EXPLAINING CHANGE IN BIOMEDICAL POLICY

Many different sorts of people helped promote the new inclusionary policies described in this book, or worked to implement them, or opposed them, or have had to grapple with their implications. To research this book, I interviewed past and present DHHS officials, clinical researchers, experts on pharmacology, biostatisticians, medical journal editors, drug company scientists, health advocates and activists, bioethicists, members of Congress, congressional aides, lawyers, representatives of pharmaceutical company trade associations, experts in public health, and social scientists.[40] I also analyzed an enormous number of print and electronic materials in which notions of inclusion and difference have been discussed or debated. These included government documents and reports; archival materials from health advocacy organizations; materials from pharmaceutical companies and their trade organizations; articles, letters, editorials, and news reports published in medical, scientific, and public health journals; and articles, editorials, letters, and reports appearing in the mass media. Finally, I attended conferences at which issues of inclusion and difference were discussed. Juxtaposing different kinds of evidence coming from different occupational groups and "social worlds" concerned with these issues has helped me to acquire the depth and breadth needed for an informed historical account and a fair analysis.[41]

Analyzing the many issues raised in this book also obliged me to delve deeply into a wide range of academic literatures and develop new approaches from their intersections. In chapter 1, I build the theoretical foundations for this book by drawing on various fields, including science studies, political sociology, and critical studies of gender and race. This fruitful mix of approaches, and the hybrid concepts that arise from it, provide me with the tools I need to piece together the story—which begins in earnest in chapter 2.[42]

In terms of their goals, the empirical chapters then divide roughly into two. Chapters 2 through 7 trace the making of the inclusion-and-difference paradigm. They consider how an unlikely set of reforms made their way into common sense, despite heated opposition from those who saw them as political correctness run amok, and how abstract ideas about bodies, truth, and equity were "operationalized" and took institutional form. Chapters 8 through 12 take the story further by exploring the various social and medical consequences of the adoption of these reforms— for government agencies charged with enforcing them, for medical researchers and pharmaceutical companies who have to comply with them, and for the social groups under study, such as racial minorities and women. More specifically, in telling the story, I proceed by addressing the following questions:

To what degree was there a "standard human" in biomedical research, prior to the recent reform wave (*chapter 2*)? This chapter argues that the recent debates over who gets studied in biomedical research must be located within a longer history of the selection of humans as experimental objects in biomedicine. While certain questions—such as the precise demographics of research participation in the past—are not fully answerable given available data, I suggest that we can learn much from that history about changing medical notions of sameness and difference. I examine the variety of ways in which medical researchers have selected their research subjects—often from among those most socially disadvantaged—as well as the shifts over time in the perceived desirability of generalizing conclusions across groups. I emphasize the point that, until recently, medical emphases on differences—such as those between women and men or between black people and white people—were closely linked with social notions of superiority and inferiority. In other words, there is a deep irony in the current attempts to use claims about biomedical difference as the basis of a liberal and egalitarian social policy.

What was the nature of the reform coalition that developed to challenge a reliance on the "standard human"? What were the distinctive ways in which reformers framed their arguments (*chapter 3*)? Here I analyze the ways in which critics of the medical reliance on the "standard human" launched a loosely related series of "antistandardization resistance movements" that insisted on the importance of differences. This chapter analyzes the political rhetoric of a diverse group of reformers—health advocacy organizations, health professionals, grassroots social movements, members of Congress, insiders within the DHHS, and others. I trace how these reformers questioned the legitimacy of current biomedical practice and how they brought political and ethical arguments about representation and citizenship together with scientific arguments about the importance of studying difference.

How did reformers achieve their first successes? What accounted for the potency of their critiques (*chapter 4*)? In this chapter I tell the story of how reformers targeted two key state agencies, the NIH and the FDA, and how they achieved their first important victories in the early 1990s. I present the concept of "categorical alignment"—the merging of social categories from the worlds of medicine, social movements, and state administration—to shed additional light on reformers' successes. I also examine the special characteristics of the reformers' political alliances, their complex "multirepresentational" work, and their claims for a new kind of citizenship as manifested by biomedical inclusion.

How did controversy develop around the proposed reforms, and how was this controversy settled (*chapter 5*)? Having tracked the reformers' actions and arguments, I next examine the claims of opponents of the new policies mandating inclusion and the measurement of difference. In addition to researchers, politicians, and pharmaceutical companies, these opponents included statisticians and experts on clinical trial design, who maintained that the policies made no medical sense and that reformers simply failed to comprehend the logic of scientific generalization as employed in the arena of clinical research. I then analyze the roles of DHHS employees in finding creative ways of institutionalizing the reform mandate and, to a substantial degree, settling the controversy. These officials performed crucial "boundary work"—reestablishing an accepted divide between the realms of science and politics, with the new policies located on the "science" side of the boundary.[43] This work was critical not only for the legitimacy of science, but also for the ability of DHHS agencies to defend their jurisdiction and autonomy.

What is the nature of the "new regime"? And what has become of the "standard human" (*chapters 6 and 7*)? The inclusion-and-difference paradigm is no abstract idea; it is undergirded by an infrastructure of procedural standards, encoded in regulations, and enforced and overseen by new bureaucratic offices. Here I sketch the various policies that came to constitute the inclusion-and-difference paradigm over the course of the 1990s and into the twenty-first century, and I analyze how the paradigm has become institutionalized within the DHHS. I also examine the new standard operating procedures that govern biomedical knowledge production.

I then extend my analysis of the workings of the inclusion-and-difference paradigm by considering the abstract debate between universal, standardized approaches to medicine and policy (treating everyone the same as everyone else) and individualized approaches (recognizing the uniqueness of each person). I argue that the inclusion-and-difference paradigm is a form of what I call "niche standardization" that bypasses this polar opposition between universalism and individualism in order to standardize at the level of the social group.[44] I describe how DHHS officials developed policies, procedures, and classification schemes that have shored up this niche standardization. These officials, along with researchers, played a central role in "operationalizing" sex, gender, race, ethnicity, and age for biomedical purposes—transforming these dimensions of social reality into "variables" whose effects can be measured in quantitative terms. However, this work of formalizing, standardizing, and operationalizing has not been able to paper over the extraordinary difficulties that may sometimes arise when researchers or federal health officials attempt to sort human beings into categorical boxes.

How has the work of government agencies been affected by the new policies? How successful have officials been in monitoring and enforcing the policies? To what degree has enforcement brought about real changes in medical research practices (*chapter 8*)? In this chapter I examine how DHHS agencies such as the FDA and the NIH have trained their attention on ensuring compliance with inclusionary policies. At the same time, I use the debates about the success of these enforcement efforts to investigate some of the real-world effects of the paradigm. I examine various measurable effects of the paradigm on academic research and pharmaceutical drug development, and I consider the complaints both of those who think the changes have gone too far and those who think they have not gone far enough. In examining the mixed success of reform, I explain why neither of these sets of critics is likely to be satisfied. However, I also consider some of the other—direct and indirect—ways in which the new policies have affected the world of biomedicine, including medical journals, medical education, and the pharmaceutical industry.

What are the implications of the inclusion-and-difference paradigm for the task of recruiting people to serve as research subjects (*chapter 9*)? Because the new policies create strong pressures for researchers to diversify their study populations, they have prompted a renewed interest in the practical problem of finding and convincing different sorts of people to participate in medical experiments. Not only must researchers find willing subjects, not only must those subjects be diverse, but the groups which researchers must represent include those, such as African Americans, that routinely are considered among the most difficult of all to convince to participate. The historical ironies are also profound. The new mandates enjoin researchers to study groups that, in some cases, were horribly exploited by medical researchers in the not-so-distant past—for example, in the infamous Tuskegee study of "untreated syphilis in the Negro male."[45] In this chapter I trace the origins of what might be considered a new field of empirical study—I call it "recruitmentology"—that seeks to develop scientific evidence about the best ways successfully to enroll so-called hard-to-recruit populations for clinical studies. In evaluating the success of recruitmentology, I consider the inability of the inclusion-and-difference paradigm to resolve the tension between the increased pressure to recruit and the longtime, vexing problem of establishing trust in the relationship between researchers and research subjects.

What are the implications of this reform wave for how difference is understood within biomedicine? What, therefore, are the effects of reform on those most directly targeted by it, such as women and racial and ethnic minority groups (*chapters 10 and 11*)? In these two chapters, I argue that biomedical research does not, in neutral fashion, simply absorb and reflect ideas about sex, gender, race, and ethnicity that are prevalent in society. Rather, biomedicine is a domain in which conceptions of identity and difference actively get worked out in practice. In this sense, the policies that make up the inclusion-and-difference paradigm play a role in refashioning and redefining the very meanings of social categories and attributes. In chapter 10, I advance this argument by examining the heated debates over "racial profiling" in medicine—prescribing treatments to patients on the basis of their racial membership—and I argue that this practice may work to the detriment of the health of individual patients.

Then, in chapter 11, I examine the case of sex and gender, analyzing the emerging philosophy known as "sex-based biology" or "gender-specific medicine." Here I present a double argument: On one hand, sex/gender is a different case from race/ethnicity, because the biological and the social intertwine in different ways, and that means that the tendency for various forms of difference to be "handled" in the same ways by the inclusionary policies may be problematic. But on the other hand, much of the critique directed at racial profiling may also apply to sex profiling—which raises interesting questions about why the former has been the subject of much debate while the latter has not.

What is the trajectory of the paradigm? What other groups may "qualify" for inclusion? Will the paradigm be extended or rolled back (*chapter 12*)? In this chapter I raise questions about where the paradigm may be heading, including whether it will be extended to encompass other identities. A primary case that I consider in this chapter is the attempt by lesbian, gay, bisexual, and transgender health advocates to include sexual orientation and gender identity as dimensions of difference whose salience is authorized by federal health policy. I also examine how well the paradigm holds up in hostile political climates, as well as to what degree it is creeping into the discourse and practice of nations other than the United States.

Finally, in the conclusion, I summarize my findings on the meanings of these reforms and their consequences, both intended and unintended, as well as the implications of this case for the study of biomedical politics. I then consider alternative pathways: How might things be otherwise? What are other ways of conceiving of the problem and its solutions? I address the issue of alternatives with reference to conceptions of clinical research, notions of public participation in biomedical debates, debates over identity politics, and the fundamental issue of inequality in the domain of health.

CHAPTER ONE

How to Study a Biopolitical Paradigm

This book tells a story about the politics of how human beings are known, classified, administered, and treated. At the center is the idea of what I call the "inclusion-and-difference paradigm"—the research and policy focus on including diverse groups as participants in medical studies and in measuring differences across those groups.

The word *paradigm* has become ubiquitous in recent years, and my use of it requires explanation. My goal is not to resurrect historian and philosopher of science Thomas Kuhn's familiar (but oft-criticized) account of decisive shifts over time in how communities of scientific practitioners look at the world.[1] "Inclusion-and-difference" is not a paradigm in the strict Kuhnian sense, because it does not constitute the central set of assumptions guiding any scientific specialty group, nor is it restricted to any single such group.[2] Neither am I claiming (as the use of Kuhn's term might lead some to imagine) that the new emphasis on inclusion and difference is a thoroughgoing medical "revolution," marked by ideas that are radically incommensurable with those they replaced.

Instead, the inclusion-and-difference paradigm should be understood as an example of what I term a "biopolitical paradigm." Building on Peter Hall's concept of the policy paradigm[3] and Michel Foucault's characterization of biopolitics,[4] I define biopolitical paradigms as frameworks of ideas, standards, formal procedures, and unarticulated understandings that specify how concerns about health, medicine, and the body are made the simultaneous focus of biomedicine and state policy. The inclusion-and-difference paradigm is one such biopolitical paradigm, both because it reflects the presumption that health research is an appropriate and important site for state intervention and regulation and because it infuses the life sciences with new political import. While some might see the inclusion-and-difference paradigm as an example of how biomedicine (for better or for worse) gets politicized, it might just as well be taken as evidence of the converse—how, in the present period, governing gets "biomedicalized." Medical research thereby becomes reconceived as a domain in which a host of political problems can get worked out—the nature of social justice, the limits and possibilities of citizenship, and the meanings of equality and difference at the biological as well as social levels.[5]

The label "inclusion-and-difference paradigm" is my own invention, and no one within the DHHS, the pharmaceutical industry, or the academic world of clinical research uses the term. But this distinctive approach to health research policy can be seen as built into the standard operating procedures, discourse, and organizational structure of the DHHS, and it stretches out from there into a wide range of biomedical contexts. As a biopolitical paradigm, the inclusion-and-difference approach hybridizes scientific and state policies and categories. Specifically, it takes two different areas of concern—the meaning of biological difference and the status of socially subordinated groups—and weaves them together by articulating a distinctive way of asking and answering questions about the demarcating of subpopulations of patients and citizens.

STUDYING KNOWLEDGE, POLITICS, AND DIFFERENCE

Describing and analyzing biopolitical paradigms is impossible except by carefully amalgamating academic literatures that are more typically kept apart. Yet bringing these literatures together is a crucial task for scholars concerned with key features of the modern world. The issues raised in this book point to the intersections among three broad arenas of scholarly investigation: *knowledge formation* (how medical truths about human beings are uncovered), the *politics of institutional change* (how social movements and other political actors transform scientific, governmental, and corporate practices), and the *making of identity and difference* (how the human population is divided and what meaning is assigned to stratifying terms such as race and gender). In this chapter, I assemble my toolkit for studying these three arenas jointly.

As an analysis of how medical knowledge is made and how the population of humans and its relevant subgroups come to be known, this book is rooted in social and cultural studies of science, technology, and medicine. Science studies (for short) has focused attention on how scientific practitioners organize their work activities; make claims about knowledge and strive to endow those claims with credibility; and defend, or extend, the boundaries of their practice.[6] Increasingly, scholars working from this framework have turned their attention to understanding biomedical research,[7] as well as the ways in which human bodies, in all their organic, cellular, and genetic distinctiveness, appear to take on an ever more central role in defining our selves, our identities, and our places within the society and the polity.[8]

At the same time, especially since the mid-1990s, the field of science studies has moved decisively "beyond the lab" to analyze—in all their complexity, variability, and volatility—the broader dimensions of public engagement with science and technology. Recently this shift has found expression under quite a number of different banners: the "new political sociology of science," which unites science studies with sociological approaches to the study of power, the state, and organizations;[9] "co-production," which proposes "that the ways in which we know and represent the world (both nature and society) are inseparable from the ways in which we choose to live in it;[10] a focus on the "knowledge society," and study of "epistemic cultures" and their "machineries of knowing"[11]; studies of the participation of social movements or other "concerned groups" in questions relating to science and technology;[12] and work that tracks the forging of various new forms of citizenship.[13] (The list of new approaches could easily be extended.) Although these diverse reformulations or extensions of the project of science studies are by no means entirely compatible, I rely on them collectively to orient me in certain important directions—especially, an institutional focus, and a concern with questions of participation and citizenship.

Institutional Focus

Because this book is a study of how policies, practices, and facts emerge out of conflict and compromise, I am especially interested in understanding both the broader structuring of conflict and the processes by which social and scientific changes come to take an institutionalized form. I attend, therefore, to what Kelly Moore and Scott Frickel have called the "rules and routines, meanings, organizations, and resource distributions that shape knowledge production systems."[14] Such an approach takes seriously the enabling and constraining effects of social structures on those whose work involves or intersects with biomedical science.[15]

My entry point to these concerns is less immediately at either the macro level of abstraction ("the state," "the market," "science") or the micro level of particularity (the realm of face-to-face interaction or embodied practice) but is located more at what Diane Vaughan has called the "meso" level of the organization[16]—for example, the government agency, the pharmaceutical company, the advocacy group, or the research institution. As Vaughan has emphasized, organizations function as powerful machineries of knowing that "can complicate and manipulate the entire knowledge-production process"—changing how people and objects are understood; discouraging certain domains of inquiry while encouraging others; and "requiring classification systems and standardized documents that regiment, restrict and reduce experience and understanding into easy digestible and communicable abstractions from more complex, dynamic interactions and situational logics."[17]

The analytical approach that I describe here—a structural and cultural analysis of the "rules and routines, meanings, organizations, and resource distributions that shape knowledge production systems"[18]—is also consistent with particular ways of analyzing the state, social movements, and social institutions that have emerged in recent years. Taking my cue from others who have called for the "disaggregation of the monolithic entity of the state," I approach "the state" through attention to particular agencies and offices and with an understanding that the practices carried on within them may sometimes merge seamlessly with ones conducted "outside" the state.[19] This formulation, which challenges the accepted notion of a sharp dividing line between state and society, is consistent with work that reveals the inextricability of science and the state in the modern West and traces the history of technoscientific activity within processes of state formation.[20] It is likewise consistent with a number of ways of approaching the study of social movements as they interact with the state: recognizing that social movements are sometimes inside as well as outside state agencies;[21] appreciating that social movements challenge many institutions and not simply the state;[22] and observing the powerful effects of social movements in transforming organizational behavior.[23] All of these approaches are helpful in thinking about a sequence of changes in biomedical research practices that are, at the same time, changes in the administrative and classificatory practices of state and market organizations.

Lay Participation and Citizenship

The stunning advances in the life sciences in the twentieth century have paved the path for what Nikolas Rose has called "vital politics," where matters of health, illness, risk, suffering, and life itself move to center stage.[24] In recent years, as questions of health and illness have been recast as thoroughly political matters, more and more ordinary citizens, often organized into patient advocacy groups or broader social movements, have demanded a say in how scientists and health professionals go about their work, tossing aside the presumption that technical matters are best left up to the experts.[25] I will argue that the creation of the inclusion-and-difference paradigm reflects this participatory impulse to some degree—though I also will show that these policy changes were not brought about by a lay social movement, pure and simple, but rather by a hybrid coalition linking health advocates with experts, bureaucrats, and policymakers.

The language of citizenship—understood here to refer to differentiated modes of incorporation of individuals or groups fully or partially into the national polity through the articulation of notions of rights and responsibilities—is also relevant in understanding this case.[26] The program for inclusion of previously underrepresented groups in biomedical research reflected more than a desire for "representation" in a purely statistical sense: it also suggested a demand for *political* representation and for inclusion in the polity and society more generally. Therefore, I will treat this case as an instance of a broader class of phenomena to which science studies scholars increasingly have been devoting attention—a cluster of concepts labeled variously as "biological citizenship," "genetic citizenship," "therapeutic citizenship," and "sanitary citizenship," but that might all be characterized as "biopolitical citizenship."[27]

As Adriana Petryna described it in her analysis of Ukrainian survivors of the Chernobyl nuclear disaster, such terms apply to moments when the "biology of a population has become the grounds for social membership and the basis for staking citizenship claims."[28] This concept calls attention to what Paul Rabinow has called "biosociality": the ways in which various sorts of classifications created, or given a transformed meaning, by the life sciences—for example, all those who share a disease, a treatment, a genetic risk factor, an exposure, or even a sex or a race—provide a basis for affiliation.[29] But the concept of biopolitical citizenship also points to the politically contested nature of claiming those groupings and saying what they "really mean." Finally, by emphasizing the varying degrees to which different people or groups actually are able to lay claim to the full rights and prerogatives of citizenship, the concept impels a consideration of the role of biomedical authorities and technologies in reproducing or transforming practices of social stratification and exclusion—as well as the role of others in resisting those authorities.[30]

PROCESSES

The amalgam of theoretical and conceptual resources that I bring to bear in this book—including the institutional approach and the concern with lay participation and citizenship described above—is suited to the study of a diverse set of actors, objects, or entities: bodies, groups, populations, citizens, movements, coalitions, researchers, professionals, firms, politicians, and state agencies. However, it may be easier to grasp my use of these tools through a shift in focus from nouns to verbs—that is, to the kinds of *processes* that the above-named entities are engaged in and emerge out of. Three such processes—simultaneously scientific, political, and cultural—are at the crux of the concerns in this book: *classifying*, *generalizing*, and *standardizing*.[31] I take these up in turn.

Classifying

Science studies scholars, along with many others, have had much to say about the broader phenomenon of classification—the practices that establish the boundaries of "being the same as" and "being different from," so that we know what belongs where. The work of Geof Bowker and Susan Leigh Star is exemplary in calling attention to the centrality of classification to modern science and, indeed, nearly every domain of modern life. Building on the contributions of Mary Douglas and Michel Foucault, Bowker and Star have analyzed how systems of classification reflect prevailing hierarchies of power and serve to shape both moral and social order.[32] These analyses dovetail nicely with those of scholars from other fields. As Paul Starr has observed, official classifications "are sewn into the fabric of the economy, society and the state" and provide incentives for action of all sorts.[33] In modern, formally democratic polities, governments are often placed in the business of designating "corporate identities," to use Seyla Benhabib's term—those group identities that come to be "officially recognized, sanctified, legitimized, and accepted by the state and its institutions."[34] Determining such identities inevitably remakes the map of political opportunities to the extent that benefits are distributed on the basis of categorical membership.[35]

Even more emphatically, Pierre Bourdieu referred to systems of social categorization as "the stakes, par excellence, of political struggle";[36] and he emphasized the tremendous power of the modern state "to produce and impose . . . categories of thought that we spontaneously apply to all things of the social world" and to assert "common principles of vision and division."[37] However, as others have insisted, no state can fully monopolize the power to classify, and "the literature on social movements . . . is rich in evidence on how movement leaders challenge official identifications and propose alternative ones."[38] Indeed, work on modern, identity-oriented social movements has suggested that self-naming and self-classifying are among their most consistent preoccupations.[39] And in other settings of everyday life, ordinary people constantly " 'perform' their differences and similarities" in ways that define and redefine group classifications.[40] Thus, a wide range of actors and institutions—including scientists studying difference, activists asserting identities, policymakers monitoring practices, and firms marketing products—may participate, collude, or compete in projects of human classification.

Ultimately, many of the most contested and socially resonant classifications—"race" being a prominent example—have taken their meaning historically through the complex interplay among scientific, administrative, and popular definitions and practices, and have become irreducibly hybrid as a consequence. In Ian Hacking's terms, these categories are "interactive kinds"—that is, "classifications that, when known by people or by those around them, and put to work in institutions, change the ways in which individuals experience themselves—and may even lead people to evolve their feelings and behaviors in part because they are so classified."[41]

Generalizing

Of particular relevance to this case is the investigation by science studies scholars into the problem of generalizability—extending conclusions beyond the confines of the experimental situation. Whenever one conducts a clinical trial on a set of individuals, the assumption is that knowledge gained from a few can be extended to the many. But what sorts of extrapolations are appropriate? Is it warranted, for example, to generalize medical findings across categories—to claim that the findings from a study of adults applies equally to children, or that a treatment shown to benefit white people will also be efficacious in other racial groups? Empirical work in the sociology of scientific knowledge has shown that the contention that an experimental test has succeeded presumes the forging of collective agreement on the substantial similarity between the test situation and those real-world situations for which the test is putatively a stand-in.[42] Alternatively, Bruno Latour has described how scientists' capacity to generalize reflects their ability to, in effect, dissolve the boundaries between what is inside and outside the laboratory.[43] Thus, science studies scholars call attention to the practical work and acts of persuasion that make generalization possible.[44]

Practices of generalizing are consequential for this book in another way as well. Generalizing can refer to the extension of a political solution from one case to another that appears similar—for example, when programs for biomedical inclusion designed to apply to one set of groups in society then get extended to incorporate new constituencies. Or, some-times, particular ways of approaching problems are transposed to new circumstances—for example, when the notion of affirmative action is "lifted" from the setting of employment policy and introduced into the domain of health policy. As William Sewell has emphasized, generaliza-tions ("stating [a rule] in more abstract form so that it will apply to a larger number of cases") and transpositions ("a concrete application of a rule to a new case, but in such a way that the rule will have subtly different forms in each of its applications") are not trivial practices: they are the bases of the "cultural schemas" that orient human action in distinct settings, and therefore they are central to the very maintenance and transformation of social structures.[45] Generalizations and transpositions take a number of concrete forms studied by sociologists, including the extension of policies through "domain expansion" and analogical reasoning,[46] the diffusion of protest repertoires from one social movement to another,[47] and the feed-back effects by which social problems spread across social arenas.[48]

Standardizing

Scholars in science studies and other fields increasingly have become attentive to the centrality in modern life of standardizing—constructing uniformities across time and space, through the generation of agreed-upon rules for the production of objects.[49] The conduct of science is crucially dependent on the availability of standardized instruments, tests, and protocols; and the conduct of governance is likewise impossible with-out standardized forms, procedures, and measures.[50] Nils Brunsson and Bengt Jacobsson have gone so far as to claim that "standardization is a form of regulation just as crucial as hierarchies and markets."[51] As Bowker and Star have emphasized, while standards often have a formal or even legal definition, they have a way of sinking below the level of social visibility, becoming part of the taken-for-granted technical and moral infrastruc-ture of the modern world.[52] In this regard, standardization enhances what Michael Mann has described as the "infrastructural power" of the modern state—"the institutional capacity of a central state, despotic or not, to penetrate its territories and logistically implement decisions."[53]

Standards also have a way of enduring. As Bowker and Star have ob-served, because successful standards "have significant inertia," changing them or ignoring them can be difficult, time-consuming, and costly.[54] Similarly, John Kingdon has noted that "establishing a principle is so im-portant because people become accustomed to a new way of doing things and build the new policies into their standard operating procedures. Then inertia sets in, and it becomes difficult to divert the system from its new direction."[55] Numerous political sociologists, using terms such as "path dependence," "policy legacies," and "policy feedback," have emphasized the durability of standard ways of doing things, examining how "decisions at one point in time can restrict future possibilities by sending policy off onto particular tracks."[56]

But despite the inertial and resistant character of standards, sometimes standardization comes under powerful attack. Uniform, one-size-fits-all approaches to problem solving are often unpopular, perhaps especially in cultures that prize individuality, and not infrequently in domains like medicine, where (at least at the rhetorical level) much is made of the unique qualities of each patient.[57] In the case considered in this book, the rise of a reform movement was premised on an important critique of standardization, encapsulated in the notion of resistance to the "standard human." The result has been the creation and substitution of a new regime of standards, complete with new conceptions of standard human subtypes, along with new standardized procedures for studying those subtypes as well as documenting that one has done so.[58]

THE POLITICS OF SOCIAL CATEGORIES

This book positions the general social processes of classifying, generalizing, and standardizing at the center of an analysis of how a biopolitical paradigm gets made, how it functions, and what its consequences are. However, in the story that I tell, these three abstract processes come down to earth in relation to specific forms of social identity and difference: those based on sex and gender, race and ethnicity, and (to a somewhat lesser extent) age. These are the categories that have proved most significant to the debates on inclusion and difference in U.S. biomedicine and that have been most explicitly represented in new policies and practices. In analyzing these categories, I draw on the growing and important bodies of work on gender and science[59] and race and science,[60] as well as on other approaches to the study of these categories from diverse fields.

I conceive of sex, gender, race, ethnicity, and age as intersecting attributes of identity, markers of difference, and dimensions of social hierarchy and power.[61] I adopt a number of principles in thinking about these categories. First, Michael Omi and Howard Winant's theorization of race applies to the other classifications as well: each should be understood not as a fixed essence but as "an unstable and 'decentered' complex of social meanings constantly being transformed"—by political struggles as well as by a wide range of social activities (including, for instance, biomedical ones). Rather than seeing their meanings as stable, we should be attentive to the historical processes by which categories come to be imbued with significance—what Omi and Winant, in the case of race, refer to as "racial formation."[62] And we should likewise track the efforts by which differently situated social actors seek to control the production, circulation, and reception of public and mass media discourses about difference— what Charles Briggs, writing about race and health, has called the politics of "communicability."[63]

Second, the operations of state organizations crucially reflect and reshape the social dynamics of these forms of difference. We should consider how distinctive gender and racial regimes become crystallized within state agencies, as well as how the state actors help to regulate the operations of gender and race.[64] Third, as Joan Scott has claimed about gender, these phenomena all need to be studied at multiple levels simultaneously: making sense of them means examining cultural symbols, normative judgments, social institutions and organizations, and subjective identity.[65] Fourth, at the interpersonal level, identities and differences of all kinds should be seen as what Candace West and Sarah Fenstermaker describe as "an ongoing interactional accomplishment": the very meanings of terms such as *female* or *elderly* emerge out of social interactions and the practices of everyday life.[66]

Fifth, categorical terms are crucially relational: *white* takes its meaning in relation to *black*, *male* in relation to *female*—these categories literally have no meaning when they stand alone. Finally, identities and hierarchies intersect in complicated ways. Because they infuse one another with meaning—for example, the sense of what it means to be a man or a woman varies across ethnic groups—the effects on an individual of laying claim to multiple identities are more than simply additive.[67] With these general principles in mind, let me now briefly discuss, in turn, the dimensions of difference that are most central to this book:

Sex and Gender

In reaction against the hegemonic, everyday understanding of men's and women's differences as natural, academics influenced by feminism in the 1970s developed a now familiar distinction between sex and gender. By this reading, "sex" referred to the biological "bedrock" (the anatomical, hormonal, and chromosomal differences between males and females), while "gender" referred to a cultural "overlay" (the various meanings associated with femaleness and maleness in a society, such as ideas about women's and men's work, women's and men's roles, and so on).[68] In recent years, however, academics from fields such as feminist studies and science studies have cast doubt on the adequacy of this way of distinguishing sex and gender and have rejected the approach of treating sex as a biological given. For example, through studies of scientific research into sex hormones and the scientific and social management of intersexuality and transgenderism, they have argued that a good deal of cultural work is necessary to shore up the notion of an ineradicable biological divide between males and females.[69]

Therefore, in this book I use the term *sex differences* to refer to socially, culturally, and historically specific understandings of anatomical or biological differences between women and men; and I use the term *gender differences* to refer to understandings of differences between men's and women's places in society, their roles, or their social identities. That is, rather than treat "sex" as a biological category and "gender" as a social category, I analyze them as two different sets of ideas about how men and women are different, one of which links that difference to biology and nature, and the other to society and culture.[70]

Race and Ethnicity

The relation between "race" and "ethnicity" is also complex and perplexing. In the second half of the twentieth century, as scientific evidence mounted that the so-called continental races—such as Africans, Caucasians, and Asians—simply cannot be demarcated by any scientific means and that the terms do not correspond to any sharp genetic divisions in the human species, many analysts proposed that the term *race*, in all of its invidious history, be discarded. Some have proposed that *ethnicity*, understood as a marker of cultural difference with no specific biological referent, can perfectly well replace *race* in our conceptual vocabulary.[71] While admirable in some respects, these strategies are impractical in the short run insofar as they ignore the incredible salience of racial categories in the politics of everyday life. Moreover, as I will discuss in detail in chapter 10, there continues to be heated debate within biomedicine over the potential usefulness of racial categories for medical purposes. Historical evidence of the transmutation of categories also provides grounds for retaining "race" and "ethnicity" as distinct concepts: some of the groups now called ethnicities in the United States, such as Irish Americans and Italian Americans, were understood in the nineteenth century as constituting separate "races."[72]

Therefore, in these pages, I use both terms, adopting the framework of Stephen Cornell and Douglas Hartmann in viewing ethnicity and race as "distinct but often overlapping bases of identification." In their analysis, a race is a "a human group defined by itself or others as distinct by virtue of perceived common physical characteristics that are held to be inherent."[73] An ethnic group is "a collectivity within a larger society having real or putative common ancestry, memories of a shared historical past, and a cultural focus on one or more symbolic elements defined as the epitome of their peoplehood."[74] It follows from these definitions that a race may or may not also be an ethnic group, and vice versa. In neither case, however, are we speaking of differences that are predetermined by human biology. Rather, ethnic and racial groups emerge out of processes of collective attribution.

Age

Because it is fastened to a chronological measuring scheme that has all the virtues of numerical precision, age is perhaps the most naturalized of all the categorical attributes considered here. However, there is evidence to suggest that the tendency of individuals to know and assert their ages with exactitude is a relatively recent historical development.[75] More importantly for my purposes, the social meanings of categories such as "childhood," "maturity," or "old age" have changed significantly over time and vary across societies, while concepts such as "adolescence" may be quite historically and culturally specific.[76] In our society, as a result of a tight interplay between medical advances and demographic developments, new age groupings, such as "newborns" or "the oldest old," have emerged into prominence within biomedicine. Thus, while age may often seem like a straightforward attribute of identity, the set of age categories that are salient at any given place and time are by no means obvious. Neither is it obvious which age categories will serve as bases for political mobilization or as objects of scientific scrutiny, and, therefore, it is worth paying attention to the work that people do to move particular categories into the spotlight.

Terminology

A final note about the use of categorical terms in this book: Anyone writing about social categorization confronts an obstacle that is simultaneously terminological, definitional, and conceptual—not to mention political. Several of the basic terms of analysis—such as *gender* and *race*— are both categories of social and political *analysis* and categories of social and political *practice*.[77] They are key concepts in the architecture of my own analysis, but they are also buzzwords in the vocabularies of individuals whom I study. Of course, many other terms that show up in my account, such as *science* or *policy*, also have this dual character. But identity categories—what we call ourselves and others—are terms that ordinary people are particularly intent on laying claim to and whose histories (as I have said) especially reflect the complex interactions between popular and expert definitions.

When it comes to categories of practice, my approach is purely pragmatic: I report the terms employed by the actors I studied, in all the ambiguity of everyday usage. For example, throughout much of the period under consideration here, policymakers and commentators tended to use the term *gender* to refer to both biological and cultural aspects of the differences between men and women and avoided the term *sex* altogether, often out of fear of confusion with sexuality. (One NIH employee described to me how a conference on male/female differences in the experiencing of pain that was to be called "Sex and Pain" ended up bearing the word *gender* in its title instead, lest anyone suppose that the NIH was showcasing sadomasochism.) In recent years, however, NIH documents have begun to use the hybrid term *sex/gender* in an attempt to gesture at both the biological and the cultural simultaneously. Therefore I will use *gender* when those who figure in my story said "gender" and *sex/gender* when they said "sex/gender"—but I will also consider the implications of these different terms. Another example of the particularity of discourse is the adoption, by DHHS agencies, of the U.S. Census Bureau's conception of ethnicity as meaning just "Hispanic or Latino" or "not Hispanic or Latino"; still another is the difference between the NIH and the FDA in how a child is defined for medical research purposes. Here again, rather than impose my own conceptual framework on these varied and interesting instances of naming and categorizing, my approach will be to let people and organizations speak for themselves, but also to analyze their linguistic production.[78]

CHAPTER TWO

Histories of the Human Subject

An oft-repeated claim from the mid-1980s onward is that the field of medicine has long presumed a "male norm" and that various groups, especially women, have been invisible to researchers and clinicians.[1] Critics of the underrepresentation of women, children, the elderly, and racial and ethnic minorities as research subjects have suggested that privileged white males in their twenties through their fifties were, for too long, taken to be the "standard human"—the reference point from which knowledge about human health and illness flowed. This was precisely Bernadine Healy's argument, as described in the introduction: the former NIH director blasted "the orthodoxy of sameness and the orthodoxy of the mean" and described how the 35-year-old white male had long served as the "normative standard" in medical research.[2] Or to quote the blunt assessment of an "outreach notebook" distributed by the NIH in 2002 to assist researchers with the recruitment and retention of women and minority research subjects: "Historically, the typical and usual research participant was a white male."[3]

Like any influential representation of history, this one merits scrutiny. Have other groups besides middle-aged white men simply been overlooked by medicine? To the degree that they have been overlooked, was it because they were seen as so similar to the "standard human" that specific study wasn't deemed necessary? Or was it because they were seen as fundamentally different yet socially inferior—in which case specific study was no one's priority?[4] And to the degree that groups such as women and racial and ethnic minorities *have not* been overlooked and instead have been the object of explicit study, what have been the motivations for such studies, and what generalizations about humanity have been drawn from them?

In this chapter, I lay the groundwork for understanding recent changes in clinical research practices by investigating how medical researchers at earlier historical moments decided on which people to study. Addressing this issue demands attention to three crucial sets of oppositions that surface in the history of medical experimentation:

- *Privilege versus vulnerability*: Under what historical conditions do socially advantaged groups become the objects of researchers' attention? Conversely, when do researchers find it more convenient to subject marginalized, vulnerable, or captive populations to the risks inherent in medical experimenting?
- *Sameness versus difference*: From a medical standpoint, how alike or unlike are different social groups imagined to be?
- *Generalizability versus specificity*: When do researchers believe that results from experiments conducted on one group can be extrapolated to other groups, and when are they hesitant to make such generalizations?[5]

The basic claim of this chapter is that there is no single set of answers to these questions that universally captures or characterizes Western medical thought or practice in recent centuries or even decades. Using examples and arguments drawn primarily from the work of historians, I will show how medical experts have arrived at varied responses to these questions at different historical moments, and I will demonstrate that, even at a given point in time, researchers often have not been unanimous or consistent in their views. Therefore, it is important to examine the distinctive and sometimes idiosyncratic ways in which medical authorities have resolved these different debates. But in order to do so, we need to sketch the outlines of several intertwining histories—of medical philosophies, methodologies of testing, and understandings of the ethics of experimentation on humans. As I review these histories, I will consider the implications of each for the representation, underrepresentation, or exclusion of various groups from medical research.

What will this review of the historical record allow us to conclude about reformers' claims concerning inclusion and the standard human? Were the advocates of social change accurate in their portrayal of history, or have they gotten the history wrong? The question is difficult to answer for several reasons, not least because the rhetoric of the movement in favor of inclusion is rather imprecise about *when* these claims are meant to apply. Is the argument supposed to be that medicine *always* has taken adult white men as the standard human? Or are we speaking of a twentieth-century phenomenon? Or is this tendency deemed to be characteristic of the modern era of the clinical trial—a method of formal experimentation that became prominent only after World War II? Or, perhaps, is the underrepresentation of groups something that emerged only in the 1970s, as an unintended consequence of other reforms that sought to protect "vulnerable populations" from the risks of research? One can find statements by critics of biomedicine over the past two decades that are consistent with each of these conceptions of the historical period under consideration, while many statements are simply too vague to be associated with any specific epoch.

It would be reasonable to imagine that the validity of claims about underrepresentation could be assessed through hard numbers—statistics on precisely who has populated medical studies in the past. I consider numbers of this sort in later chapters, but I defer doing so until then for several reasons. First, even in the period of modern clinical research, the numbers are hard to come by, because researchers were not always careful about collecting or presenting data concerning the social characteristics of their research subjects. (Indeed, one of the benefits of the recent emphasis on inclusion and difference is that federal health agencies are now gathering much more precise aggregate data on research participation—especially in NIH-funded studies, but also in clinical trials leading to drug approvals by the FDA.[6]) As a result of this lack, the available data provide selective and sometimes contradictory views of who was studied, even in the relatively recent past. Second, proponents and opponents of the inclusion-and-difference paradigm have presented competing quantitative analyses of such matters as whether women actually were underrepresented in clinical research in recent decades. Debate on these points has been tightly interwoven into the larger controversy over the desirability of the new policies mandating inclusion. It therefore makes more sense for me to present the numbers in the context of the controversy itself, locating the data within the argumentation of different parties to the debate, so that they may be considered in that context.

Most importantly, when we consider the characteristics of research practices in the past, what is at issue is more than just numbers. The concepts that underlie medical judgments about the use of human subjects—concepts such as sameness, difference, standards, generalizations, vulnerability, ethics, and justice—all have their own complex histories. My goal in this chapter, then, is to excavate some of the meanings of these concepts in order to better situate the analysis of controversy that follows. In doing so, I also mean to develop three points. First, medical researchers have operated with a considerable range of ideas about who constitutes the ideal, the appropriate, or the acceptable research subject, and these sensibilities also have shifted over time. Second, while therefore it is incorrect to say that white men always have been the "typical and usual" experimental subject, it is true that certain historical developments have encouraged that tendency. And third, given the troubling history of medical conceptions of race and gender, there is a sharp irony associated with the new attention to difference. Recent reformers assume that a medical insistence on difference necessarily advances the interests of historically disadvantaged groups; but the old medical theories of group difference had just the opposite effect, reinforcing oppression and helping to consolidate the very disadvantages we now hope to overturn.

THE HUMAN SUBJECT AS WORKING OBJECT

A key problem confronted by medical experimenters is one that, to a certain degree, faces every practitioner of an experimental science. As analysts in the field of science studies have shown about science generally, the production of trustworthy knowledge out of laboratory settings invariably presumes the creation of standardized "working objects" whose essential characteristics can be claimed to vary little from one laboratory to the next.[7] "No science can do without such standardized working objects," note Lorraine Daston and Peter Galison, "for unrefined natural objects are too quirkily particular to cooperate in generalizations and comparisons."[8] While such working objects are often inanimate, such as scientific instruments and procedures, they may sometimes be living things. For example, Robert Kohler has described how the natural variability of the fruit fly had to be reduced before it could become a reliable experimental object.[9] However, creating a standard human for research purposes is potentially more problematic than standardizing other living things. Whereas scientists could construct a variety of the fruit fly for laboratory purposes, clinical researchers studying humans are obliged to take those humans essentially as they find them. Researchers seeking a standard human "working object" therefore have several options: they may assume that differences between humans are irrelevant for their purposes, they may seek out only those individuals who have chosen characteristics, or they may subject different subpopulations of humans to separate or comparative study.

Of course, researchers may seek to bypass this dilemma—and simultaneously solve the practical problem of finding willing subjects—by substituting experimental animals drawn from other species in place of the standard human. This solution is as old as the history of medical experimentation, and it continues to be both common and important in many biomedical contexts today. But it, too, may engender controversy over the generalizability of findings.[10] First, it is not always the case that other animals are more easily standardized than humans, and attempts to employ them in medical testing have sometimes run afoul of significant intraspecies variation.[11] Second, there often may be considerable uncertainty about the implications for *Homo sapiens* of findings in other species. For example, a culture like ours today, which has been growing suspicious of extrapolating findings from men to women, adults to children, or white people to people of color may have little patience with the notion that "rats are miniature people."[12] In practice, many medications that appear promising and many findings that appear compelling when tested in animals simply fail to pan out when the experiment is repeated in humans. Thus, most important domains of present-day clinical research, particularly including the clinical trials required by the FDA for the licensing of new drugs, frequently begin with animal testing but ultimately require experimentation in humans for findings to be seen as scientifically adequate and publicly credible.

Let's assume, then, that medical experimentation designed to benefit human beings does require human subjects and that experimenters must, at least in some measure, aim to standardize their practice and the objects of that practice. How have such necessities been made consistent with medical understandings of the human body and human differences?

Medical Theorizing and the Hierarchy of Bodies

In some respects, standardizing the human is a concept foreign to the history of Western medicine. Rather than dealing inevitably in universals, Western medicine has often been preoccupied with differences, both between individuals and between social groups. From a present-day vantage point, this history is both ironic and disturbing. While today's presumption is that medical attention to difference is a beneficial and enlightened response, more typically such attention has both presumed and reinforced a social hierarchy that placed heterosexual European men at the pinnacle. By treating variations between genders and races as something fixed in the body, medical theorists helped to reinforce the perception that social inequalities were a straightforward reflection of the natural order of things.

Western medical theorizing about differences between men and women has a long history. As Londa Schiebinger has noted, the ancient Greek physician Galen "believed that women are cold and moist while men are warm and dry; men are active, women are indolent."[13] Yet for Galen the female body was essentially a variation on the theme of man: female sex organs were just male organs "turned inward."[14] In eighteenth-century Europe, however, while ideas about male and female sameness did not disappear, strong notions of fundamental medical differences between men and women—of men and women as "opposites"—were used by some medical authorities to breathe new life into claims that women were destined to be socially subordinate to men. As Thomas Lacquer has expressed it, whenever Enlightenment ideas about democracy and equality threatened to erode the old distinctions between men's and women's places in society, "arguments for fundamental sexual differences were shoved into the breach."[15] From a biological and anatomical standpoint, women were often understood to be inalterably different and were portrayed as dissimilar from men in essential and thoroughgoing ways. "The essence of sex," argued the French physician Pierre Roussel in 1775, "is not confined to a single organ but extends, through more or less perceptible nuances, into every part."[16]

These conceptions of female difference did not vanish with the passing of the eighteenth century. In the nineteenth-century United States, physicians seeking to understanding an epidemic of "women's maladies" tended to construe femaleness as almost inherently unhealthy and viewed women as essentially controlled by their reproductive organs. Barbara Ehrenreich and Deirdre English quote one physician who, "addressing a medical society in 1870, observed that it seemed 'as if the Almighty, in creating the female sex, *had taken the uterus and built up a woman around it.*' "[17] Moreover, by the nineteenth century, measurements of European women's skulls and pelvises had led some scientists to conclude that women ranked below men in terms of evolutionary development.[18]

As this history of conceptualizing women's differences suggests, it is important to note that, at least in the nineteenth century, women by no means were "ignored by" or "invisible to" medical practitioners. Carol Weisman has pointed out in her analysis of the history of the women's health movement: "In contrast to the current view that medicine ignores or neglects women, the recruitment of women patients was critical, historically, to physicians' practices, and the development and control of medical treatments for women played a key part in the profession's attempts to establish itself both economically and socially." Indeed, Weisman cites the medical historian W. F. Bynum's claim that, in the nineteenth century, "more often than not, the abstract patient was referred to as female"—either because women were more likely than men to turn to doctors, or because physicians were more inclined to pathologize women's bodies than men's.[19]

Claims about biological differences also were invoked in nineteenth-century Europe and the United States to justify racial hierarchies in general and the practice of slavery in particular.[20] Samuel Cartwright, chairman of a committee appointed by the Medical Association of Louisiana to report on the "diseases and physical peculiarities of the Negro race," described in a medical journal in 1851 how the skin color of the black man reflected a difference that went all the way inward: "his bile, . . . his blood, . . . the brain and nerves, the chyle and all the humors" were "tinctured with a shade of the pervading darkness." Cartwright argued further that blacks suffered from a deficiency of red blood caused by "defective atmospherization"; but since hard exercise could cure this condition, it followed that slavery improved them "in body, mind and morals."[21] Others argued similarly that rates of insanity were demonstrably higher among freed blacks than among those who remained slaves.[22] Thus, not only did medical beliefs reflect social preoccupations with racial superiority and inferiority, but medicine also played an active role in constructing those very notions of racial character and shoring up the boundaries between races.

Some historians have argued that Cartwright's views may have been somewhat out of the mainstream and that other medical authorities believed that "sickness among blacks and whites differed in terms of degree rather than kind."[23] Still, the arguments of Cartwright and his contemporaries were generally consistent with a broader medical philosophy that was dominant among nineteenth-century U.S. physicians in both the North and the South, which has been called the "principle of specificity." According to this principle, medical therapy "was to be sensitively gauged not to a disease entity but to such distinctive features of the patient as age, gender, ethnicity, socioeconomic position, and moral status, and to attributes of place like climate, topography, and population density." As John Harley Warner has described, "admonitions to heed the various elements encompassed by the principle of specificity permeated therapeutic instruction. . . . Professors routinely taught that [these various] individuating factors . . . modified the character of the disease and the operation of drugs."[24] Thus, notions of racial differences in health and disease were just one dimension of a general insistence on specificity.

As I discuss below, in the late nineteenth century the principle of specificity mostly gave way to notions of medical universalism. Nevertheless, notions of medically inferior races persisted well into the twentieth century in the United States. A turn-of-the-century work entitled *The Surgical Peculiarities of the Negro* was, according to David McBride, a standard medical reference throughout World War I. In 1910, the *Journal of the American Medical Association* (*JAMA*) published an article by Dr. H. M. Folkes of Mississippi that was entitled "The Negro as a Health Problem."[25] Also writing in *JAMA*, Dr. Seale Harris observed in 1903 that the "[lesser] development of lung tissue and the accessory muscles of respiration among the negroes than for the whites" reflected the fact that "the negro, a century or two ago, was a savage, perhaps a cannibal. . . . [With] the warm, humid atmosphere, less oxygen was required to maintain body temperature, so there was a corresponding lack of development of the lungs of the native African."[26] Allan Brandt has described how physicians pointed to the comparative anatomies of blacks and whites in order to support their claims that emancipation had led to the declining health of the black population.[27] Physicians also were obsessed with the sexuality of black people, who were viewed as "a notoriously syphilis-soaked race," in the words of one early-twentieth-century physician. This presumed susceptibility later provided some of the justification for the infamous Tuskegee Syphilis Study, which was crucially premised on a hypothesis of difference: the study, which denied treatment to black men in rural Alabama in order to track the progression of the disease, sought to investigate whether syphilis might take a different course in blacks than in whites.[28]

Often, white physicians conceived of nonwhite races as posing a special risk of infection to the mainstream U.S. population. Some argued that blacks were, "like the fly, the mosquito, the rats, and mice, an arch-carrier of disease germs to white people."[29] (As Vanessa Gamble has noted, black physicians, by contrast, attributed ill health to poverty and discrimination—not to innate characteristics.[30]) Similarly, in the late nineteenth and early twentieth centuries, public health authorities in cities such as San Francisco conceived of the "alien" Chinese element as a special source of risk to the health of the society and blamed the Chinese for diseases such as syphilis and the bubonic plague.[31] But infectiousness was not the only dimension of racial risk. Under the influence of the eugenics movement, nonwhite racial groups were portrayed as genetically inferior, and intermarriage as a threat to the human gene pool.[32]

Two points are worth emphasizing in considering these troublesome histories of medical conceptions of racial difference. First, while physicians' beliefs reflected the dominant values of the societies in which they lived, their medical arguments were not just passive vehicles for the transmission of racist ideas. Through a specification of difference as rooted in biology, and by means of the cultural authority invested in the medical and scientific professions, physicians and researchers actively reshaped social understandings of race. For example, in the early twentieth century, when sickle-cell anemia became understood as a disease of "Negro blood," clinicians argued that it was impossible for whites to contract the condition. As both Keith Wailoo and Melbourne Tapper have described, the discovery of apparent cases of sickle-cell anemia in whites led to classificatory dilemmas that were resolved by inferring the existence of some hidden African ancestor in the "white" individual's family tree. In this way, medical theorizing helped not only to shore up the racial divide, but also to give new meaning to what it meant to be black: part of the very definition of black identity was the susceptibility of "Negro blood" to illnesses such as sickle-cell anemia.[33]

The second point is that invidious notions of biomedical racial differences persisted in some quarters in the United States past the formation of a scientific consensus, in the interwar years, that notions of racial superiority and inferiority lacked any scientific basis.[34] Indeed, even the association of Nazism with eugenics and racialized medical science failed to dispel completely the notion that racial hierarchies were "in the blood."[35] In 1942 a committee of physical anthropologists complained that the maintenance of segregated blood banks under Jim Crow laws was embarrassingly reminiscent of practices "based on the Nazi theory of race."[36] Blood plasma was also kept segregated in the U.S. military throughout World War II, though apparently less because military physicians perceived a medical necessity to do so than because some members of Congress thought that "the argument that the blood of whites and blacks was interchangeable [was] a Communist plot to 'mongrelize America.'"[37]

The residue of nineteenth-century biological conceptions of race is also evident in the antiquated terminology that was used in the United States until 2004 in the indexing codes for medical journal articles. The National Library of Medicine's "Medical Subject Headings" included the indexing term "Racial Stocks," which was subdivided into "Australoid Race," "Caucasoid Race," "Mongoloid Race," and "Negroid Race." A search of the medical literature reveals that from 1990 through 1999, nearly 13,000 medical journal articles about human populations were coded with the indexing term "Racial Stocks," and thousands bore the more specific codes. Beginning with articles published in 2004, these subject headings were eliminated and replaced with "Continental Population Groups."[38]

Experimentation and Difference: Sex, Age, Class, and Race

The preceding section provides a schematic overview of the significance of certain kinds of difference for medical theory and practice in the eighteenth and nineteenth centuries. But it mostly leaves to one side a consideration of the more specific issue of medical experimentation. In fact, during this period, many physicians were active experimenters, eager to test new substances for their therapeutic properties. As David Rothman has noted, "the idea of judging the usefulness of a particular medication by actual results goes back to a school of Greek and Roman empiricists," but it was in the eighteenth century that human experimentation began to make "its first significant impact on medical knowledge . . . , primarily through the work of the English physician Edward Jenner."[39] On whom did doctors perform such experiments? Although it was common to try out such substances first on animals, physicians considered it necessary to proceed to experiments with humans. In many cases, physicians then experimented initially on themselves.[40] But medical patients often found themselves serving as experimental subjects whether that was their choice or not.

In a recent article, Schiebinger provides an illuminating look at how understandings of difference and conceptions of the natural body affected experimenters' selection of subjects in eighteenth-century Europe. She notes: "To some extent, the choice of subjects was simply arbitrary. As with dissection, physicians and surgeons used any bodies they could lay their hands on (perhaps legally and morally, perhaps not)." Prisoners, hospital patients, orphans, and soldiers were among those most likely to be experimented upon, and "from a medical point of view, there was nothing special about these bodies, except their availability." At the same time, conceptions of sameness and difference were sometimes important to experimental practice. Schiebinger presents evidence that many physicians routinely recorded the age and sex of those experimented upon, reflecting beliefs that therapies might have different effects on children and adults and on women and men. But despite the extraordinary importance attached to social class distinctions in the eighteenth century—and the extent to which class differences were seen as inherited—experimenters in that case "assumed an interchangeability of bodies among Europeans" and were content to trust that experiments conducted on the poor held medical relevance for the rich. Neither was race considered a barrier to extrapolation throughout most of the eighteenth century. By the end of the century, however, as strong biological notions of race became more widespread, experimenters began to worry whether the bodies of Africans were representative of humankind. Such worries did not, however, prevent physicians from continuing to experiment on slaves, whose "availability" for such purposes was simply too appealing to be ignored. Thus, in the eighteenth century, certain differences were seen as barriers to generalization while others were not (and these distinctions themselves varied somewhat over time), but practical exigencies concerning the supply of experimental bodies often overrode all other considerations.[41]

As the work of other historians has suggested, by the nineteenth century, conceptions of racial difference had become so entrenched in medical practice that those who wanted to experiment on slaves—and many did, once again for the simple reason of their availability[42]—were obliged to make arguments about human similitude that challenged the conventional wisdom. A case in point is the surgical experimentation conducted by Dr. J. Marion Sims, the nineteenth-century, South Carolina—born "father of gynecology." Sims developed an important and revolutionary surgical procedure—a remedy for vesico-vaginal fistula—through experimentation on slave women. These women were provided to him by their owners, though in at least one case Sims purchased a slave specifically in order to experiment upon her. That Sims's choice of subjects was dictated by expediency and the social organization of power in the antebellum South is obvious enough. Yet it was crucial to the larger success of Sims's work that he be able to argue that the procedures that he elaborated on the bodies of black women would be equally efficacious when applied to white female patients. From an intellectual standpoint, Sims thus found himself in direct opposition to contemporaries such as Cartwright who emphasized the "peculiarities" of the Negro race. Instead, as Deborah McGregor has noted, "Sims assumed that female anatomy was homologous between whites and blacks" and that extrapolations could therefore be made from the latter to the former.[43]

A similar example would be the use, in the antebellum South, of black corpses for purposes of anatomical dissection. At a time when medical institutions resorted to contracting with grave-robbers to obtain corpses, black bodies were simply more vulnerable to expropriation. "In Baltimore the bodies of coloured people exclusively are taken for dissection," a visitor to the United States from France commented in 1835, "because the Whites do not like it, and the coloured people cannot resist."[44] But the interesting outcome is that nineteenth-century physicians developed ideas about human anatomy based largely on the study of African Americans. As Robert Blakely and Judith Harrington have observed: "It is one of the ironies of medical history that, although blacks were generally regarded as 'inferior' or even 'subhuman,' their corpses were considered 'good enough' to use in the instruction of human anatomy."[45] Here again, the "availability" of black people for medical purposes resulted in the fact that, in specific contexts, they, rather than whites, effectively served as the standard human.

There are also plenty of more recent instances of medical experimentation on racial and ethnic minorities that have resulted in the extrapolation of findings from people of color to whites: for example, the use of women in Puerto Rico for some of the early studies of the Pill in the 1950s and the present-day interest of some geneticists in studying African Americans because they possess some of the genetic mutations that are the "oldest" and hence the most universally distributed.[46] Who, then, is the "standard human"? These latter cases seem to contradict the claims of those who say that only the most socially privileged groups have served as the standard and that others either have been invisible or have been studied only in terms of their difference. These examples demand attention to those moments when researchers not only have (for whatever combination of sensible and dubious reasons) placed women and minorities front and center, but also have been willing to say that results thereby obtained will apply to humans generally.

Captive Populations, Abuses, and the Rise of Protectionism

The use of specific groups as "captive populations" for research purposes merits further consideration. While it is rightly assumed that captive populations typically come from socially disadvantaged or exploited groups, this is not always the case. Occasionally, availability has meant the study of relatively socially advantaged groups. In an article aptly titled "Using the Student Body," Heather Munro Prescott has described the ubiquitous reliance on college students as samples of convenience for academic researchers. As Prescott notes, "the assumption that undergraduates are natural research subjects is so deeply embedded in both the history of and present-day thinking on human experimentation that it is difficult to separate discussion of student subjects from that of other healthy volunteers." Studies of students have been used to establish a range of "baseline" physiological measures and standards of normality, including "the normal ranges for blood pressure, lung capacity, pulse rate, basal metabolism, and other physiological processes." For these purposes, students have been considered "ideal" in the double sense: a handy "captive population," but also ideal specimens of human normality. In this case, "captive" does not necessarily mean "vulnerable"; as Prescott makes clear in considering patterns of research at schools such as Harvard in the first half of the twentieth century, student research subjects may have treated their professors with deference, but they were not their social inferiors, and they did have a capacity to look out for their own interests. And researchers interested in making claims about "normality" often preferred students from privileged backgrounds, who were perceived to be "the best representatives of normality by virtue of their race, class, and gender."[47]

As interesting as this case of "the student body" may be, it should be emphasized that the captive populations that have served as the basis for medical generalization typically have consisted not of the socially privileged but of the relatively disadvantaged. Institutionalized populations of various kinds—soldiers, incarcerated prisoners, the mentally ill, retarded children—along with the poor in general, continued to provide much of the human raw material for medical studies at least through the mid-1960s.[48] After World War II, with a huge influx of funds to the NIH, the scope of medical experimentation in the United States increased enormously. But from 1945 to 1965—a period that David Rothman has called "the Gilded Age of research" in ironic recognition of the laissez-faire attitudes that prevailed—this expansion sparked little reflection on the rights of research subjects.[49] Indeed, although the Nuremberg trials after World War II had provided graphic evidence of the horrific uses to which medical experimentation could be put, only in the 1960s, with the publication of reports of widespread abuses of patients in high-profile, U.S. medical experiments, did many policy makers begin to assert that stricter measures were needed to safeguard human subjects in the United States.

Rothman has chronicled the impact of the appearance in the *New England Journal of Medicine* in 1966 of a whistle-blowing article by a doctor named Henry Beecher, who compiled a list of twenty-two examples of studies published since World War II that struck him as patently unethical: withholding penicillin from soldiers with streptococcal infections in order to study alternative means of preventing complications; feeding hepatitis virus to residents of a state institution for the retarded; injecting live cancer cells into elderly and senile hospital patients without telling them the cells were cancerous; and so on. As Beecher emphasized, these examples did not come from the fringes of medicine; they were conducted by well-established researchers at prominent institutions, and the results had been written up in all the best journals.[50]

Six years later, in 1972, Associated Press reporter Jean Heller broke the story of the U.S. Public Health Service study of "Untreated Syphilis in the Negro Male"—commonly known as the "Tuskegee Syphilis Study" because government researchers collaborated with physicians at the Tuskegee Institute in Alabama. A 1929 survey by the U.S. Public Health Service had found an exceptionally high prevalence of syphilis in Macon County, Alabama—a rural county with high rates of poverty and low rates of education among its heavily black population. Therapies consisting of mercury and arsenic compounds, though dangerous, were known to be of at least limited benefit to patients with syphilis, but these medications, like many others, did not typically find their way to rural Alabama. Therefore, as James Jones has described the rationale, because most of those with syphilis in Macon County went untreated anyway, it seemed sensible to researchers to observe the consequences.

After recruiting 399 men with syphilis and 201 controls, investigators tracked the progression of the disease over four decades, minutely recording its devastation in the form of skin ulcers, deterioration of the bone structure, problems in motor coordination, blindness, and death. Incredibly, even after the discovery in the 1940s that syphilis could be treated effectively with penicillin, participants were never given antibiotics for their condition, and they were actively discouraged from seeking medical attention from other doctors, lest they inadvertently gain access to such drugs. In the end, somewhere between twenty-eight and one hundred of the men died as a direct result of syphilis or its complications. To complete the picture of abuse, participants mostly were unaware even that they were subjects in an experiment; they were led to believe that they were receiving treatment for their "bad blood." Invasive tests such as spinal taps, designed only to gather data for the study, were presented to research subjects as "special" treatments intended for their medical benefit.[51]

The story of the Tuskegee study is crucial to the arguments in this book for several reasons, two of which need to be emphasized here.[52] First, as mentioned previously, Tuskegee was justified in part through the logic of racial difference. As untreated syphilis had already been studied in a white population in Norway, researchers claimed that part of the goal of the study was to determine whether the progressive course of syphilis in black people was similar to, or different from, its known trajectory in whites.[53] Thus, from the vantage point of the present era, in which it is frequently claimed that racial minorities will benefit from research that does not presume that whites and people of color are medically equivalent, the episode serves as yet another troublesome reminder that medical research premised on racial differences can sometimes serve stigmatizing and dangerous ends.[54]

A second aspect of the significance of the Tuskegee Study is that the reaction to it in the 1970s was emblematic of a shift in "common sense"

on the part of medical professionals and the broader society—a transformation that held important implications for the study of "vulnerable
populations." The Tuskegee study was in some respects an extreme case,
but, as Beecher's article had made evident (and as more recent revelations,
ranging from radiation experiments to novel treatments of the mentally
ill, also have underscored[55]), it was by no means unique in the annals of
experimentation in the twentieth-century United States. Moreover, the
study had never been a secret. Although news of the study was greeted
with horror and disbelief when Heller "exposed" it, reports from Tuskegee
had appeared in the pages of medical journals on a regular basis since 1936.
As late as 1969, a CDC committee had reviewed the study and determined
that it should be permitted to continue. Therefore, Tuskegee was not a
"dark secret" that was suddenly brought to light. Rather, the publicizing
of Tuskegee marked, and further propelled, a changed understanding
of legitimate practice with regard to experimentation on the socially
disadvantaged—a new moment in what Sydney Halpern has described
as the ever-evolving formation of researchers' "indigenous moralities," as
well as a new phase in public debate.[56]

In the 1970s in the United States, the public attention drawn to the
ethics of human experimentation swelled into a wave of governmental
reform. This wave crested with the enactment of formal, legal protection
of the rights of experimental subjects, along with a new conception of participation in research as a burden which, therefore, must be distributed
as equitably as possible in society.[57] With the passage of the National
Research Act of 1974, researchers became obliged to comply with procedures established by the NIH's new Office for Protection from Research
Risks, to submit their protocols beforehand to local "institutional review
boards" (IRBs) that would ensure that human subjects were not placed at
undue risk, and to document the process of obtaining informed consent
from their subjects. The new thinking was further enunciated in the "Belmont Report" published by the National Commission for the Protection
of Human Subjects of Biomedical and Behavioral Research in 1979, which
outlined the ethical principles that ought to guide medical research with
human subjects: justice, respect for persons, and beneficence.[58]

A distinguishing feature of this regime of regulation was its emphasis
on the protection from harm at the hands of the research enterprise of
what were now officially defined as "vulnerable populations," including
children, prisoners, the poor, and the mentally infirm.[59] In the wake of
severe birth defects in the children of women (mostly in Europe) who received the drug thalidomide during pregnancy, U.S. regulators increasingly came to view women, or at least their potential fetuses, as yet

another vulnerable population meriting protection. In 1977 the FDA instituted a rule formally excluding women "of childbearing potential" from many drug trials, out of concern that an experimental drug might bring harm to a fetus if a woman became pregnant during the course of a clinical trial.[60]

It is easy to see how this new regulatory climate, designed to protect against abuse of subjects, may have resulted in the reduced representation of women, children, and racial and ethnic minorities in biomedical research. But it is important to observe how relatively recent these reforms were at the time that complaints about underrepresentation became rampant in the late 1980s. Like many reforms, they may inadvertently have created a new set of problems to which a subsequent generation of reformers then found themselves obliged to respond. But it would be incorrect to attribute any long-term tendencies in medical knowledge-making practices (in terms of who gets studied or who serves as the standard) to procedures that were introduced only in the 1970s.

FROM THE PRINCIPLE OF SPECIFICITY TO *L'HOMME MOYEN*

In attempting to make sense of the complexity of historical beliefs and practices with regard to medical theory and experimentation, this chapter has examined several interlocking historical trajectories: the evolution of medical conceptions of difference, ideas about drawing generalizations from experiments on human, the exploitation of captive populations, and the rise of modern notions of protecting human subjects. One additional but equally crucial history remains to be discussed: the entry of modern statistics into medicine and, more broadly, the role of quantification, measurement, and standardization in promoting notions of medicine as a science.

When the French mathematician Adolphe Quetelet announced the new science of "social physics" in 1831, its central concept was what he called *l'homme moyen*, the average man. This man would have not just an average height, weight, education, and length of life, but also an average propensity to marry, commit suicide, or engage in criminal acts. As Gerd Gigerenzer and coauthors have noted, Quetelet fully understood that *l'homme moyen* was an abstraction who existed nowhere in reality: "But abstraction was essential to social science. Real individuals were too numerous and diverse for psychological study to contribute much to an understanding of the social condition."[61]

Under the logic of the "principle of specificity" that I described as prevailing in U.S. medical practice much of the nineteenth century, statistical constructs of this sort would have found little place. As proper medical treatment was presumed to be different for men and women, Northerners and Southerners, the rich and the poor, and so on, few physicians would have been comfortable diagnosing or prescribing for *l'homme moyen*. However, in the latter part of the nineteenth century, with the increasing adoption of European theories of scientific medicine, U.S. physicians gradually abandoned the notion that treatments should be tailored to the idiosyncratic constitutions of patients, in favor of the idea that each specific kind of illness required a distinctive treatment that might be applied universally to sufferers.[62] Increasingly, medical practitioners began to adopt conceptions of the human individual that were influenced by the rise of the sciences of statistics and probability.

The move away from the principle of specificity and the importation of statistical conceptions of humanity into medicine presaged a broader tendency. Over the course of the twentieth century, a host of developments converged to encourage a thoroughgoing, though often resisted, standardization of medical practice: the rise of modern methods of pharmaceutical drug testing and drug regulation, the development of epidemiological studies based on notions of statistical risk, the codification of international classification systems for morbidity and mortality, the increased reliance on standard protocols and expert systems, the rise of evidence-based medicine as a social movement within biomedicine, and the growth of managed care as a system of rationing and surveillance. All these developments have privileged a conception of medicine as "science" (consistent, predictable, and transparent) over a competing conception of medicine as "art" (dependent on intuition, experience, and embodied skills, and respectful of the particularities of individual patients).[63] By no means have conceptions of artful medicine disappeared, and physicians may often invoke the idea when defending their professional autonomy against bureaucrats or insurance companies. But the significance of standardization to present-day medical practice would be hard to deny.

The standardization of medical practice has often carried with it a strong presumption that the object of medical attention—the patient— could likewise be conceived of in relatively standard and universal terms. In spite of resistance, such views have informed medical education and training in various respects. It is telling that the actors who are trained to simulate disease symptoms for the benefit of students in medical school classrooms are referred to as "standardized patients." Now used in medical schools across the United States to provide students with "real-life" experience, standardized patients are labeled as such because the actors endeavor to present a consistent simulation each time they perform.[64]

Mechanical simulators of patients—such as the virtual reality surgical simulators currently used in some medical teaching settings—carry this standardization to an even greater degree, helping thereby to standardize the practices being taught by means of the simulators.[65]

Importantly, such standardization has implications for the key question of which sort of person actually proves to be the focus of biomedical attention. In particular, the standardization of the patient in medical training has sometimes coincided with a privileging of the male body over the female, precisely as recent critiques of biomedicine would suggest. For example, in a study of the classic medical reference book *Gray's Anatomy* from 1858 to 1998, Alan Petersen found remarkable consistency, over 140 years, in the manner by which "the male body has been . . . posited as the standard or norm in both illustrations and textual descriptions." Petersen's point was not, however, that the female body was absent or invisible in *Gray's Anatomy*. Rather, Petersen found that the volume appeared to call attention to women's bodies precisely insofar as they differed from men's. These comparisons emphasized "the superiority of the male body, which is seen as stronger, more fully developed and more active than the female body."[66] Similarly, in her analysis of the mechanical simulators used for teaching purposes, Ericka Johnson found that "the male body is used as the norm and the female body represented only when it differs from the male, and then only in the 'parts' which are 'importantly' different."[67]

In considering the trend toward standardization in medicine, one might well object that the modern notion of the "risk factor"—itself also a product of the statistical revolution in medicine and epidemiology—complicates any simple story of the standard patient. After all, it has become increasingly well understood that each patient may have a distinctive risk profile that makes him or her more or less susceptible to particular diseases.[68] Yet the development of risk guidelines in practice often has reflected a tendency to universalize in potentially inappropriate ways. A classic case is that of the famous Framingham Study, an observational study of heart disease conducted in a small community near Boston that began in 1948 and has continued for more than half a century. Framingham data have had an extraordinary impact on medical practice, and they are the basis of the standard risk assessment tools for gauging the impact of high blood pressure, blood lipids, smoking, physical activity, and obesity on the risk of developing heart disease.[69] But Framingham was hardly America, even in 1948 when the research began. As one of its directors observed in 1980: "There were virtually no blacks or Orientals, and the composition of the white population was not necessarily that of white populations elsewhere."[70] Moreover, because participants were aged 36–68, investigators missed many cases of heart disease in women, who tend to develop it later in life.[71] Thus, even tools designed to differentiate within populations (by distinguishing those at higher and lower levels of risk) may inappropriately homogenize the population to which they are applied, if developed on the basis of unrepresentative samples.[72]

The Randomized Clinical Trial and the Problem of Variation

A crucial stage in the standardization of the patient, the quantification of medical research, and the increased reliance on the human subject as an experimental object was the emergence of the randomized, controlled clinical trial as a distinctive kind of medical experiment. Formally adopted by medical authorities after World War II, and subsequently made part of the legal process of regulatory decision making about the safety and efficacy of drugs, the methodology of the randomized clinical trial has sought to place clinical practice on a solidly scientific footing; it is often called the "gold standard" for establishing the effect of any medical treatment on humans, and it is considered more reliable than observational methods.[73] By comparing results in two (or more) groups of patients—divided typically into a "treatment arm" and a "control arm"—investigators could determine with greater confidence whether the apparent outcomes of a medical intervention were genuinely due to that intervention rather than to some other cause or to chance. Randomization—the random assignment of each study participant to either the treatment arm or the control arm of the study—decreased the possibility of investigator bias in placing patients into groups, while also making possible the use of statistical tests to assess the significance of results. Randomization also was the prerequisite of the successful use of another important technique to avoid bias: "double blinding," in which neither the investigator nor the subject knows which subjects have been assigned to which arm of the study.[74]

How did the development of the randomized clinical trial affect who served as the experimental subject of choice in medical research? In fact, this innovation in medical knowledge-making held a variety of consequences for the demographics of human experimentation. As clinical research became more scientifically grounded and more central to the image of modern medicine, and as more and more funding poured into clinical trials from both the government and pharmaceutical companies, it is reasonable to imagine that researchers wanted to use the new techniques to address problems affecting mainstream or socially privileged groups, such as a perceived epidemic of heart disease in men. Similarly, it is reasonable to suppose that drug manufacturers wanted to study those groups in society with the greatest ability to afford their remedies. At the same time, the methodological advances themselves obviated some of the need to worry about precisely who was in one's study. Specifically, the technique of randomization provided at least a partial solution to the problem at the heart of the discussion in this chapter: how to deal with the fact that patients vary. In theory, at least in trials with large numbers of subjects, any factor that might, unbeknownst to investigators, cause certain patients to respond differently—say, a patient's age or previous medical history—would end up being more or less equally represented in both arms of the trial after randomization and therefore would not affect the trial's overall results. Thus, randomization could solve some of the difficulties associated with human variability without requiring any additional efforts on the part of researchers to recruit particular kinds of individuals.[75]

As researchers and statisticians refined the rules governing randomized trials, they developed additional procedures with implications for who ends up populating a study. Importantly, the protocols for all trials came to specify "inclusion/exclusion criteria"—formal rules designating eligibility for participation in a trial. All trial protocols must state some such criteria, but the question is just how specific they need to be in any given case. Strict inclusion/exclusion criteria are sometimes used to create a more standardized and homogeneous research population for a study, on the argument that the more researchers reduce the number of variables that might affect a study, the easier it will be for them to distinguish "signal" from "noise." On the other hand, experts on clinical trials who are concerned with the "external validity" of a trial—the significance of its findings for large numbers of people in everyday life settings, and not just for the smaller number of people who happened to participate in the clinical trial—often tend to favor more relaxed entry criteria. These experts argue that heterogeneous research populations are better models of actual conditions and that studies with homogeneous populations may result in scientifically elegant experiments that lack much real-world significance.[76] There is no solution, in principle, to the problem of how to resolve this trade-off between experimental rigor and generalizability of findings. As late as 1983, one authority on clinical trials, Dr. Alvan Feinstein, writing in the *Annals of Internal Medicine*, described an ongoing war between these two conceptions of clinical trials, which he labeled "fastidious" and "pragmatic," respectively.[77] Others have used the terms *efficacy* and *effectiveness* to distinguish between two different, potential goals of clinical trials—on one hand, establishing a statistically significant finding through experimental procedures; on the other hand, demonstrating the worth of medical interventions on a large scale, outside the experimental situation.[78]

Once again, it is worth considering the implications of these innovations in technique for the issue of who has been most or least likely to be represented in biomedical research populations. In the next chapter, I return to the question of homogeneity versus heterogeneity in subject populations and consider the implications for debates about the underrepresentation of racial and ethnic minorities, the elderly, children, and women in medical research. For the moment, it is enough to observe that, to the extent that researchers adopt the goal of recruiting a homogenous subject population, the possibility clearly exists that some social groups will find themselves excluded from studies.

Complexities

This chapter has emphasized a consistent medical preoccupation over several centuries with a set of problems: how to assess the medical relevance of differences between groups; how and whether to make generalizations about human health and illness; and how to decide which human beings are appropriate, or preferred, or deserving, or exploitable as experimental objects. It is important to observe the continuities in these preoccupations. But it is equally crucial to chart the impact of historical changes and the continued evolution of various relevant notions—of what a proper medical experiment looks like, of what we imagine group differences to signify biologically, of what rights we consider human beings intrinsically to possess. Shifts in such sensibilities, combined with scientific and technological advances in medical and statistical capacities, have held important implications for experimentation on humans—or particular subpopulations.

Let us take stock of the arguments developed in this discussion. First, though one can certainly find examples reaching into the past of cases in which medical professionals and researchers have presumed a standard human, significant standardization of the human for medical purposes is mostly a development of the twentieth century. Indeed, much of the history of Western medicine is a history of difference-making, importantly including gender difference and, by the late eighteenth century, racial difference. In the nineteenth-century United States, doctors by no means ignored women or people of color, nor were such groups medically invisible—to the contrary, physicians and researchers were often preoccupied with making claims about them. However, while in present-day discourse a medical attention to difference is considered progressive and liberatory, the past history more typically suggests a much more deeply problematic tendency—the attempt to inscribe notions of superiority and inferiority, and normality and pathology, on the bodies of different races and sexes.

Second, practical issues governing the availability of subjects for medical experiments often have overridden medical concerns about extrapolation: when the only subjects available were those from captive or vulnerable populations, then experimenters many times have been willing to "take what they could get" and, moreover, to maintain that the information thereby gleaned is of some general relevance. However, recent concerns with the rights of human subjects have inspired moves to protect "vulnerable populations" from the risks of medical experimentation; and while such protection may have lessened the tendency to rely on "available" subjects, it also may have resulted in reduced representation of women, children, the elderly, and racial and ethnic minorities (among others) as subjects in clinical research.

Third, with the importation of statistics into medicine, standardized notions of the medical patient and the research subject gradually have taken hold within medicine, especially in the twentieth century—potentially promoting a bias in favor of seeing white male adults as the standard type of human. But this standardization has proceeded unevenly and in the face of resistance and contrary tendencies. Also, some techniques associated with the modern clinical trial, such as randomization, appear to bypass the problem of confronting variation among research subjects. However, at least some investigators have sought to use strict inclusion/exclusion criteria as a way of ensuring a more homogeneous study population; and this also has the potential to contribute to the underrepresentation of particular groups as research subjects.

In short, this chapter has identified several paths by which various groups, such as women and racial and ethnic minorities, have sometimes come to be underrepresented as research subjects. But at the same time, the notion that the heterosexual, middle-aged, white male has served as the biomedical standard and that all other groups have been essentially invisible, is simply too sweeping when posed in universal terms. Claims such as Healy's—about "the orthodoxy of sameness and the orthodoxy of the mean," about treating "the average American male" as the "normative standard" and extrapolating from him to others—need to be qualified and placed in context.

The more, it seems, that we examine diverse instances of medical experimentation in the past, the less confident we may feel about making general claims about who has been included, who has served as a standard, and when the extrapolation of findings across groups has been deemed reasonable or advisable. By reviewing this history and cataloguing various examples, my point is not to doubt the observation that the adult white male frequently has been taken as the standard human type in medical thinking and practice. But the broad-brush assertion that the adult white male had become the universal human subject fails to do justice to the varying particularities of research designs, the competing ideas about human sameness and difference, and the creative and sometimes troubling ways in which researchers have responded to practical exigencies in order to carry out their work. Nor has this whole past history of contingency and particularity been unearthed by medical historians in a systematic or comprehensive way. A more adequate understanding of the diverse imaginings of the human subject awaits a good deal more scholarly investigation.[79]

This historical review sets the stage for a consideration, in the next chapter, of the rise in the 1980s of "antistandardization resistance movements" that demanded greater inclusion of underrepresented groups in medical research. First and foremost, the preceding discussion is meant to provide helpful context for thinking about this movement's claims with respect to medical standardization, representation, and generalization. But in addition, many of the examples presented here provide an important and ironic counterpoint to the argumentation of reformers: In the past, claims about differences between men and women and between whites and other racial groups were used to bolster conceptions of the innate superiority of white men. By contrast, the reformers of recent decades have sought to use evidence of biological differences precisely as a grounding for antisexist and antiracist political activism.

CHAPTER THREE

The Rise of Resistance: Framing the Critique of the Standard Human

A HETEROGENEOUS AND TACIT COALITION

No one precisely set out to create a set of policies and offices regulating the inclusion in biomedical research of a diverse set of social groups. Instead, many people's strategic action in pursuit of various individual reforms culminated in the emergence of this general approach to the problem of difference in biomedicine. No organization or leader took up the banner of biomedical inclusion on behalf of all those who ended up pursuing it, nor did everyone get together under one organizational "big tent." Representatives of the various groups covered under the umbrella of the inclusion-and-difference paradigm mostly went about their own business, sometimes borrowing one another's rhetoric or seizing common political opportunities, sometimes building on one another's successes.

In effect, reformers comprised a mostly "tacit" coalition, one marked less by direct and sustained cooperation than by a certain unity of purpose that is observable mainly in hindsight: to call for increased attention by researchers to specific groups in society and to warn against extrapolating onto those groups medical findings derived from the study of others. In this chapter and the next, I will examine how the various reformers articulated their critiques of medical research practices in a range of venues, from scientific journals to the mass media to the floor of Congress. This chapter introduces the reformers and then describes the primary ways in which they constructed their arguments about why change was necessary. I place particular emphasis on how claims about bodily differences were brought together with other kinds of political and ethical rationales for reform. The following chapter then traces the history of the practical work of individuals and organizations who brought the first set of new laws and policies into being.[1]

What Is "It"?

How do we characterize this eclectic and tacit coalition? Several points are worth making from the outset. First, although there was no unified "Movement," pressure for reform was promoted by a number of individual social movements. These included the women's health movement, the AIDS activist movement, the breast cancer advocacy movement, and movements promoting the health of racial and ethnic minorities. In other words, some of the contributors were "disease constituencies"—a long tradition in U.S. health politics—and others were organized around social identities.[2]

Yet this observation immediately requires a second point of clarification. It is misleading to attribute social change in this case simply to a collection of social movements, if by that we mean the "usual suspects" of groups that are disenfranchised and that mount their opposition from "outside" the mainstream political process. In fact, many of those who participated would have to be counted among the elites of U.S. society. The reform wave was pushed forward by supporters from within DHHS agencies, sympathetic physicians and scientists, professional organizations (such as the American Academy of Pediatrics and the National Medical Association), politicians (including members of the Congressional Caucus for Women's Issues and the Congressional Black Caucus), and specialized advocacy groups (such as the Society for Women's Health Research), and it received indirect support from some pharmaceutical companies. Therefore, it would be mistaken to understand the new biomedical policies and emphases as the product solely of a grassroots movement of the dispossessed. The tacit coalition was doubly hybrid—not just in terms of the diverse social interests that were represented within it, but also in the way that its composition traversed boundaries between laypeople and experts, or between ordinary people and elites.[3]

A third point of clarification concerns the reasons why representatives of different social interests—women, racial and ethnic minorities, children, the elderly, and so on—adopted similar strategic goals and social critiques. As Ann Swidler has observed, "many movements may invent simultaneously what seem to be common cultural frames (like the many rights movements of the 1960s or the identity movements of the 1980s)." While these kinds of convergences may reflect a "cultural contagion," they also may be "common responses to the same institutional constraints and opportunities."[4] In other cases, however, what matters most in the creation of similar outcomes is the establishment of precedent. Once a critique is mounted and an organizational solution is engineered to address it, the path is cleared for other challengers to call for the extension of that same solution to their own predicaments.[5] In practice, the consolidation of the inclusion-and-difference paradigm has depended on both of these general processes by which similarities are forged. For example, while advocates fought more or less simultaneously for policies promoting inclusion of women and racial and ethnic minorities, the policies on behalf of children mostly followed afterward, and advocates for them gained strategic advantage by invoking the precedent that was in place.

Finally, it is important to note that the various members of this tacit coalition all pursued diverse goals that often extended beyond issues of research inclusion. For example, female members of Congress who promoted the greater representation of women in medical research presented their demands under the rubric of a wide-ranging "Women's Health Equity Act" that, among other things, called for the creation of a research center on infertility and Medicare coverage for screening mammography.[6] However, the common characteristic that united the individuals and groups that I study here was a concern with research underrepresentation and the biomedical scrutiny of differences. Out of this interest, which cut across the individuals and organizations that comprised the tacit coalition, the policies and practices that I call the inclusion-and-difference paradigm gradually fell into place.

Women Take the Lead

Among the range of constituencies encompassed by the coalition, advocates of women's health played a special role in launching the reform wave. The concern with women's health has been the driving wedge for a number of important reasons. Of course, women as a class are simply the largest social category invoked in these debates, and any failure on the part of biomedicine to attend satisfactorily to more than half the U.S. population seems especially egregious. There is also a history of women's health activism in the United States going back well into the nineteenth century. As Carol Weisman has noted in her account of that history, the recent attention by women to questions of health research policy can plausibly be read as simply "the latest installment in a long American tradition of organized efforts by groups of primarily middle-class women to draw public attention to their health problems and to reshape health care institutions."[7]

But in addition, feminist movements of the 1970s and 1980s helped create new possibilities for social change in this arena. Indeed, different political "lines" within feminism had different effects, all contributing, directly or indirectly, to the concern with research on women's health.[8] On the more left-leaning end of the movement, radical feminists and socialist feminists had promoted a thoroughgoing critique of patriarchal practices and assumptions. Activists within the feminist women's health movement had adapted this critique to address sexism within the medical profession and the health-care industry specifically.[9] Foundational texts, such as *Our Bodies, Ourselves*, first published by the Boston Women's Health Book Collective in 1971, had delivered a multilayered critique: not only were women excluded from the ranks of the medical profession (the second edition noted in 1979 that only 7 percent of U.S. physicians were women and that only in South Vietnam, Madagascar, and Spain was the percentage lower), not only was the doctor-patient relationship shaped by the paternalism of male physicians, but also medical training and practice were permeated through-and-through with sexist assumptions.[10] As one commentator noted in a 1978 article entitled "What Medical Students Learn about Women": "Many of the obstetrics and gynecology textbooks used in medical schools focus more on how neurotic women might be than they do on the etiology and treatment of disease. . . . The medical student is taught to believe that many symptoms of illness in pregnancy (excessive nausea, headache) are really a result of her 'fear of pregnancy' rather than any physical condition he . . . need test for."[11]

The legacy of the feminist women's health movement, then, was a deep skepticism toward the mainstream medical profession, a critique of many of its characteristic practices (including the overuse of such procedures as hysterectomies and Caesarean sections), and a strong emphasis on women's personal autonomy and control over their bodies (reflected in the concern with reproductive rights, but also actualized through practices such as the pelvic self-exam). These sensibilities were important not only for their direct impact on women who grew to care about the politics of biomedical research, but also because they were absorbed by many activists who became involved in organizing around HIV/AIDS or breast cancer and whose concern with these medical conditions led them to focus on research politics and practices.

On the more moderate end of the broader women's movement, liberal feminists had pushed for the mainstreaming of women within all branches of U.S. society, with results that are consequential for the developments I describe here: because of the relative successes of this project of mainstreaming, women—at least in limited numbers—had risen into positions of prominence in government, the medical profession, and the world of scientific research.[12] As Cynthia Pearson, longtime women's health activist and director of the National Women's Health Network, observed in reference to reformers within the establishment, "this was the first generation of women who had been young adults at the time of women's liberation." And some of these women, influenced by feminist ideals, have been especially inclined to use their positions of influence to press for reforms of biomedicine. Some of them also had witnessed firsthand the obstacles placed in the way of female professionals in medical and scientific institutions: in her biographical reflections, Bernadine Healy, who became the first female director of the NIH in 1991, commented on the unofficial quotas that limited admission of women to medical schools in the 1960s. Others, such as Sherry Sherman at NIH's National Institute on Aging, noted the gendered assumptions that seemed to be inculcated in medical research practices at various levels. Describing her return to school for graduate training in biochemistry in the 1980s (after ten years at home raising children), Sherman recalled: "About that time when I began to do research in rats, I noticed that all rat studies were done on males."[13]

To be sure, there are important tensions between these two concep- tions of feminism and women's health. In contrast with the mainstream- ing project of liberal feminism, activists within the feminist women's health movement were more inclined to stress the need to build separate women's institutions, such as clinics and hotlines, that stood apart from the health-care industry and the state. As Sandra Morgen has described, women's health activists did gradually become more sanguine about en- tering into relationships with state agencies, but even in doing so they retained fears that movement goals would be co-opted.[14] Later in this book (in chapter 11), I will return to the question of competing visions of how to pursue women's health, and I will consider how the new focus on research representation has affected the trajectory of the women's health movement. For the moment, it is enough to note that different groups of women, influenced by varying conceptions of feminism, were primed to criticize research practices that appeared to favor men.[15]

Moreover, once women put forward their critiques, they opened up a space of possibility that others could occupy. Racial and ethnic minorities immediately followed with arguments that they, too, were underserved by modern medicine and underrepresented in study populations. These advocates drew strength from traditions of health activism within those minority communities as well as from advocacy organizations within the women's health movement that represented the interests of women of color. In addition, here as well, the recent successes of the challeng-

ing group in gaining entry into the medical profession made a difference, as did their political organization. In the case of African American
physicians, for example, their representative organization, the National
Medical Association, had grown from 5,000 members in 1969 to 22,000
members in 1977.[16]

Advocates on behalf of children and the elderly (particularly including
pediatricians and geriatricians) also joined in with similar claims soon
thereafter. This sort of historical sequence—in which a common set of
political demands is adopted by a series of challengers in turn—is a familiar pattern that sociologists have studied in other political contexts,
such as the passage of antidiscrimination policies and hate-crime legislation.[17] In this case, it is reflected in the employment of a more-or-less
common set of "frames" by all of the constituencies concerned about their
treatment at the hands of biomedicine.

KEY FRAMES

A number of scholars who study social movements, including David Snow
and Robert Benford, have used the concept of framing to call attention to
the ways in which groups with political agendas actively seek to shape representations of reality and say what the world is like. Such groups "frame,
or assign meaning to and interpret, relevant events and conditions in ways
that are intended to mobilize potential adherents and constituents, to garner bystander support, and to demobilize antagonists." Frames provide a
diagnosis of a social situation, they propose solutions, and they can serve
as a call to arms. However, in order for frames to work, they must resonate:
they must be empirically credible, consistent with personal experience,
and congruent with larger cultural heritages.[18] As Francesca Polletta has
argued, frames are both enabling and constraining: they permit strategic
cultural work on the part of activists who manipulate frames and move
them about from one setting to another, but they also shape or even limit
what activists deem to be the strategic options open to them.[19]

The biomedical reformers who promoted greater research inclusiveness consistently framed their arguments in five distinctive ways. The
first frame—"underrepresentation"—made the basic case for inequity by
focusing attention on inclusion statistics. Two other frames—"misguided
protectionism" and "false universalism"—extended the critique by suggesting two causes of this underrepresentation, both of them worthy
of concern. The final two frames—"health disparities" and "biological
differences"—added further weight to reformers' arguments by pointing
to serious negative consequences of inadequate inclusion.

Underrepresentation

As analyses of the politics of affirmative action in the workplace and in higher education have shown, a common strategy for groups pursuing social equality is to demonstrate that they have been numerically underrepresented in some important domain in society.[20] Similarly, the underrepresentation frame has been central to the argumentation of the new biomedical challengers. Indeed, by claiming numerical underrepresentation, reformers have been able to construct an analogy between their cause and the successful (if contested) struggles to institute affirmative action measures in other social domains.[21]

It is important to say from the outset that any discussion of quantitative analyses of underrepresentation demands attention to a number of complicated issues, including how underrepresentation is to be defined, what methods are most appropriate for demonstrating it, and what kinds of data are available for analysis. I will examine the debate over this issue in chapter 5, when I consider opposition to the new politics of inclusion. For the moment, it is sufficient to emphasize that highlighting underrepresentation was an important move on the part of advocates of change in biomedicine. As Jerome Karabel has shown in his critical history of admissions to elite colleges, institutions that under- or overrepresent groups often seek to maintain the status quo and maximize their own discretion by preserving the opacity of their own decision-making practices.[22] Thus, a key strategy for challengers is precisely to bring numbers and practices into the light of day.

As might be expected, a considerable portion of the emphasis on numerical representation focused on women, whose underrepresentation was described as causing a "gender gap" in medicine knowledge. Quantitative analyses arguing that women were underrepresented as subjects in biomedical research had appeared in the medical literature as far back as 1981. However, such reports received relatively little notice until the latter part of the decade, when, suddenly, they seemed to become ubiquitous. The 1981 study, by Evlin Kinney and coauthors, writing in the *Annals of Internal Medicine*, examined recent issues of two key pharmacology journals and found that, out of forty-five published studies, only eleven explicitly indicated that women had been included as subjects.[23] Writing ten years later, Barbara Levey similarly reported that many studies in pharmacology journals continued to be male-only; comparing the January issues of *Clinical Pharmacology and Therapeutics* from 1981 through 1991, she found that substantial percentages of the studies in the sample each year contained no women, while very few contained no men. (Although the trend in male-only studies was downward overall, this decline was not statistically significant.) In 1993, using a similar approach but a more expansive sample, Douglas Schmucker and Elliot Vesell found that the percentage of trials restricted to men actually increased between 1969 and 1991 in two journals of clinical pharmacology.[24]

One area of particular concern was cardiovascular disease, a disease that killed both men and women in large numbers but tended to strike down men at earlier ages. Here it seemed that differences in the timing of disease within the life cycle, combined with social perceptions of men's and women's differing "worth," had contributed to a significant research disparity. The basic point, as Claude Lenfant, director of the NIH's National Heart, Lung, and Blood Institute (NHLBI), later expressed it, was that "the devastating effects of coronary heart disease on men in their prime working years was viewed as a national emergency."[25] From the 1920s onward, rates of heart disease among men had soared, and in the early 1970s, at the time of the inception of several major NIH studies, this perceived "epidemic" of heart disease in men was at its peak. Norman Lasser, an investigator on the NHLBI-funded Multiple Risk Factor Intervention Trial (a study later singled out by critics as a textbook case of one that excluded women, not least because of its suggestive acronym, MR FIT), recalled the "mindset" that prevailed "in the days when women were mostly at home": "I still remember my internship days. It was very dramatic when you saw a man in his forties come in and die of an MI [myocardial infarction, or heart attack]. In the prime of his life, and he was the only breadwinner in the family. So men were thought of as having the premature heart disease."[26]

As Lenfant noted in a 1998 public lecture on women and heart disease: "The message to middle-aged men was clear: coronary heart disease can kill you. . . . In contrast, the message sent to women at that time was that coronary heart disease can make you a widow. . . . These reminiscences may make you cringe but they were, indeed, the facts of the time."[27] The problem with the prevailing logic, as many critics have pointed out, is that cardiovascular disease remained the leading cause of death for women; they simply tended to contract it at later ages, on average, than did men.[28] The assumption, then, that the leading cause of women's death was less of a public health emergency than the leading cause of men's death just because men were more likely to be affected at a younger age was, ultimately, a value judgment, though one consistent with the cost-benefit logic often used in the health-care arena, which emphasizes the years of "productive" life lost to illness. (It also raised the interesting question of how much of the underrepresentation of women in heart disease research was actually a consequence of the tendency to underrepresent the elderly.)

By the late 1980s, reformers were also citing statistics on the under-representation of racial and ethnic minorities in research samples. An article published by Craig Svensson and coauthors in a special issue of the *Journal of the American Medical Association (JAMA)* devoted to the health of black Americans analyzed a major pharmacology journal from 1984 through 1986. The researchers found that only ten of fifty published studies provided any data on the racial composition of the research subjects. After tracking down the investigators and obtaining demographic data for an additional twenty-five cases, Svensson and coauthors reported that only twenty of the thirty-five clinical studies included any black subjects. Moreover, in many cases where black people *were* included, their representation as a percentage was much lower in the study than in the city where the study was conducted. Another analysis, examining articles published in the *American Journal of Epidemiology*, appeared in the pages of that journal in 1991. Jones and coauthors found "an increasing trend," since 1970, "toward the explicit exclusion of 'nonwhite' subjects and the selection of predominantly 'white' base populations for study."[29]

By the early 1990s, it also became routine to cite statistics on the underrepresentation of children. Decades before, in 1963, one physician had referred to children as "therapeutic orphans" because medications in routine use had never been studied in them. Although the FDA began requiring drug manufacturers to provide pediatric information in drug product labels and package inserts in 1979, the policy had little effect in encouraging the industry to study children. In 1983 Sumner Yaffe, a pediatrician who played a leading role in bringing attention to children's underrepresentation in research, reported that more than 75 percent of drugs marketed in the United States could not be advertised as safe and effective for infants and children, because of the failure to study the drugs in those populations. This "75 percent" figure became a staple in public debate and media commentary in the 1990s.[30]

The AIDS epidemic, which cast a spotlight on nearly every aspect of health care and health research in the United States, brought further attention to the numbers of women, people of color, and children in drug trials. As a 1989 front-page *Los Angeles Times* exposé by Robert Steinbrook revealed, "blacks, Latinos and intravenous drug users, the groups increasingly afflicted with AIDS virus infections, are significantly underrepresented in federally sponsored AIDS clinical trials." Using documents obtained from the NIH under the Freedom of Information Act, Steinbrook showed that while blacks and Latinos accounted for 42 percent of adult U.S. AIDS patients, they made up only 20 percent of the research subjects in the AIDS Clinical Trials Group, the government-sponsored network of drug trials that had received $57 million in federal funds in 1989 alone. A later study by New York activists that was presented at an international AIDS conference in 1991 showed that women made up only 6.7 percent of the AIDS Clinical Trial Group participants. (While women accounted for only 9.8 percent of overall AIDS cases by the CDC's statistics, activists argued that many actual cases of women with AIDS were not captured by the CDC's surveillance definition.)[31]

Of course, critics of the biomedical status quo were inclined not simply to quantify underrepresentation but also to account for it. How could medical researchers possibly be ignoring—or, at least, inadequately studying—what, after all, amounted to the greater part of the U.S. population? Reformers offered a wide variety of explanations, beginning with simple biases on the part of white male researchers about who was worthy of study.[32] Many also pointed to researchers' reliance at times on samples of convenience—such as Veterans Administration patients or the inhabitants of single city—that were highly unrepresentative of the U.S. population.[33] But some also acknowledged that many of these populations were hard to recruit—especially African Americans, who were said to reject the role of medical "guinea pig" out of suspicion of the long history of medical experimentation on black people that dates to slavery and includes the infamous Tuskegee study of "untreated syphilis in the Negro male."[34] In some cases, circumstantial factors seemed to explain a lack of representation. For example, the fact that, at the time of Steinbrook's article, the federally funded AIDS Clinical Trials Group had no presence in five of the thirteen cities that contributed the greatest numbers to the CDC's statistics for U.S. AIDS cases—Houston, Philadelphia, Atlanta, Dallas, and San Juan, Puerto Rico—certainly didn't help ensure a high representation of racial minorities.[35] But in addition to all these explanations, reformers placed special emphasis on two causes of underrepresentation that were central to the overall framing of the problem: "misguided protectionism" and "false universalism."

Misguided Protectionism

In the preceding chapter, I described how the U.S. government in the 1970s introduced a series of measures designed to protect the rights of research subjects, especially those belonging to "vulnerable populations." According to this logic, experimentation was something that vulnerable populations were to be *protected from.* Children, for example, were generally not to be the subjects of clinical trials until after a drug had been proven safe and effective in adults. Ironically, in little more than a decade, aspects of these same well-intentioned policies came to be denounced as paternalistic by activists and reformers, who portrayed women and children as victims of medical neglect. The shift in perceptions is not entirely surprising: as Harold Edgar and David Rothman have pointed out, the emphasis on protectionism that arose in the 1970s ran counter to dominant trends in medical politics of the time: "In a period when autonomy and rights were the highest values in almost every aspect of medical and health care delivery, this was one particular area in which heavy-handed paternalism flourished."[36] By the 1980s, however, patients began to insist on their right to assume risks—indeed, their right to serve as "guinea pigs." Some of the same groups that had been singled out for protection in the earlier era were now portrayed as victims of substandard care, stemming from researcher indifference to the particular manifestations of illness in those groups and inadequate access to potentially lifesaving drugs.

The AIDS activist movement proved to be an especially significant source of pressure to change the protectionist or paternalistic emphasis in the approach toward human subjects and research risks. Activists demanded the inclusion of more women, children, and racial minorities in clinical trials of experimental drugs, arguing that clinical trials served as an important means of access to otherwise unobtainable and theoretically helpful new therapies. If, as activists claimed, access to experimental drugs should be considered a social good (rather than simply as a risk from which vulnerable populations should be protected), then it was only right to distribute such access fairly across the population. While many researchers and ethicists deplored the perception that medical experimentation with unproven therapies should be viewed as a drug distribution system, it was hard to refute the bald logic behind the claim that a new treatment, however risky, might be preferable to certain death. "Drugs into bodies!" became the activist manifesto. "Since virtually every drug used to fight HIV, or the concomitant opportunistic infections of AIDS, is experimental, very often one must be *in a drug trial to get the drug*, noted members of the New York City branch of ACT UP (AIDS Coalition to Unleash Power) in 1988: "Yet [AIDS] drug trials exclude many of those infected with the virus," including women, people of color, children, injection drug users, people with hemophilia, and others.[37] The history of AZT, the first antiviral drug shown to have efficacy against HIV, seemed to validate activist complaints about children in particular: AZT was not widely distributed to children with AIDS in the United States until October 1989, more than three years after adults had gained broad access to the drug.[38]

Not just AIDS activists, but many others concerned about women's health, pointed out that women seemed to be bear an extra burden from regulatory protectionism. As a result of a 1977 FDA guideline, women "of childbearing potential" were formally excluded from many drug trials, whether they were pregnant or not, or had any intention of becoming so, out of concern that an experimental drug might bring harm to a fetus (as, for example, the drug thalidomide had done, especially to Europeans). This exclusion of "pregnant, pregnable, and once-pregnable people (a.k.a women)"—to cite Vanessa Merton's telling phrase in the title of a 1993 article critical of the FDA guideline—had clear implications for the testing of new medications as well as for how women framed their critique. Whereas other groups protesting underrepresentation could argue only that their numbers were lower than they should be, women were in a position to point to a policy that explicitly excluded them.[39]

In intent, the FDA guideline restricting women's participation as subjects applied only to early, so-called Phase 1 and Phase 2 trials of new drugs, whose potential for causing birth defects was still unknown; and it was not supposed to apply to later, large-scale (Phase 3) efficacy trials or, for that matter, to any trials of drugs for life-threatening conditions. In practice, however, the broad and automatic exclusion of premenopausal women from new drug development had become commonplace. This largely was because of drug companies' desires to minimize the risk of legal liability in the case of birth defects, though also because the FDA was making no special efforts to prevent the exclusion of women who did have life-threatening illnesses.[40]

Reformers criticized these tendencies as well as the apparent underlying "natalist" logic—that women's fetuses were to be privileged over women themselves. They also disputed the implicit claim that only women had an effect on fetuses, pointing to evidence that men's exposure to chemicals and toxins affected their sperm.[41] "It's like *The Handmaid's Tale*," reflected women's health activist Cynthia Pearson, in a reference to Margaret Atwood's dystopian novel of a future world in which a class of women function only as breeders: "Your eggs were your purpose in life. And regardless of . . . what you say about how you're making sure that you're not going to get pregnant if you're having sexual intercourse with men, it doesn't matter. . . . The eggs must be protected at all costs."[42]

However, Pearson also acknowledged the irony that, at an earlier juncture, it had been women's health advocates, horrified by women's experiences with DES and the Dalkon shield, who had pressed for greater federal regulation of drugs and devices used by women. Indeed, as several commentators have noted, the rise of a broad-based reaction against regulatory protectionism constituted a remarkably rapid "pendulum swing" away from an equally vociferous emphasis in the 1970s on protecting subjects from research risks.[43] Gary Ellis, director of the NIH's Office for Protection from Research Risks, which oversaw the protection of human subjects, described this shift in sensibilities as nothing less than a "sea change."[44]

Indeed, it is entirely conceivable that institutions and organizations deeply invested in the protectionist reforms that developed in the 1970s— such as the national institutional review boards (IRBs) structure overseen by Ellis, which was created at that time—might have been especially resistant to the new calls for inclusion. For example, Richard Klein, the HIV/AIDS program director in the FDA's Office of Special Health Issues, recalled encountering "an awful lot of resistance" on the part of IRB members to the idea of doing a "180 degree turn and saying now you should be including these groups of people, particularly women." Said Klein: "Even if companies were willing to have . . . that particular population represented in the study, the IRBs might have been the barrier."[45] Because the whole raison d'être of the IRB system is the protection of human subjects, institutional leeriness toward the new inclusionary philosophy would not be surprising.

False Universalism

Another frame that helped the reform coalition to account for—and denounce—the inadequate inclusion of groups in research could be called "false universalism." A familiar complaint in identity politics, this term describes situations in which the experience of the dominant group in society (such as white men) is taken to be the universal experience—the norm or standard—rather than the particular experience of that group alone.[46] False universalism seemed capable of leading to the underrepresentation of subordinate social groups through various routes. One possibility was that researchers who happened to find themselves studying men for reasons of convenience—say, because they conducted their studies in Veterans Administration hospitals or military settings—might not even notice that their representation of humanity was incomplete.[47] Another possibility was that researchers who viewed the male or white or adult body as the standard deliberately sought to avoid any bodies that seemed different.

Indeed, many anecdotal reports attributed the underrepresentation of women to biomedical researchers' belief that women were "complicated" research subjects: their monthly fluctuations in hormone levels, it was felt, could confound the effects of the medical regimes or therapies under investigation. Men's bodies, by this reasoning, were simpler to study, as there were fewer "variables" to control for.[48] Somewhat similarly, researchers presumed not just that elderly patients deserved protection from the risks of biomedical experiments, but also that the tendency for the elderly to suffer from multiple health problems and consume many medications simultaneously would muddy the results from clinical trials. Most generally, some researchers believed that trials with a homogeneous subject population constituted a quicker route to medical knowledge, while the "noise" of variation would introduce heterogeneity that would inevitably complicate the interpretation of findings and make them more difficult to publish in medical journals.[49] Left unstated, of course, were the presumptions about who constituted "noise."

Rebecca Dresser nicely captured the logic of these various assumptions in a critique published in 1992:

> NIH officials and biomedical researchers have, consciously or unconsciously, defined the white male as the normal, representative human being. From this perspective, the goal of advancing human health can be achieved by studying the white male human model. Physical differences between males and females, or between whites and people of color, are unacknowledged or irrelevant in this world view. Including women and people of color would simply complicate the work, thus making it more difficult and costly, which would detract from the researchers' mission of improving human health and welfare. According to this world view, "special money" must be raised to study women and people of color, so that the "regular money" can be reserved for "normal" research.[50]

In effect, specific identities were falsely taken as universals, much as the term *Man* was once commonly used to refer to the species as a whole.

As suggested by the historical review in the preceding chapter, any blanket accusation that biomedical researchers and their sponsors had equated "white" and "male" with "normal" was somewhat of an overstatement. Still, it was easy for reformers to point to specific instances in which false universalism was at work. Hence, it proved to be a potent mobilizing frame, one that aligned closely with broader and well-known critiques of how a false universalism can disguise institutionalized sexism and racism.[51] Critics suggested that this narrow conception of the standard human had thoroughly penetrated medical theory, practice, education, and training. Its signs ranged from the anatomical images used in medical textbooks, which "present male anatomy as the norm which must be understood before the student can comprehend female structures," to the presumptions about which sorts of people could best work as doctors or scientists.[52]

Opposing false universalism, some physicians took aim at the notion that any group in society could be deemed "simple" for purposes of study in comparison with the "complexity" of others. Jerry Avorn, a geriatrician and professor of social medicine at Harvard, told a reporter for *JAMA* that the idea that white men's bodies offer fewer confounding factors to the experimenter is "an assumption made very glibly, and only because white men run the country."[53] Critics of the status quo also pointed out the obvious inconsistency in the rationales put forward in defense of studying homogeneous populations. On one hand, women's differences were taken to mean that they were unsuitable research subjects; on the other hand, women's membership within the universal category of "Man" meant that results, once obtained from experiments on men, were presumed to be applicable to women. Challenging this shaky logic, reformers responded that if sex differences didn't matter, then there were no grounds for excluding women; but if women's differences were indeed medically significant, then it only made sense to study them. Genuine equality between the sexes should be based not on a false assertion of sameness, but rather—at least sometimes—on a proper acknowledgment of difference.[54]

Importantly, some pharmaceutical company representatives concerned about ensuring the broadest possible marketability of their products joined the criticism of using narrow or homogeneous research samples. At a 1993 workshop on the "relevance of ethnic factors in the clinical evaluation of medicines," Leigh Thompson, the chief scientific officer for Eli Lilly, argued that "estimations of efficiency in general use are best made from large global trials that admit widely diverse patients, with the results analysed by many defined factors." Indeed, Thompson suggested that studying the "average" patient proved deceptive in gauging proper drug doses, and he noted that Lilly had adopted policies of "ensuring minimal exclusion of patients, early incorporation of women, and inclusion of all ages that are safe for study (often with no age limit)."[55]

In promoting the false-universalism frame, reformers adapted for their purposes the widespread commitment to diversity as a social goal, and they rejected the Procrustean limitations of a one-size-fits-all approach to health care. At the same time, reformers leaned on popular discomfort with the notion that humanity ought to be subjected to standardization. The literary critic Raymond Williams observed an interesting tension in everyday language use: "standards" are often applauded as things to be upheld, but "standardization" is often viewed skeptically as an unfortunate byproduct of modernization that suppresses choice and beneficial variation.[56] And there seems to be something especially troubling about the notion of standardizing *people*: the concept is jarring to popular sensibilities, especially in an individualistic society such as the United States.[57] As I described in the preceding chapter, modern scientific medicine and systems of managed care have ushered in a considerable degree of medical standardization, but not without resistance from both consumers and health care professionals. Opponents of a reliance on the standard human as the subject of medical experiments were able to tap into that resistance. Moreover, they could point to the particular inequities associated with the reliance on what might be called a "typological" standard human: singling out a sociodemographic group as the ideal specimen of humanity—the ones most worthy of study—and then treating knowledge derived from the study of that group as universal truth, applicable without modification to all other groups in society.[58]

Health Disparities

In framing the problem of inadequate inclusion, advocates focused not only on the causes of underrepresentation but also on its consequences. To that end, in the case of at least some of the groups in question (particularly, racial and ethnic minority groups), advocates invoked abundant documentation of "health disparities" collected by epidemiologists and health services researchers. This concept encompassed a range of inequalities between groups in the domains of health and health care, including the degree of access to medical care; the differential utilization of specific medical procedures, treatments, and technologies; differences between groups in the rates of disease incidence and prevalence; and outcome differences such as infant mortality rates and survival rates after diagnosis of illness.[59] Perhaps the most eloquent indicator of the racial gulf in health was the simple statistic of life expectancy: on average, a white baby born in 1980 could expect to live about six years longer than a black baby.[60]

At the federal level, a 1985 report from a committee established by DHHS Secretary Margaret Heckler (the Secretary's Task Force on Black and Minority Health) placed the issue of disparities squarely on the nation's health agenda. In her cover letter, Heckler lamented the continuing disparity for "blacks and other minority Americans"; and much of the report itself emphasized the importance of collecting better data on minority health trends in order to generate clearer comparison across racial and ethnic groups. The report's title clearly reflected the tendency, at the time, to treat racial issues in the United States as fundamentally a black/white matter, but the report itself did address health disparities among other groups, which it named as Hispanics, Native Americans, and Asian/Pacific Islanders.[61] (Although included here, the concerns of American Indians often have been addressed somewhat separately by DHHS for historical reasons; in 1955, responsibility for their health needs was transferred from the Department of the Interior's Bureau of Indian Affairs to the Indian Health Service, a distinct Public Health Service agency reporting directly to the Assistant Secretary for Health.[62])

Evidence of disparities pointed to fundamental inequalities in U.S. society. But in addition, such findings presented strong presumptive grounds for greater biomedical attention to underrepresented groups and, hence, inclusion in higher numbers in studies. If, for example, blacks and Latinos had worse health outcomes and higher mortality rates than other racial and ethnic groups, then it seemed manifestly problematic for researchers to be studying them *less*. (Of course, in the case of women, who experience higher rates of morbidity than men in the United States but also have longer life expectancies, such arguments potentially cut both ways.)

Biological Differences

A fifth—and important—frame remains to be discussed. Advocates of change placed particular emphasis on the argument that underrepresentation matters because of medical differences across groups—differences generally understood in biological terms. This frame linked the politics of inclusion to the science of extrapolation: it was crucially important to include women, people of color, children, and the elderly as subjects in research because the findings from studying middle-aged white men simply could not be assumed to be generalizable. While this emphasis on bodily difference was pivotal in making the case for reform, I will argue in the latter chapters of this book that the appeal to biology was a problematic way of grounding the call for reform.

Those who emphasized biological differences relied in part on commonsense understandings, but advocates were also quick to argue that science was on their side. Beginning in the early twentieth century, investigators had reported findings of differential responsiveness to medications. Initially, these reports mostly concerned sex differences in other species—differences in the responses of male and female cats to ether, mice to morphine, rats to strychnine, and rabbits to alcohol.[63] In recent decades, however, and especially with the rise of new techniques to study genetic variation in human metabolic processes, reports of findings of difference in humans had become quite frequent.[64]

Many studies have analyzed the unequal distribution by sex and race/ethnicity of genetic variants of the cytochrome P450 enzymes that metabolize many pharmaceutical drugs, and researchers argued that such differences cause a standard dose of these medications to have different effects in different groups. In a 1989 article in the *New England Journal of Medicine*, Werner Kalow and coauthors reported that "about 90 percent of whites have a form of alcohol dehydrogenase in their liver that metabolizes ethanol in vitro more slowly than does the corresponding liver enzyme found in approximately 90 percent of Orientals." A 1990 news report in *JAMA*, entitled "Examples Abound of Gaps in Medical Knowledge Because of Groups Excluded from Scientific Study," noted a range of such findings—including that "Asians have much faster metabolism and elimination rates for propranolol, which lower plasma concentrations"—and discounted the possibility that they could be due to average differences in body weight or size.[65]

Some pharmacologists suggested that the ultimate significance of findings related to differences in how people metabolized drugs was often less than it appeared at first, because such differences really would matter only in the minority of cases where medications have a narrow "therapeutic index"—where the margin of safety between the effective dose and the toxic dose is relatively small.[66] However, studies appeared to indicate that the same medications did actually have different therapeutic consequences for different groups. For example, Douglas Schmucker and coauthors cited FDA data to the effect that women aged 20 to 39 suffered twice as many adverse drug reactions as males of the same age, perhaps as a result of "differences in body fat, lean mass, body water content, liver volume," and other factors affecting drug metabolism.[67]

Another widely cited example concerned the drugs commonly used to treat hypertension. As early as 1966, reports in the medical literature had suggested that reduced improvements from antihypertensive drugs in African American patients as compared to whites might be due not just to lesser access to drugs on the part of African Americans but also to actual physical differences in how the drugs affected the two groups. By the 1990s, it had become conventional wisdom that African American patients respond better to diuretics than to other drugs such as beta-blockers, perhaps because of biological differences in how the kidneys process sodium.[68] In light of such findings, advocates for minority health increasingly expressed reservations about medical treatments that had been tested only in white populations. As Vivian Pinn—at that time the president of the National Medical Association, but later the director of the NIH's Office of Research on Women's Health—told a reporter from *JAMA* in 1990: "Some of our physicians are a little leery" of some drugs because "we can't be certain whether minorities have been participants" in clinical trials.[69]

In addition, pediatricians—whose medical specialty is, in some sense, premised on the insistence that a child is not simply a "miniature adult"[70]—also put forward difference arguments. They noted that not just children's size, but also the maturational process itself, affects the course of disease and the physiological responsiveness to medications.[71] As evidence of the gravity of their concerns, pediatricians invoked the classic example of the "gray baby syndrome" in the 1950s, which was determined to have been caused by the administration of the drug chloramphenicol to treat nursery infections. Physicians of the time had calculated a dosage based on body weight or body size—failing to recognize that newborns had a much-reduced capacity to metabolize the drug. Thus, a medication that had a tissue half-life of four hours in children had a half-life of twenty-six hours in newborns, and the accumulation of the drug in the bodies of newborns had resulted in vomiting, an ashen color, cyanosis, vascular collapse, and death.[72] Only the actual testing of medications in children of different ages, pediatricians contended, could forestall such tragedies in the future.

Analogously, geriatricians pointed to differences in how the elderly respond to medications. For example, age-associated physiological impairments and reduced rates of drug clearance (that is, removal of the drug from the blood by the kidneys) make it more likely that the elderly will suffer from adverse drug reactions.[73]

Thus, a range of findings by certain groups of biomedical researchers and physicians gave weight to notions of biological differences. Moreover, these findings both suggested and presupposed that key identity categories of everyday life—gender, race, ethnicity, and age—were also the relevant categories for biomedical purposes.

To be sure, the proportion of medical research reporting on differences according to these categories was by no means substantial. For example, from 1970 to 1979, only 2,915 Medline articles were indexed with the Medical Subject Heading "Blacks"—just 0.21 percent of all articles on human beings. From 1980 to 1989, despite a small increase in absolute numbers to 3,080 articles, the percentage of journal articles indexed as referring to "Blacks" actually fell to 0.15 percent.[74] But the fact that these reports were a relatively minor current in the vast flow of medical journal articles did not prevent reformers from calling attention to them.

In fact, advocates of inclusion used these findings strategically to bolster their arguments about the inequities of underrepresentation. For example, at the same time as AIDS activists stressed the ethical principle of equal access to experimental therapies, they also put forward a scientific argument: they noted that, because AIDS had different clinical manifestations in women, it made good scientific sense to study the disease separately in women and not to assume that therapies would have the same efficacy or toxicity across groups.[75] A number of physicians treating AIDS patients voiced similar views about the importance of studying both women and racial and ethnic minorities. The same *Los Angeles Times* article that reported on underrepresentation in AIDS trials quoted the director of the AIDS service at the Johns Hopkins Hospital in Baltimore: "Drugs may behave differently in different racial and ethnic groups and in women. . . . Consequently, you can't generalize from studies done in middle-class gay white men."[76] (Indeed, although the hypothesis was later rejected, well-publicized preliminary findings from one large study of the drug AZT suggested in 1991 that the drug was less efficacious in "non-whites" than in "whites."[77]) The failure to investigate such differences consistently, and the consequent inability of doctors and patients to speak with confidence about health and illness across populations, therefore constituted an interesting example of what Robert Proctor has, in a different context, described as the "social construction of ignorance."[78]

Not all reports of treatment differences across groups presumed that such differences were strictly biological in nature. Sometimes researchers targeted cultural differences in diet, attributing, for example, the differences in how Mexican Americans metabolize certain medications to the effects of a chemical found in chili peppers. Other researchers were simply more interested in other questions, such as how the different likelihood that women or minorities would receive specialized medical procedures might be attributed to conscious or unconscious racism on the part of health-care providers. However, it is perhaps not surprising that, in a society that so often tends to understand social difference as something rooted in biology, sex/gender, racial, ethnic, and age differences in response to medications seemed quite plausibly to be located in physiological and genetic processes.[79]

Indeed, what is striking is that proponents of the biological-differences frame appeared to be relatively unbothered by the risk, well suggested by the historical studies of biology and medicine reviewed in the preceding chapter, that difference might be conceived of in pejorative terms and used to bolster arguments about social inferiority. In past centuries, to be called medically "other" was to be considered a lesser sort of human being; but by the late 1980s, reports of biological differences seemed strategically advantageous to those who sought better health care for socially disadvantaged groups.[80]

Moreover, calling attention to biological differences in the domain of pharmacology also sometimes suited the financial interests of pharmaceutical companies. A 1993 report on "ethnic and racial differences in response to medicines" issued by a trade group called the National Pharmaceutical Council made this logic explicit. Various "cost containment tactics" that had become common with the advent of managed care—including the mandatory use of generic drugs or the requirement that drugs be selected from an approved list called a formulary—functioned to restrict physicians' and patients' choices of medications in cases where several drugs were marketed for the same condition. But the presumption "that related medicines having the same general effect are almost identical in their actions and are therefore interchangeable" failed to take into account the ethnic and racial differences that had been demonstrated in the literature. Such restrictions could therefore "lead to inappropriate or suboptimal therapy for minority groups." Here the logic of recognizing group differences went hand in hand with a desire to ensure the continued marketability of the widest possible range of pharmaceutical company products and not just the ones with the least expensive price tags.[81]

Diverse Critics, Diverse Arguments

What is striking about the framing of the politics of biomedical inclusion is the multiplicity of arguments that these various critics put forward. The five frames described above identified—and sometimes joined together—analyses of disparate causes and consequences. These frames traversed a great deal of intellectual distance, from the statistics of inclusion to the politics of the standard human to the fine details of pharmacology and drug metabolism. Some of the frames rested primarily on the language of ethics and social justice; others, like the biological-differences frame, took a more scientific tone. But all of them in some measure blended ethical, political, and scientific arguments. I now turn to the story of how reformers, relying on these arguments, went about changing federal research policies.

CHAPTER FOUR

The Path to Reform: Aligning Categories, Targeting the State

How to bring about biomedical change? "Biomedicine" encompasses a highly diverse set of institutions spread around the country and around the world, and reformers concerned about the politics of inclusion needed a more precise target—at least initially—if they were going to be effective. The sensible choice proved to be the U.S. federal government—specifically, the DHHS, especially the wing of it called the Public Health Service (PHS), which includes such agencies as the NIH, the FDA, and the CDC. Focusing on the state made sense because of the control it exerts over medical research. At the same time, state agencies lay within the sphere of influence of activists and politicians—more so than research centers, pharmaceutical companies, or other biomedical institutions.[1] Moreover, as already emphasized, some of the advocates of change were positioned *within* the state, as DHHS employees, and therefore were able to press for reform from the inside.

Taking up the story begun in the previous chapter and following it forward into the early 1990s, I will trace the process by which reformers achieved their first key victories: new policies guaranteeing greater inclusion of women and minorities in clinical trials and in pharmaceutical drug development. I then conclude the chapter by analyzing this tacit coalition's successes in bringing about policy change. Beginning with an issue described previously—the hybrid composition of the reform effort—I go on to define and highlight two techniques that reformers employed adroitly: what I call "multirepresentational politics" (the linkage of numerical, political, and symbolic forms of representation) and "categorical alignment" (the merging of social categories from the worlds of medicine, social movements, and state administration).

TAKING ACTION

In the 1980s, questions relating to group differences and health disparities began to surface within DHHS agencies. The National Institute of Mental Health (NIMH) was perhaps the first agency to create, in 1983, a special office devoted to underserved groups—or "special populations," as they came to be termed.[2] (At the time, the NIMH was not yet part of the NIH; it was part of a separate PHS agency called the Alcohol, Drug Abuse, and Mental Health Administration [ADAMHA].) Delores Parron, the director of this office, has described special populations as "all those groups who were de facto treated as second-class citizens."[3] With some justification, Parron refers to that office as the "mother cell" that helped to inspire the creation of many of the offices for underserved groups that emerged subsequently within the DHHS.[4]

In the mid-1980s, the DHHS responded to public scrutiny and internal pressure by creating task forces to study its efforts in aiding specific communities. As already mentioned, DHHS Secretary Margaret Heckler's Task Force on Black and Minority Health presented its report in 1985. That same year, another commission, the Public Health Service Task Force on Women's Health Issues, created by Assistant Secretary for Health Edward Brandt, issued its own report. Urging the expansion of biomedical and behavioral research "to ensure emphasis on conditions and diseases unique to, or more prevalent in, women in all age groups," the task force recommended that oversight of women's health issues be assigned to a specific office within the DHHS.[5]

As Judith Auerbach and Anne Figert have noted in their account of the politics of women's health research in the 1980s and early 1990s, this document had considerable strategic benefit: it "provided the 'proof'—in the form of a legitimate scientific report—that women's health activists, scientists, and members of Congress needed in order to push for further reform."[6] In 1986, in response to the Task Force on Women's Health Issues, the NIH, along with ADAMHA, issued guidelines that, for the first time, recommended including women in research studies funded by the agencies. Upon the urging of Delores Parron (who had served on both the Task Force on Women's Health Issues and the Task Force on Black and Minority Health), the two agencies extended the emphasis on inclusion the following year by issuing parallel guidelines urging the inclusion of racial and ethnic minorities.[7] Importantly, however, these guidelines stopped short of actually *requiring* anyone to do anything, and they had no specific enforcement mechanism. Furthermore, there does not appear to have been much effort to communicate these guidelines to the research community. Nor is there any evidence that the institutional review boards (IRBs) around the country that review the ethics of research protocols were instructed to pay attention to the issue of inclusion.[8]

Over the next few years, a growing number of prominent women sought to bring attention to the problem of underrepresentation as well as the broader question of women's health. Female scientists at the NIH, such as Florence Haseltine, the director of the Center for Population Research at the National Institute of Child Health and Human Development (NICHD, one of the NIH institutes), worked behind the scenes to call attention to the low profile of women's health issues at the agency. Influenced by the example of the "AIDS lobby" and breast cancer advocacy groups, Haseltine, in her words, "began to work with women who knew how to affect legislation."[9] As a federal employee, Haseltine was forbidden from lobbying Congress, but she encouraged a lobbying group called Bass and Howes that specialized in women's issues to found a new, Washington, D.C.–based, advocacy group called the Society for the Advancement of Women's Health Research (SAWHR).[10] Emblematic of a new wave of women's health advocacy—more professionalized than the women's health movement of the 1970s, more focused on research issues, less critical of pharmaceutical companies, and willing to sidestep divisive issues such as abortion—SAWHR explicitly took up the cause of inclusion of women in clinical research as its priority issue. The group worked to raise the issue with female legislators and others who might be sympathetic.[11]

Congress and the NIH

At the same time, the broad issue of women's health became a galvanizing one for women in Congress, even as the topic of health reform edged toward the top of the policy agenda in Washington.[12] Women in Congress, especially Rep. Patricia Schroeder and Rep. Olympia Snowe, cochairs of the Congressional Caucus for Women's Issues, seized upon the issue of inclusion as a means to bring broader attention to women's health needs. "Every time you picked up the paper, there was something," recalled Schroeder, a Democrat from Colorado, thinking of the news reports in the 1980s that trumpeted the findings of medical researchers conducting clinical studies—reports about "men eating fish, men riding bikes, men drinking coffee, men taking aspirin. And we were just wondering whether 'men' was an all-encompassing word, or whether it was truly just men."[13] Schroeder had become acquainted with Florence Haseltine at the NIH, and Haseltine took the opportunity to cart her slide projector to meetings with the Caucus, teaching them the basics about the "structure and function" of the NIH.[14]

Schroeder and Snowe (a Republican from Maine) took their concerns about women's health to Henry Waxman, chair of the Health and Environment Subcommittee in the House of Representatives. Ruth Katz, who served as counsel to the subcommittee, working along with Leslie Primmer, a staff member for the Caucus, then devised a "hook" to draw congressional attention to the broader issue of women's health. As Katz recalled, "I said, 'I wonder if they have any rules about making sure that women are included in clinical trials?'" Upon discovering that, indeed, NIH had already implemented a policy encouraging inclusion of women and minorities in 1986, Katz proposed: "Why don't we get GAO [the General Accounting Office, Congress's own investigative agency] to take a look at the simple question of to what extent NIH is following its own rules?"[15] Thus, the focusing of congressional attention on inclusion policies—a choice that would prove consequential—came about, in some measure, as a result of a purely strategic decision about how best to attract public attention to the broader issue of women's health.

The Caucus convinced Waxman to authorize the GAO study, and the results of that investigation only confirmed the suspicions of Katz and the Caucus members—indeed, as Primmer put it, the GAO's report was "the spark that ignited the explosion of legislative action around women's health."[16] The investigators found that the 1986 policy on inclusion had been poorly communicated even within NIH and had been applied inconsistently; moreover, "NIH has no way to measure the policy's impact on the research it funds."[17] At the June 1990 House subcommittee meeting at which the GAO report was unveiled, Schroeder declared bluntly: "American women have been put at risk."[18] As Carol Weisman has noted in her account of these events, the report's release "was carefully orchestrated for maximum public impact," with representatives of the media well in attendance.[19] But what may have caused reporters to sit up and take note was the testimony of the acting director of the NIH, William Raub.

Raub outlined steps taken by the NIH in recent years to address the issue of inclusion, and he also took exception to some misleading interpretations of funding statistics that had been bandied about in Congress: some had noted that only 13 percent of NIH expenditures were for conditions exclusively or primarily affecting women and had concluded from this figure that the remaining 87 percent of spending must be on men; in fact, only about 6 percent was on conditions exclusively or primarily affecting men. Nevertheless, in essence Raub acknowledged that the congressional criticism had merit. "He flat out admitted it," recalled Katz.[20] Indeed, Raub confessed to a reporter for the journal *Science* that at least some NIH staff members had "disdain" for the existing inclusion guideline.[21]

In communicating with the media and the public, Caucus members emphasized the false-universalism frame, citing, for example, the NIH-funded Baltimore Longitudinal Study of Aging: its final report, based on the study of more than one thousand men and no women, was entitled "Normal Human Aging." Another prominent, all-male study, the Multiple Risk Factor Intervention Trial examining cardiovascular disease, seemed even by its acronym—MR FIT—to suggest which half of humanity was deemed worthy of scientific attention. Other studies caught the attention of GAO simply because of the complete absence of women in research on topics of broad public health significance. A chief culprit was the NIH-funded Physicians' Health Study, begun in 1981, which had investigated the role of aspirin use in preventing heart attacks: the study had enrolled 22,000 male doctors. "[NIH] officials told us women were not included in the study, because to do so would have increased the cost," commented Mark Nadel, who presented the GAO's findings. "However, we now have the dilemma of not knowing whether this preventive strategy would help women, harm them, or have no effect."[22] Olympia Snowe, whose mother had died of breast cancer, also described for reporters a federally funded study on the relation between obesity and cancer of the breast and uterus; the pilot study had used only men. "Somehow I find it hard to imagine that the male-dominated medical community would tolerate a study of prostate cancer that used only women as research subjects," Snowe commented.[23]

Members of the Caucus, following up on the publicity generated by the GAO report, presented their concerns at a meeting with the directors of the NIH institutes (all but one of whom were men). Seeking to address congressional criticism, acting NIH director Raub announced that he was creating an a new Office of Research on Women's Health, to be headed initially by Dr. Ruth Kirschstein, an NIH insider.[24] However, as Schroeder recalls the meeting, the institute directors were resentful of congressional interference and "very haughty, very arrogant" in justifying the status quo: "[They told us], 'Women are in all these different metabolic states, blah-blah-blah.' So we said, 'Could those different metabolic states require different treatments?' And they said, 'Well, we really don't know because we've never tested.'" Schroeder left the meeting fearing that, given the history of gender bias in medical research, going to the doctor made about as much sense for a woman as "going to a vet."[25] The Caucus then began pressing for legislation that would force the NIH to change its ways.

Fortuitously, the NIH budget was up for reauthorization, and as Caucus staff member Leslie Primmer has observed, "The need to reauthorize NIH in 1990 proved a prime opportunity to address the issue of research on women's health. In the jargon of Capitol Hill, it is known as 'having a vehicle,' and the NIH reauthorization bill provided the congresswomen with the vehicle they needed to move their legislation."[26]

By September 1990, acting NIH director Raub had reinforced the guidelines on inclusion, warning researchers requesting federal funds that they would need to provide "compelling justification" for not including women. However, by this point, the Caucus was unlikely to be mollified by any policy that stopped short of legally requiring change on the part of the NIH and the researchers it funded. Congressional staff drafted a new section to be included in the NIH Revitalization Act that obligated the NIH to ensure that women were included as subjects in NIH-funded research—transforming the NIH's existing inclusion policy from a recommendation into a requirement and giving it the force of law.

As legislators began building support for these additions to the NIH Revitalization Act, African American members of Congress called for a further extension of the legislative mandate. The Congressional Black Caucus was somewhat less focused on health issues than the Congressional Caucus for Women's Issues—for example, they did not have a staff member specifically working on the topic. However, the Black Caucus had for some time kept an eye on any legislation concerning health through the activities of its "health brain trust," an advisory group of health professionals established by Rep. Louis Stokes.[27] Once members of the Black Caucus expressed interest in the new NIH initiative, members of the Congressional Caucus for Women's Issues were receptive: as Schroeder recalled, "NIH actually collects from every taxpayer equally," so "when they put these studies together, they ought to be looking at what America looks like."[28] Consequently, the phrase "and minorities" was added to the wording about inclusion of women in research.

Twists and Turns in NIH Reform

Along the way to eventual passage, the NIH Revitalization Act followed a path that was anything but linear. The first version of the Act died in the House of Representatives in 1990. After its reintroduction, the Act was passed by Congress in 1991 but vetoed by President George Bush, who objected to an unrelated provision of the legislation that would have overturned a ban on fetal tissue research. As congressional staff member Ruth Katz recalled, had it not been for the fetal tissue issue and its complex relation to abortion politics, passage "wouldn't have been a snoozer, but I believe the bill would have passed overwhelmingly, and President Bush would have proudly proclaimed, 'Look at what I'm doing for women's health.'"[29] After President Bill Clinton was inaugurated in January 1993, he issued an executive order removing the fetal tissue research ban. With that issue off the table, the Act then moved quickly through Congress and thence to Clinton's desk. Clinton signed the bill on June 10, 1993, with members of the Congressional Caucus for Women's Issues standing at his side. (When I visited Schroeder in her office in 1998, the official photograph of the signing was hanging on her wall.)

However, these changes to NIH research policy were only one dimension of the women's health agenda promoted by the Caucus in the form of an omnibus Women's Health Equity Act. This legislative package contained twenty-two bills addressing not only research issues, but also health services and prevention; although many of these measures never were enacted, some were, including Medicare coverage for mammography screening.[30] A separate omnibus bill, the Minority Health Initiative Act, died in the Senate. Thus, congressional discussions of inclusion of women and minorities in health research were tied together not only with other issues related to NIH funding, but also with a range of health concerns affecting women and racial and ethnic minority groups. However, inclusion in research—a goal originally selected largely for strategic reasons, as a hook to attract attention to women's health—ultimately proved more sellable than many of the other specific issues deemed important by health advocates.

Support for the NIH Revitalization Act in Congress grew out of the convergence of political opportunities and circumstances. As Carol Weisman has noted, although the political climate during the Bush administration was not especially friendly to women's issues, in the early 1990s women's health became a popular bipartisan issue—a way for members of both parties to demonstrate a commitment to women. This became especially true after the 1992 elections, which nearly doubled the number of women in Congress. Moreover, the charged and bitter confirmation hearings for Supreme Court Justice Clarence Thomas (accused of sexual harassment by Anita Hill) left many members of Congress anxious to demonstrate that they did care about women's issues, and the health arena was a generally safe one in which to make a statement. And Schroeder and Snowe promoted bipartisan support by deliberately avoiding any issues relating to abortion.[31]

Health care in general moved to the forefront of public concern after Clinton began work on his health care reform plan. In addition, a powerful breast cancer advocacy movement, seeking to emulate the successes of AIDS activists, fostered "an unprecedented spate of consumer advocacy and government action." Not only did breast cancer advocates achieve considerable success in increasing federal research funding for the disease, but they also helped keep the whole question of women's health on the front burner.[32] Caucus staff member Primmer also noted the ways in which female members of Congress shared personal stories with colleagues on the Hill in order to gain their support for women's health-related legislation: Snowe spoke of her mother's death to breast cancer, Rep. Mary Rose Oakar described her sister's breast cancer, Rep. Rosa DeLauro recounted her personal battle with ovarian cancer, and so on.[33] All these factors help explain the support that gradually formed behind the NIH legislation.

Meanwhile, officials in the executive branch of government continued to take steps to appease congressional critics. In 1991 Dr. Bernadine Healy, a Harvard Medical School–trained cardiologist, former director of the American Heart Association, and deputy director of the White House Office of Science and Technology, was appointed by President Bush as the new director of the NIH—the thirteenth director in that agency's history, but the first woman to hold the position.[34] Days later, Healy told Congress that the NIH would fund the Women's Health Initiative, a huge, cross-institute study of cardiovascular disease, cancer, and osteoporosis.[35] Writing in the *New England Journal of Medicine* about the study, Healy declared, "it is now time for a general awakening" with regard to women's health. She complained, "Decades of sex-exclusive research have reinforced the myth that coronary artery disease is a uniquely male affliction and have generated data sets in which men are the normative standard. The extrapolation of these male-generated findings to women has led in some cases to biased standards of care and has prevented the full consideration of several important aspects of coronary disease in women."[36]

Healy also reinforced Raub's actions to coordinate women's health issues at the NIH. In what a reporter described as "one of the only known examples in NIH history of the old girl network in action," Healy appointed one of her former instructors at Massachusetts General Hospital, Vivian Pinn, to head the NIH's recently created Office of Research on Women's Health. A former president of the National Medical Association, Pinn had been both the only woman and the only African American in the University of Virginia's medical school class of 1963.[37]

However much these actions were applauded in Congress, they did not slow the determination of Caucus members to promote their legislative agenda. Moreover, Healy's relationship with the Caucus was not always smooth. When Healy, presumably under pressure from the Bush administration, wrote to Congress in 1992 expressing her opposition to the NIH Revitalization Act and accusing Congress of meddling in health research, women in Congress felt they had been "double crossed" by the NIH Director.[38] "That really got some of the members just boiling mad," recalled Susan Wood, who served as deputy director of the Caucus.[39]

The Devil in the Details

What actions did the NIH Revitalization Act compel? In a new section entitled "Inclusion of Women and Minorities in Clinical Research," the legislation required that women and "members of minority groups" be included as research subjects in NIH-funded studies beginning with fiscal year 1995. (This requirement applied both to "extramural" research—the bulk of NIH-funded research, performed by scientists based at universities and elsewhere who applied to the NIH for funds—and to the "intramural" research conducted in-house by NIH scientists.) Inclusion might be waived in cases where it would be "inappropriate with respect to the health of the subjects; . . . inappropriate with respect to the purposes of the research; or . . . inappropriate under such other circumstances as the Director of NIH may designate." However, issues relating to increased cost were explicitly ruled out as a possible example of what might determine inappropriateness. The bill also formally established an Office of Research on Women's Health and an Office of Research on Minority Health within NIH. Reporting to the NIH Director, these offices were charged with identifying women's health and minority health research projects worthy of support and promoting collaborative work on these topics across the various NIH institutes. (Though the NIH had already created these offices, the passage of the legislation ensured their continuation as a statutory requirement.)[40]

Perhaps the most controversial aspect of the NIH Revitalization Act, however, was its unabashed intrusion into questions of scientific research methodology. In this regard, the legislation went well beyond the simple issue of inclusion. Consistent with the biological-differences frame, the legislative language required that NIH-funded clinical trials be "designed and carried out in a manner sufficient to provide for a valid analysis of whether the variables being studied in the trial affect women or members of minority groups, as the case may be, differently than other subjects in the trial."[41] That is, it would not be enough just to ensure that there were some women and racial and ethnic minorities in the study. Researchers would have to design their studies in order to be able to report, at the end of the day, whether there were sex/gender, racial, or ethnic differences in the results. This demand on the part of Congress would serve as a lightning rod for criticism by many of the opponents of the measure. Importantly, however, the legislation left it up to the NIH to develop formal guidelines specifying when inclusion might be inappropriate, how outreach programs should be designed to recruit women and minorities as subjects, and exactly how clinical trials should be structured in order to "provide for a valid analysis" of differences.

The FDA Gets Its Turn

As the distributor of significant amounts of taxpayers' money, the NIH bore the brunt of congressional scrutiny with regard to inclusion. By contrast, as Karen Baird has noted, less pressure was placed on the FDA initially, both because that agency was not funding research with tax dollars and because many politicians had motivations that cut the other way: committed to a probusiness, deregulatory agenda, they believed that the FDA already was placing too many roadblocks in the way of drug approvals and that the last thing needed was additional bureaucracy.[42] However, during the early 1990s, the FDA increasingly became a target as well.

Like the NIH, the FDA had been moving to address issues of inclusion and difference in the late 1980s and early 1990s.[43] In 1988 the agency had requested that drug manufacturers provide analyses of subpopulation differences (by gender, age, and race/ethnicity) in new drug applications, and in 1989 the agency had called for the inclusion of elderly patients in clinical trials leading to drug approvals. However, the agency had shown little inclination to police these recommendations. And most importantly, the 1977 guideline restricting the participation of women of childbearing potential as research subjects was still on the books. Thus, when Congress commissioned another GAO study in 1992, which surveyed all manufacturers of drugs that had been approved by the agency in recent years, investigators concluded that "for more than 60 percent of the drugs, the representation of women in the test population was less than the representation of women in the population with the corresponding disease." Even when women were included, drug companies typically were not analyzing the findings from clinical trials "to determine if women's responses to a drug differed from those of men." Nor were all manufacturers equally scrupulous about testing whether their products interacted with female hormones, including the hormones found in oral contraceptives.[44] In light of these findings, members of Congress considered taking legislative action to change FDA policies and began drafting legislation—though in this case they lacked the "hook" that was provided them, in the case of the NIH, by the fact that the agency was up for reauthorization.[45]

To be sure, even FDA officials who supported including women took exception to these numbers. Ruth Merkatz (the first director of the FDA's Office of Women's Health), along with coauthors from the agency, argued in 1993 that the GAO study actually had confirmed the results of internal FDA investigations conducted in 1983 and 1988, which found that the proportions of women and men in studies leading to FDA approvals were roughly *similar* to the proportions of women and men *of the same age* who had the disease in question. The reference to age was an important qualifier, because women tended to contract some conditions, such as heart disease, at a later age than men. (Thus, arguably, an apparent underrepresentation of women was actually a consequence of the underrepresentation of the elderly in clinical trials.) Furthermore, the FDA maintained that the underrepresentation of women was most likely to be found just where it was most appropriate: in Phase 1 trials (small studies of drug safety) and Phase 2 trials (initial studies of efficacy). In the case of Phase 3 trials (large studies leading to drug approval), women's numbers were much higher. However, FDA officials did agree with the GAO investigators that even when women were being included, pharmaceutical manufacturers were failing to perform analyses of differences between men and women—despite the 1988 FDA guideline requesting the industry to do just that.[46]

The Pharmaceutical Manufacturers Association was happy to inform its members that the FDA had "debunked" the "myth of too-few-women in clinical trials."[47] But, gradually, some pharmaceutical companies were moderating their positions with regard to studying women—indeed, some sensed it might be profitable to do so. By 1993 one female executive at Merck Research Laboratories had observed an "increasing interest and sensitivity within the pharmaceutical industry" to studying women and noted that several companies recently had established female health-care research departments.[48] Companies interested in positioning themselves in the vanguard of women's health research often were sympathetic to reformers; for example, many of them became dues-paying members of the Corporate Advisory Council of the SAWHR.

In some domains, however, the 1977 guideline hit hard. One of these was AIDS research, and AIDS activists kept up their pressure on the research establishment. In June 1990, just days after Schroeder and Snowe held their press conference to announce the GAO study on inclusion of women in NIH studies, more than five hundred protesters blocked the streets outside the international AIDS conference being held in San

Francisco, protesting the inadequate inclusion of women in AIDS drug trials.[49] Inside the convention center, women sprang to the stage to dramatize how researchers' interest in women with HIV seemed to extend solely to the question of how to prevent transmission of the virus to women's fetuses. "Women with AIDS can't wait till later," the protesters chanted: "We are not your incubators."[50] The NIH-funded AIDS research program was responsive to pressure and gradually increased the numbers of women and people of color, not only in the high-profile AIDS Clinical Trials Group program (which added new cities to its roster of sites), but also through a parallel program that funded community-based research.[51] By contrast, pharmaceutical companies testing AIDS drugs seemed much slower to adapt their practices or even to acknowledge a problem.

Indeed, activists complained that when women did seek entry into many AIDS trials, they faced extraordinary obstacles. Terry McGovern, director of the HIV Law Project, a New York City—based advocacy group, described the not atypical case of a homeless woman who tried to enroll in a clinical trial in New Jersey in 1991 for an antiviral drug she saw as her last chance for survival. The woman was told she would be eligible only if she obtained an IUD, but because of her history of AIDS-related gynecological problems, "there was no way that the doctor was going to give her an IUD." Noting that sex was "the last thing [she] was even thinking about" given her state of health, the woman showed up at McGovern's office in a rage.[52] Some women with AIDS charged that even after they had offered to undergo sterilization, they still were told they would be unable to join the clinical trials for drugs they considered promising.[53]

In 1992 the HIV Law Project, in conjunction with a number of other advocacy groups, filed a "citizen petition" demanding that the FDA rescind its exclusionary guideline. In restricting women's participation in research, the petitioners argued, the FDA "foster[ed] and, indeed, actively encourage[d] unconstitutional gender-based discrimination."[54] Significantly, the U.S. Supreme Court recently had ruled in another case where the goal of protecting women and their fetuses from harm seemed to consign women to second-class citizenship. In its 1991 verdict in *International Union, UAW v. Johnson Controls*, the court maintained that corporations could not use the risk of birth defects as justification for keeping women out of jobs they desired. The HIV Law Project's petition argued that the issue of women's participation in research was "analytically similar" to that of women's employment.[55]

With the citizen petition pending and the eyes of Congress upon them, it behooved the FDA to take action. Moreover, pressure for change was also bubbling up through the ranks of the agency itself, and it acquired support from FDA Commissioner David Kessler, who was appointed to head the agency in 1990.[56] Reversing the 1977 restriction on women's participation, the FDA issued new guidelines in 1993 that permitted the inclusion of women even in the early phases of drug testing, provided that female subjects used birth control. Furthermore, the agency called upon drug companies to submit data on the effects of new drugs in both men and women.[57]

As the new policy acknowledged, "the 1977 guideline, seen from the viewpoint of the 1990's, has appeared rigid and paternalistic, leaving virtually no room for the exercise of judgment by responsible female research subjects, physician investigators, and IRB's." Although the policy stopped short of requiring companies to include women, the FDA expressed its confidence "that the interplay of ethical, social, medical, legal and political forces will allow greater participation of women in the early stages of clinical trials."[58] Moreover, in promoting the changes, agency insiders stressed the importance of "sex-specific differences" in the body's absorption of, or response to, medications. Reviewing the new policy in the *New England Journal*, Ruth Merkatz and coauthors from the agency acknowledged that the FDA's 1988 request for reports of drug differences by sex, race, or age was not being heeded by manufacturers about half the time. Henceforth, the authors promised, "the FDA will review all new drug applications shortly after submission to ensure that they include appropriate analyses by sex. If such analyses are lacking, the FDA will call for their submission and may consider refusing to initiate review of the application if sex-specific analyses are not provided within a reasonable period."[59]

Battle Lines

By 1993, with the passage of the NIH Revitalization Act and the replacement of the FDA's exclusionary guideline, reformers had won two significant and unprecedented victories; these victories had important implications especially with regard to women's inclusion, though also for racial and ethnic minorities. Proponents of inclusion and attention to difference had also achieved considerable success in getting their views out into public discourse. According to a study by Anne Eckman of five major newspapers and newsmagazines, in the three years following the GAO report, "coverage of 'women's health' in the popular and mass media more than doubled."[60]

A series of news segments presented on ABC News in April and May of 1994 also attested to the broader resonance and growing circulation of reformers' analytical frames. Describing the changes at the NIH and the FDA and quoting various members of the Congressional Caucus for Women's Issues, the series observed that "medical science has almost always used white males as standard, the model for everyone else." Reporters cited "decades of neglect" and "lingering discrimination" as the causes and complained that even now, in medical schools, "the 70-kilogram man remains the norm." DHHS Secretary Donna Shalala was quoted as observing: "We have not paid as much attention to women's health, to issues that involve women's bodies, as we have to men's bodies."[61]

Of course, not everyone agreed that the criticisms of the reformers had merit, and not everyone approved of the recently announced remedies. To the contrary, as might well be expected, these proposals to transform the operations of medical research and drug development drew heated opposition. The chapter that follows this one begins by investigating the arguments and actions of these opponents. First, however, I want to analyze the strengths of the reform coalition: What accounts for its impressive success in placing its concerns squarely in the public agenda?

UNDERSTANDING THE REFORMERS' STRENGTHS

Hybrid Composition

Certainly, some of the successes of reformers in raising their concerns can be attributed to broader circumstances. By the 1980s, in the wake of several decades of struggles for equality and civil rights by women, racial minorities, and others, and in a climate where commitment to some notion of multiculturalism was taken for granted by at least some sectors of the public, political demands couched in the language of equity and social justice on behalf of important groups in U.S. society were likely to attract attention. Still, there was no guarantee that such demands would be seen as making sense in the specific domain of research inclusion.

Just as clearly, some aspects of reformers' successes in framing the debate reflect their own distinctive characteristics. In particular, the power of the tacit coalition was enhanced because it traversed boundaries. Membership spilled across the normally recognized divides between state and society, experts and the laity, science and politics, "insiders" and "outsiders," and the powerful and the disenfranchised. To be sure, styles of activism and organizing varied considerably. On the one hand, there was, for example, the AIDS activist who, at a noisy protest outside the FDA in 1988, held up a mock tombstone reading, "As a person of color

I was exempt from drug trials."[62] On the other hand, we have Florence Haseltine's description of how she began working with Pat Schroeder on the inclusion issue: "And then one day I was [returning home from] a meeting, and I saw Pat Schroeder sitting in first class. And fortunately I had upgraded. So I just sat next to her. . . . And Pat and I talked, and she said, 'How many gynecologists are there [working at the NIH]?' And I said, there are three permanent ones . . . and there are thirty-nine veterinarians. And she was aligned [with us] from then on."[63] Literally but also metaphorically, some advocates rode in "first class," while others traveled in "economy." However, because no members of this loose coalition were obliged to agree on tactics, these differences in social location proved a form of strength.

Indeed, thinking about the composition of this coalition should cause us to reflect critically on some of the typical assumptions about how social movements bring about change. This is not a simple story of how "outsiders" to biomedicine forced that institution to change its ways. Outsiders certainly were important to the story, but they acted in concert with well-placed members of the biomedical establishment to promote reform. Recently, several analysts of social movements have pointed to an array of cases that suggest that this is by no means unusual—that insiders (or what Kelly Moore has termed "mediators") frequently prove central to the political processes by which institutions become forced to change.[64] Neither is this a simple story of how challengers from outside the state moved in, disrupted the status quo, and transformed the state's operations. Instead, the case demonstrates what Jack Goldstone has called the "fuzzy and permeable boundary between institutionalized and non-institutionalized politics" and underscores the risk (described by John Skrentny) of assuming that "social movements are discrete entities that exist *outside* of government."[65] As Mark Wolfson noted in his analysis of a comparable case, the tobacco control movement, too often analysts of social movements tend to see the state simply as a movement's "target," "sponsor," or "facilitator," or as the provider or denier of "opportunities" for activism. But in many cases, "fractions of the state are often allied with the movement in efforts to change the policies of other fractions." In such cases—for which he has proposed the label "interpenetration"—"it is hard to know where the movement ends and the state begins."[66]

The Multiple Politics of Representation

Another way of understanding reformers' success is to examine their complex representational work. In effect, specific representatives had to position themselves as credible speakers for each group in order to bring it into being as a political actor. After all, change in this case was brought about *not* by research subjects themselves, nor, in any simple sense, by the downstream users of medical knowledge and services (that is, patients). Nor, of course, was action accomplished by any sort of comprehensive, collective effort on the part of the groups whose interests were constantly invoked. ("Women" as a class did not fight for biomedical reform.) Instead, specific individuals, organizations, and professional groups—the Congressional Caucus for Women's Issues is perhaps the clearest example discussed so far—had to claim to speak on behalf of such entities as "women," "children," and "people of color." This success in plausibly representing the health needs of substantial groups in U.S. society was central to the reformers' ability to get their agenda on the table.[67] Such an accomplishment should not be taken for granted. In a recent analysis of a failed scientific endeavor, the Human Genome Diversity Project, Jennifer Reardon has shown how this project—similarly concerned with inclusion and difference—came to be doomed when geneticists' desires to sample the diversity of the human genome in an inclusive way clashed with the desires of indigenous groups to represent themselves.[68]

By contrast, in the case of the new politics of inclusion in medical research, scientific and political spokespersons from each of the affected communities successfully positioned themselves as representing the interests of underrepresented groups. Moreover, these spokespersons hardened their claims by bridging or conflating different meanings of "representation" in medical research. In their frames and rhetoric, at least four different representational goals can be discerned:

1. Representation in the *statistical* sense: Different groups should be included in clinical research populations relative to their proportion of the overall U.S. population or of the incidence or prevalence of the disease. (For example, if blacks and Latinos made up 42 percent of U.S. AIDS cases, then roughly 42 percent of AIDS clinical trial subjects should be black or Latino.)
2. Representation in the sense of *social visibility*: Different groups should be represented within subject populations (or, for that matter, within the research community), so that medical research—to borrow a phrase used by President-elect Clinton in describing the Cabinet he hoped to appoint—"looks like America."
3. Representation in the sense of *political voice*: Different communities of stakeholders have a right to demand that researchers (especially those receiving federal funding) study their particular needs and conditions and not just those of more privileged social groups.
4. Representation in the *symbolic* sense (that is, how ideas are represented

through the use of language and symbols): Biomedicine must make a positive contribution to the shaping of the ideas and imagery that surround our cultural understandings of what different social groups are like.[69]

Thus, there was nothing simple about the claim that a group should be "represented" in research studies, and the coalition sought change in biomedical knowledge-making practices by successfully fusing different representational strategies. They simultaneously articulated how groups should be numerically included in studies (What numbers of research subjects were required by the dictates of good scientific practice and equitable science policy?), how groups should put forward demands (Who speaks for them and articulates their collective interest?), and how groups should be imagined (What were their relevant social, political, biological, and medical characteristics?). What might be termed "multirepresentational politics" facilitated a complicated project of transforming biomedical science.[70]

In essence, what reformers were demanding went well beyond the demographics of research populations: what they sought was full citizenship. Biomedical inclusion was not just a matter of counting up bodies; it also was a broader indicator of "who counted." Thus, as biomedical research increasingly came to be viewed as a domain in which social justice could be pursued, questions of scientific method became fused with questions of cultural and biopolitical citizenship—of the incorporation of groups into the national polity and its scientific institutions through the articulation of notions of rights and responsibilities. These were high-stakes claims, but ones that resonated with many people who might not otherwise have concerned themselves much with the fine details of research methodology.[71]

Categorical Alignment and the Politics of Classification

When we speak of how "groupness" is constructed, we are also calling attention to the practice and politics of classification. And the classification of human populations is a consistent preoccupation of many institutions in society. Classification is central to scientific practices of description and generalization.[72] At the same time, governments often are empowered to decide which categories will count as legitimate and to provide benefits on the basis of categorical membership.[73] (The politics of affirmative action policies is an obvious example.) Yet classification projects also emerge from below: as Rogers Brubaker and Frederick Cooper have observed, "the literature on social movements . . . is rich in evidence on how move-ment leaders challenge official identifications and propose alternative ones."[74] Thus, many different sorts of people, groups, and institutions may become involved in projects of human classification.

Appropriately, a good deal of scholarly attention has focused on the ways in which different classifiers *compete* to establish their preferred classification scheme as legitimate and to institutionalize it across dif-ferent domains of society. Whose categories will rule? Which will travel beyond their worlds of origin? When will official categories provoke resis-tance from those who perceive a lack of fit between classification systems and the identities of everyday life?[75] The sociologist Pierre Bourdieu, in particular, assumed that all parties will seek a "monopoly of legitimate *naming*," employing as symbolic capital in that struggle "all the power they possess over the instituted taxonomies."[76] This sort of competition to classify is predictable, given the role of classification in maintaining the moral and social order.

However, when we consider the politics of inclusion and difference in biomedicine, it is important to consider an alternative possibility. Instead of seeking to impose a preferred classification scheme as legitimate and to displace the classifications of others, individuals may perform what I call "categorical alignment work," causing classification schemes that already are roughly similar to become superimposed or aligned with one another. In such cases, bureaucratic and scientific classifications come to be treated as functionally equivalent both to one another and to the categories of everyday life.[77] In effect, in the making of the inclusion-and-difference paradigm, categorical terms (such as *black*, *male*, or *child*) came to function as what Leigh Star and James Griesemer have termed "boundary objects"—objects "which are both plastic enough to adapt to local needs and the constraints of the several parties employing them, yet robust enough to maintain a common identity across sites."[78] The superimposition of modes of authoritative social categorization prevalent in different domains of state and society then has the effect of building bridges connecting those domains.[79]

The various opponents of the "standard human" were adept practition-ers of this sort of categorical alignment work. Reformers proceeded as if it were self-evident that the mobilization categories of identity politics, the biological categories of medical research, and the social classifications of state bureaucrats were all one and the same system of categorization. In effect, they assumed that the differences defined *politically* in our society between various "haves" and "have-nots" mapped onto the differences that emerged out of biomedical research—for example, the differences in the distribution of genetic variants of the cytochrome p450 enzymes responsible for drug metabolism. In linking together arguments about social justice and biological differences, reformers were also implying that precisely the same groupings were being invoked in both discourses. By bridging manifestly "scientific" and "political" arguments, proponents of inclusion were able to *act as if* the social movement identity labels, the biomedical terms, and the state-sanctioned categories were all one and the same set of classifications—that is, that the politically salient categories were simultaneously the scientifically relevant categories.

It followed from this presumption that political and biomedical remedies could be pursued simultaneously through a single project of reform. Categorical alignment thereby provided the operational link between the politics of identity and the project of social change. Reformers did not simply invoke their social identities to demand recognition and redress: they also made strategic use of identities, thereby tying identity politics to the politics of institutional transformation.[80]

The marker of successful categorical alignment work is that it becomes invisible in hindsight: the superimposition of political classifications with scientific ones seems natural and inevitable. But there are many bases by which claims of inequality could plausibly be put forward in the domain of health research, including by social class and geographic region; and likewise there are many ways of representing the dispersion of biological or genetic differences within the human population.[81] So it was not foreordained that medical and political categories would come to be aligned in this case—indeed, as will become clear, some of the opponents of the proposed new inclusionary policies did their best to disrupt or refute the logic of categorical alignment.

Here again, the Human Genome Diversity Project, which failed to rally supporters and get off the ground, serves as an instructive negative case. Geneticists intended to sample various cultural groups in order to construct a map of genetic diversity in the human species. But in doing so, as the anthropologist Margaret Lock has noted, the Diversity Project rested on a "category fallacy": "To make a selection of contemporary groups identified on the basis of a shared culture, and then to assume that their genetic make-up is also shared, is to conflate time and space in an entirely inappropriate way."[82] In the case of clinical research, by contrast, the proponents of inclusion and diversity were substantially successful in aligning sociopolitical and biomedical classifications.

However, proponents were aided significantly by federal health bureaucrats who, in implementing the new inclusionary mandates, greatly reinforced categorical alignment by specifying the official categories that would count for health policy purposes. The work of government officials was crucial to the story, particularly in countering the arguments of skeptics, critics, and opponents of the inclusion-and-difference paradigm. I take up these stories of opposition and federal intervention in the next chapter.

CHAPTER FIVE

Opposition to Reform: Controversy, Closure, and Boundary Work

The previous chapter traced the path to the first critical victories won by those favoring a new attention to inclusion and difference in biomedical research. Yet despite the convergence of interests behind the reform agenda, it would be a mistake to imagine that these successes were foreordained. In fact, the policies proposed in the early 1990s to change practices at the NIH and the FDA, as well as the more general emphasis on inclusion and the measurement of difference, confronted serious opposition. The various opponents were not well organized, but the ranks of dissenters and critics included politicians, representatives of the pharmaceutical industry, NIH-funded researchers, some prominent DHHS officials, and conservative writers and critics, as well as a small but influential group of statisticians who were experts on clinical trial methodology. Thus, the opposition merits attention, as does the overcoming of that opposition.

Critics of the reforms took a variety of positions regarding them. Some worried about their implications for the conduct of science, others took exception to specific claims made by supporters of the new policies, and still others disagreed with what they took to be the underlying political objectives of the reforms. Here again, it is useful to approach the rhetoric of critics by analyzing the distinctive ways in which they framed their arguments. I call these frames "renewed vulnerability," "the dangers of difference," "the bias myth," "quotas," "harm to science," and "human similarities." Although statements and actions by some opponents reflect an invocation of several of these frames, it is important to say that not everyone adopted all of them.

After describing each of these frames in turn and discussing the interventions of critics of the emergent paradigm, I will turn to the question of why opposition failed. I will place particular emphasis on the role of state agencies—specifically, the work performed by DHHS employees who interpreted legislation and policy in ways that spoke to the interests of all players. The "boundary work" performed by these NIH and FDA administrators functioned to carve out a domain of "science" that could be portrayed as somewhat protected from the intrusion of "politics." These efforts largely quelled opposition while giving further endorsement to the reforms.

OPPOSITIONAL FRAMES

Renewed Vulnerability

It is a testament to how fast the pendulum had swung away from concerns with protecting "vulnerable populations" from research risk that relatively few critics of the reforms raised objections on these grounds. Most of those who did so worried about birth defects—"another thalidomide"—as a consequence of the FDA's removal of the guideline restricting women's participation in research. However, one NIH official, Otis Brawley, an African American researcher and the director of the National Cancer Institute's Office of Special Populations Research, suggested that the NIH Revitalization Act's requirement of including minorities also left racial minority groups potentially susceptible to abuse at the hands of researchers intent on securing NIH funding. Brawley's point was that the inclusionary mandate could motivate researchers to pressure members of racial minority groups into trials at all costs. "Every investigator has been warned that his federal funding for clinical trials will cease if his or her accrual of minorities is inadequate," Brawley noted. Thus, while a researcher could "afford to accept no as an answer" from a prospective white recruit to a study, "the NIH encourages the health care professional to do everything possible to recruit the minority patient. In plain English, this is an incentive to give minorities the 'hard sell' when offering enrollment in a clinical trial."[1]

Dangers of Difference

Other remarks by Brawley exemplified a concern with the harmful social consequences of attributing biological meaning to racial differences. Clearly, as the director of an office dedicated to research on "special populations," Brawley was invested in promoting the health of racial and ethnic minorities. However, he worried that the specific requirements of the NIH Revitalization Act might "eventually do more harm than good for the minority populations that it hopes to benefit." Brawley's concerns focused in part on the treatment of race as a category rooted in biology: he suggested that the NIH Revitalization Act's "emphasis on potential racial differences fosters the racism that its creators want to abrogate by establishing government-sponsored research on the basis of the belief that there are significant biological differences among the races."[2] Thus, Brawley not only took exception to the biological-differences frame, but he also sought to disrupt categorical alignment: he disputed the implicit contention that everyday categories of racial identity and mobilization could be imported unproblematically into the realm of biomedical research and function in that realm to demarcate biological difference.

The Bias Myth

I derive the name of this frame from an article that appeared in the *Atlantic Monthly* magazine in August 1994, called "The Sex-Bias Myth in Medicine," by a physician named Andrew Kadar. In essence, Kadar took the underrepresentation frame of the reformers and turned it on its head. "One sex does appear to be favored in the amount of attention devoted to its medical needs," wrote Kadar: "The NIH . . . spends twice as much money on research into the diseases specific to one sex as it does on research into those specific to the other, and only one sex has a section of the NIH devoted entirely to the study of the diseases afflicting it. That sex is not men, however. It is women."[3] Here Kadar took up the statistic that advocates of reform had made problematic use of: the claim that only 13 percent of NIH funding was devoted to "women's health." Kadar noted that by the same definition—research devoted specifically to conditions primarily affecting one sex, such as breast cancer or prostate cancer—the percentage devoted to "men's health" was significantly smaller. And the proof of the pudding, in Kadar's view—the evidence that women were not suffering from research neglect but perhaps were benefiting from more than their fair share of medical attention—was that women on average lived longer than men. (In this sense, although Kadar did not use the term, his article suggested that men were victims of "reverse discrimination.") What Kadar failed to address, however, was the composition by sex of the bulk of NIH-funded research (on conditions affecting both women and men), and his selective examples left the implication that the numbers were roughly equal.

Many others tried to bring hard numbers to bear on the question of representation—mostly with a focus on composition by sex, but sometimes with regard to race, ethnicity, or age. Although scholarly accounts of the fights to include women in medical research have tended to take underrepresentation for granted, or have noted only in passing that some debate existed about the matter,[4] critics succeeded in throwing some doubt on the new conventional wisdom. And some analysts who appeared generally supportive of the reform agenda nonetheless reported findings that were equivocal at best.

Because no public or private agency maintained a comprehensive registry or database that could provide a definitive profile of the participants in clinical research, the direct contributors to this controversy were obliged to devise their own methodologies and determine their own samples in order to shed light on the statistics of inclusion. It was no simple matter, however, to decide which way of measuring representation was most accurate or meaningful. Some analyses (such as those discussed in chapter 3) studied subsets of articles published in pharmacology journals; these perhaps were most likely to reflect the consequences of the FDA's 1977 guideline restricting the participation of women in studies of new drugs. Others sought to examine random samples of the studies published in the leading general medical journals, such as the *Journal of the American Medical Association (JAMA)* and the *New England Journal of Medicine*.[5] Still others focused on studies approved by IRBs at major research centers.[6] In one case, the availability of a government database made it possible to tabulate the recorded races of more than one hundred thousand participants in National Cancer Institute (NCI)—sponsored trials from January 1991 through June 1994: interestingly, the results showed that the proportions of different races in clinical trial populations for cancer drugs almost exactly matched the racial breakdown of the U.S. population suffering from cancer.[7] (However, Otis Brawley, who was one of the NCI coauthors of the study, noted that the agency could hardly take credit for this outcome and acknowledged it was "a pleasant surprise" to discover it.[8])

These diverse measurement studies resist any straightforward summary; there is no single, "bottom-line" finding. It is likely that the composition of clinical research populations varied considerably, depending on funding source, the disease in question, the location of the research, and many other factors. The objectives of the investigation mattered as well. In the case of NCI-sponsored research, though racial minorities were well represented in treatment trials, they appeared to be much less in evidence in prevention trials—perhaps because prevention trials are more successful in recruiting the well-to-do, who "can afford to take time off from work twice a year to go to the doctor for a problem they do not have."[9]

Curtis Meinert, a prominent authority on clinical trial methodology who became one of the most outspoken critics of the NIH Revitalization Act, was one of those who disputed the emergent common sense regarding the history of underrepresentation. A statistician and director of a clinical trials center at Johns Hopkins University, Meinert noted the slipperiness of the very concept: "underrepresented" in relation to what? Was representation to be measured according to a group's contribution to the U.S. population? In comparison to the racial breakdown of the city in which the research was conducted (as, for example, the study by Svensson and coauthors described in chapter 3 had presumed)? In relation to the incidence of a disease in a given social group? In relation to mortality rates for that group? Or did adequate representation mean that groups had to be included in sufficient numbers to conduct statistically mean-ingful comparisons of outcome differences across groups? Each of these definitions implied different targets for inclusion and different criteria for judging the success of researchers' recruitment efforts.[10]

In any case, Meinert simply doubted that women had, in any meaning-ful sense, been under-studied. When Meinert was appointed to a special panel charged with reporting on "ethical and legal issues relating to the inclusion of women in clinical studies," he forced his fellow commit-tee members to confront the issue head-on. The sixteen-member panel was convened by the prestigious Institute of Medicine of the National Academy of Sciences in 1992, with funding from NIH's new Office of Research on Women's Health; its charge was to "consider the ethical and legal implications of including women, particularly pregnant women and women of childbearing potential, in clinical studies; . . . provide practical advice for consideration by NIH, institutional review boards, and clinical investigators; and . . . examine known instances of litigation regarding injuries to research subjects and to describe existing legal liabilities and protections." The final report, presented in late 1993 and published as a book in 1994, became a cornerstone document in the history of the new concern with inclusion of women in research.[11]

Meinert's role on the committee was, in effect, to say, "Show me the data." Ruth Faden, a bioethicist at Johns Hopkins and cochair of the panel, recalls that Meinert "had a profound effect on the committee." Labeling him a "curmudgeon" and comparing his persistence to "a dog with a bone," Faden also described Meinert as "the 'Truman' on the com-mittee [who] was responsible for integrity in the report [of a kind] that you rarely see." Similarly, Faden's cochair, Daniel Federman, the dean of medical education at Harvard University, described Meinert as the "sta-tistical conscience" of the group and its frequent tutor.[12] At least partially at Meinert's instigation, the panel conducted a thorough review of the data on women's inclusion in research, resulting in a fourteen-page table summarizing all the studies that had been conducted.[13]

In the end, the committee's judgment was surprisingly muted. In the specific cases of heart disease and AIDS research, there was reason to conclude that women had been under-studied. Overall, however, "the available evidence is insufficient to determine whether women have participated in the whole of clinical studies to the same extent as men, and whether women have been disadvantaged by policies and practices regarding their participation or a failure to focus on their health interest in the conduct of research." The report continued: "Some studies found that an appropriate number of women were included in specific study populations and that more female-only studies were being conducted than male-only studies. Others found that women were 'over-' or 'underrepresented' in certain types of studies. Others found that women—especially elderly or poor women of diverse racial and ethnic groups—are less likely to be included in studies than men."[14]

The Institute of Medicine panel also commissioned a study by a sociologist, Chloe Bird, which appeared in a companion volume. Examining all "original contributions" published in *JAMA* in 1990 and 1992, Bird found that research on sex-specific diseases tended to favor women. However, in 37 percent of the studies on diseases not specific to males or females, women constituted fewer than a third of the subjects. The "largest discrepancy" occurred in the case of cardiovascular disease, where women were absent from eleven of thirty-eight studies and men were present in all. Bird also found that only 27 percent of the articles that examined both men and women indicated that statistical tests had been performed to determine whether women and men in the study fared the same or differently.[15]

In subsequent years, Meinert has not let the matter rest, and he has pursued his own research on the question of the gender representation of subjects in clinical trials using the largest possible sample: all articles in the Medline database, which essentially includes all medical journals of note, from 1966 onward.[16] Though Meinert has gained some limited attention in the mass media for his claim to having shown that women have not been underrepresented,[17] his findings are not inconsistent with those of Bird. The points that Meinert emphasizes are that the number of female-only clinical trials has always been greater than the number of male-only trials and that "exclusionary," single-sex studies are themselves a small (and declining) portion of the total number of trials reported. But Meinert's other finding, based on counts of the actual numbers of participants of trials published in five major journals in 1985, 1990, and 1995, is that men clearly outnumbered women as participants in trials that did include both sexes. (In trials reported in 1990, there were about 63,000 men and only about 33,000 women; in 1995 there were about 217,000 men and about 145,000 women.)[18] Thus, while Meinert's research, like that of others, suggests that sweeping formulations about underrepresentation are oversimplified, neither has he found a "smoking gun" indicating that concern about underrepresentation was unwarranted.

One other argument put forward by those who questioned women's underrepresentation was that critics had singled out a few particular examples of all-male trials—the Physicians' Health Study, MR FIT—and had blown them out of proportion. The Physicians' Health Study, a double-blind, placebo-controlled trial that demonstrated a 44 percent reduction in risk of a heart attack in healthy men over age 40 who took a low dose of aspirin every other day, was an interesting case in point.[19] The study had been highlighted by the General Accounting Office in its report damning the NIH, but those involved in the study, including female researchers committed to women's health, defended the logic of the study design. Julie Buring, a co-investigator on the study, recalled her ambivalent feelings as she followed the congressional debate—on one hand, pleased that the GAO report "would really help us get studies in women done," but on the other hand, regretful that the debate failed to delve into nuances or acknowledge the scientific rationale: "It wasn't that we were unaware, and it wasn't that we were naive, and it wasn't that we were prejudiced against women—we made a carefully considered decision based on a number of scientific issues to conduct the first trial of this question in men."[20]

Indeed, what the congressional uproar obscured was that investigators intended all along to study women in a subsequent clinical trial (the Women's Health Study, completed in 2005). The decision to exclude women from the original study was a consequence of a strategic decision to study physicians. The investigators, under the direction of Charles Hennekens at Brigham & Women's Hospital in Boston, knew that they would have to follow a very large sample over a long period of time in order to determine whether aspirin had a protective effect. They came up with the idea of conducting the study entirely by mail—sending out the aspirin and placebos and having the 22,000 participants return questionnaires—and never actually seeing the participants firsthand, thereby reducing the cost of the study enormously. This decision meant, however, "that we couldn't take the general population, we had to take a medically knowledgeable group." Physicians, it was assumed, not only would be cooperative and faithful research subjects who could be trusted to take their pills on schedule, but also would be fully capable of detecting signs of the potentially serious adverse effects from prolonged aspirin use. Moreover, as a generally health-conscious group, physicians were an attractive population for testing the benefits of aspirin as a preventive measure: if aspirin helped this population, then presumably its benefits would extend to others whose risk might be somewhat higher.[21]

The problem was that women only recently had entered the field of medicine in large numbers, and only one in ten physicians aged 40 or older was female. The available population of older female physicians was simply too small to yield a reliable answer about the protective effect of aspirin in women, especially because women tend to contract heart disease at a later age than men. In fact, the investigators calculated that they would be able to recruit only one-tenth as many women as men.[22] Some critics have suggested that nurses might have served as an equally reliable and well-educated research sample and therefore could have been added to the mix to increase the representation of women. However, the investigators already had enrolled 122,000 female nurses in an observational study, the Nurses' Health Study, and, according to Buring, it seemed doubtful that another large sample of nurses could easily be found.

The investigators therefore decided to focus initially on male physicians while simultaneously applying for funding to conduct a complementary trial in women.[23] Some biomedical insiders who knew the whole story were inclined, therefore, to take the episode as evidence that claims about women's underrepresentation in research needed to be taken with a grain of salt: such claims were at least in some respects overblown and insufficiently appreciative of the practical exigencies of research design.[24] Blasting the Physicians' Health Study had made great press—but, to critics of the new inclusionary policies, it also demonstrated the dangers of letting nonscientists assess medical research priorities.[25]

Quotas

An additional way in which opponents of reforms framed their critiques was to invoke the politically explosive language of "quotas." Much as opponents of affirmative action policies in employment and higher education often have referred to these as "quota policies" in order to suggest the illegitimacy of social reforms, so too did critics of the NIH Revitalization Act contend that that it was a "quota bill": supposedly, it mandated specific numbers of women and minorities in an inflexible way as a broad-brush remedy for supposed inequities of the past. Indeed, simply by using the term *quotas*, opponents implied a tight connection between these biomedical reforms and the controversial policies of affirmative action—tarring them with the same brush, in the eyes of those who saw affirmative action as misguided policy. (Critics' frequent references to the new policies as "politically correct" served much the same rhetorical function.)

By contrast, proponents of reform mostly invoked the much more broadly palatable idea of equality of opportunity, rather than using rhetoric that would suggest that theirs was an affirmative action policy. Interestingly, the Institute of Medicine panel was a rare voice in *favor* of applying affirmative action principles to redress past underrepresentation— though they did not use the term itself. The panel's report adopted as a key principle that "where it is established that specific health interests of women, men, or other groups have not received a fair allocation of research attention or resources, justice may require a policy of preferential treatment toward these specific areas in order to remedy a past injustice and to avoid perpetuating that injustice."[26]

A key function of the quotas frame was to question the validity of what I have called categorical alignment—the implicit claim that the salient categories of identity politics were also the best categories for the study of biomedical differences. To complain of quotas was to "de-align"—to disrupt the association between social categories and biomedical categories by suggesting that the liberal remedies of affirmative action had no place in the world of biomedicine. In effect, while proponents of the reforms sought to build bridges connecting social justice arguments with biological difference arguments, conservative critics sought to widen the distance between the river banks.

Curtis Meinert was one of those who voiced concerns about quotas, arguing that "the tendency of funders to gravitate to quotas to fix perceived imbalances or as a means of fending off attack from the underrepresented is short-sighted and fraught with peril."[27] For the most part, however, invocations of the quota frame came from those whose agenda was more explicitly ideological. For example, Sally Satel, a psychiatrist and fellow at the American Enterprise Institute, a conservative think tank, blasted the Congressional Caucus for Women's Issues in an article in *The New Republic* called "Science by Quota: P.C. Medicine." Satel argued that the Caucus "managed to turn the inclusion provision into a referendum on civil rights," irrespective of scientific fact.[28]

Republican members of Congress also invoked the quotas frame. In 1991 William Dannemeyer, a social conservative from California, complained during consideration of the NIH Revitalization Act that the language requiring inclusion of women and minorities constituted "affirmative action and quotas." Similarly, in 1992 Newt Gingrich, future Speaker of the House, argued that the legislation "creates a Federal mandate for a quota system of minorities and women as subjects in clinical studies at the NIH"; he went on to use the term *quotas* repeatedly in his remarks in the *Congressional Record*. Pat Schroeder responded sharply: "Now, if the gentleman from Georgia . . . wants to stand up and call this a quota bill, listen, he sees quotas in the clouds. I want to tell you that women are paying their quota of this research."[29]

Harm to Science

Certainly the most consistent frame, and the one invoked by the most diverse set of individuals and groups, was the idea that these reforms, however well-intentioned, would bring harm to the institutions of science. The focus here was the NIH Revitalization Act because of its prescriptive language: it mandated inclusion, and it required comparisons of outcomes between women and men and across racial and ethnic groups. These demands appeared to tread on the toes of clinical researchers accustomed to making their own decisions about study design; they also constituted an invasion of the turf of the NIH, which presumed that the expertise needed to assess the importance and validity of research proposals lay with the agency itself and its appointed "study sections" (panels of peer reviewers)—not with activists or with Congress. At the same time, these demands raised questions, particularly for statisticians, about whether it would be methodologically, financially, and practically possible to comply with the guidelines. Thus, the concern about harm to science bridged a general desire to protect scientific autonomy with a more specific interest in preserving the viability of clinical research. Sometimes branding the NIH Revitalization Act as "political correctness" run amok, sometimes complaining of "bureaucracy" and "red tape," and sometimes worrying about the excessive costs and hardships that might now be associated with conducting studies, those who invoked the harm-to-science frame shared a concern that science was a fragile institution that needed protection from "politicization."

In the battles in Congress over the NIH Revitalization Act, opponents of the legislation frequently complained that Congress should not be in the business of "micromanaging" the NIH. This theme surfaced early. In October 1990, when the House Committee on Energy and Commerce submitted a report recommending that the legislation be passed, nine members of the committee signed a dissenting statement claiming that the bill "badly misdirects and micro-manages the NIH" and arguing that it was "replete with special set-asides, requirements, and unnecessary advisory committees which would harm the NIH scientific program and disrupt its management."[30]

This was also the position taken initially both by NIH Director Bernadine Healy and by DHHS Secretary Louis Sullivan. Healy's and Sullivan's comments in part may have reflected the political "line" of the Bush White House, which issued a statement in July 1991 complaining that "the bill would allow unwarranted and unwise intrusions into the authority of the Secretary of Health and Human Services and is too directive in its effort to expand certain research programs."[31] But it was certainly dismaying to reformers that Healy (the first woman to head the NIH) and Sullivan (a prominent African American in the Bush administration) would voice their opposition. While "strongly endors[ing] the need for representation of women and minorities in clinical research," Healy argued that the effect of the legislation as written would be to expand the size of studies. Given the predictable cost constraints, this expansion inevitably would result in "the conduct of only a few very large trials on a smaller number of diseases." Similarly, Sullivan argued that the "inflexible" requirement of conducting subgroup analysis was "unworkable on scientific grounds."[32]

The statistician critics added substance to these complaints. These experts on clinical trial design were painfully aware of the difficulties involved in conducting large, prospective experiments on human beings. In their view, the NIH Revitalization Act was the straw that might break the camel's back. Steven Piantadosi, a colleague of Meinert's at Johns Hopkins and the Director of Biostatistics in the Oncology Center there, recalled feeling that "the clinical research infrastructure and capabilities in the United States are slowly being poisoned and polluted in much the same way our lakes and rivers have been"; similarly, Meinert worried that he might witness in his lifetime "the rise and decline of trials."[33] The statisticians predicted the likely consequence of strict adherence to the congressional mandate to conduct subgroup comparisons—namely, the bankrupting of clinical research through the requirement of massive numbers of human subjects.

Janet Wittes, a statistician and the head of a private consulting firm in Washington, D.C., that designs clinical trials, became so concerned about this issue that she penned a short article with her son Benjamin, a writer, which appeared in *The New Republic* in 1993. The authors spelled out the enormous practical implications of a strict reading of the NIH Revitalization Act with reference to a hypothetical example:

A study designed to test whether a treatment for hypertension reduces risk of stroke requires that roughly 5,000 persons be examined regularly for five years. Showing that such treatment works in women, men, and minority groups requires an average of 5,000 *in each subgroup* (white men, white women, minority men, minority women). But if, as the bill would require, the trial designers were compelled to quantify marginal treatment differences between each of these groups, the sample size would skyrocket. The trial would have to be large enough not only to assert reliably that the treatment lowers the overall stroke rate, but also to demonstrate that differences between groups were due to more than chance. This would probably mean increasing the sample size by a factor of eight or more.[34]

The authors carried their critique even further by observing that there was no telling, in principle, how many subgroups, or sub-subgroups, might need to be compared, once one jumped on the bandwagon of difference: "Conceivably, Mexican-Americans and Cuban-Americans could display subtle differences in treatment effect and disease progression, since all people of Hispanic origin are not ethnically homogeneous. How finely must we grind?" Citing the "enormous price tags" that inevitably would result from such logic, Wittes and Wittes called the subgroup comparison requirement "the stealth bomber of American medical research: its arrival has been silent, but its explosion will be hard to miss."[35]

While statisticians were especially vocal about these issues, similar concerns about the threat to science increasingly were voiced by researchers as they got wind of the debate and began to worry about the effect of new requirements on their own work. Pat Schroeder recalled how representatives of the medical center at the University of Colorado, located in her district, "were calling me in, and they threatened [me] with everything. The entire research community went nuts. We were 'politicizing' science. We were doing this, we were doing that." Douglas Schmucker and coauthors, in a 1994 update to their study of the representation of women in clinical research, noted that "many investigators fear that 'politically correct clinical studies' can only reduce the quality of such research." Marcia Angell, the first female editor-in-chief of the prestigious *New England Journal of Medicine*, wrote an editorial in the journal's pages in 1993 (when she was executive editor) expressing her view that "the proposed amendment . . . would create worse problems than it would solve." In particular, she wrote, "to provide a valid analysis of results in subjects of both sexes and all minorities would require unreasonably large trials of new interventions." There can be little doubt that the passage of the NIH Revitalization sparked similar fears in many biomedical professionals.[36]

Though not as specific as the NIH Revitalization Act, the FDA guidelines requesting data on differences by sex, race, ethnicity, and age also imposed new obligations that, in this case, clearly had implications for drug makers. Pharmaceutical companies generally were less audible in their protests, perhaps because other FDA policies were of greater concern to companies resisting what they often saw as an undue regulatory burden. However, one representative of the Pharmaceutical Research and Manufacturers of America (PhRMA), the drug industry's main trade association, complained to ABC News: "There will now be additional requirements, additional studies that have to be done, additional analyses that have to be done, so that . . . adds to the complexity and the cost." And beyond the increased costs of drug development, pharmaceutical companies continued to worry about the risk of lawsuits if a participant in a clinical trial became pregnant and gave birth to a child with birth defects.[37]

Human Similarities

It is important to note that the biostatisticians (and others) who raised the issue of cost in relation to subgroup comparisons were not motivated by an abstract desire to economize. Their point was not just that these expenditures would crowd out other research but also that subgroup comparisons on the scale apparently mandated by the NIH Revitalization Act were simply unwarranted on scientific grounds. Their argument was that most of the time, in the world of clinical research, there was no reason to expect to find meaningful differences between sexes, races, or other social groupings. Hence, these critics directly challenged the biological-differences frame discussed in chapter 3, and they invoked understandings of fundamental similarities within the human species.

For example, Piantadosi and Wittes sent a letter to the editor of the journal *Controlled Clinical Trials*, calling upon the Society for Clinical Trials to "mount a concerted effort to wrest scientific sense from political correctness." Arguing that "people have more biological similarities than differences," the authors pointed out: "Penicillin will kill bacteria in blacks, whites, Cuban Americans, Mexican-Americans, men, women, dogs, cats, birds, and petri dishes. In the absence of plausible scientific hypotheses about subgroup differences in treatment effects, the decision concerning what subgroups to include and what subgroup analyses to perform should be made on a study by study basis."[38]

Curtis Meinert not only endorsed these arguments but began an organizing drive around them: at the 1993 annual meeting of the Society for Clinical Trials, he circulated a petition criticizing the NIH Revitalization

Act and obtained 119 signatures. Calling the requirement for subgroup comparisons "unwise, impractical, and lacking in scientific rationale," Meinert's petition complained that "it is predicated on the supposition that we, as people, are fundamentally different in the way we respond to treatments, when our collective biology and experience indicates otherwise."[39] As Meinert subsequently reflected, the "big equalizer" in treatment trials is the disease in question, and demographic considerations are usually of little consequence. Moreover, the statistician critics noted that nearly all of the known examples of treatment differences between subgroups were differences in magnitude of effect, not the direction of that effect—that is, there were hardly any cases in the medical literature of treatments or regimens that helped one group but hurt another group.[40]

As these critical comments by the dissenting biostatisticians suggest, intertwined with the question of when human differences matter is the complicated issue of extrapolation and generalizability in clinical research. In this sense, the debate over the inclusion of women and minorities as research subjects concerns a problem well studied by sociologists of scientific knowledge: when, how, and to what degree can findings obtained in a constrained experimental environment credibly be generalized and applied to a broader range of examples? As numerous case studies have shown, the contention that a test has "succeeded" presumes collective agreement on the substantial similarity between the test situation and those real-world situations for which the test is putatively a stand-in.[41] To take a not unrelated example, if it can be shown that laboratory rats administered fixed doses of saccharin develop cancerous tumors, then a decision to ban saccharin from diet foods and drinks rests on a series of assumptions that must be socially negotiated—that biological processes in humans and rats are similar in certain relevant ways, that we know how to describe comparable doses across species, and so on.

From the mid-twentieth century forward, the randomized clinical trial has epitomized the notion that medical knowledge has the potential to escape the particularities of its origin and achieve wide applicability: one can study a relatively small number of experimental subjects and then assume that the same results will hold for a much broader population of patients.[42] Despite these hopes, the problem of generalizing is intrinsic to the clinical trial and difficult to avoid. This is true in part because the subjects are not laboratory rats but human beings, whose compliance with the experimental protocol cannot easily be monitored or ensured. Thus, clinical trials are often "messy," and the true significance of their findings may sometimes be subject to considerable debate.[43] But in addition, as the biostatistician critics were at pains to point out, clinical trials do not employ random samples. Whatever its sociodemographic composition, a clinical trial is populated by those individuals who qualify for the study and who then *agree to participate*; such people, almost inevitably, are not perfectly representative of the population of patients in question.[44] Given that clinical trials, therefore, are not "perfect" natural experiments, how one goes about generalizing from the results of any trial to the real world is, according to Janet Wittes, "a matter of art, . . . a matter of clinical judgment, [and] a matter of scientific sense." And as Curtis Meinert notes, "it's always going to be a risky business."[45]

Clinical trial experts therefore relied on recognized principles to guide them in making generalizations. For example, they emphasized that research always proceeded best in stages—first, determining a basic effect of some medical intervention, and then following up with studies that clarify the fine details of how that intervention can best be employed. "There is no point in worrying about whether a treatment works the same or differently in men and women," Meinert argued in a commentary published in *Science*, "until it has been shown to work in someone."[46] Meinert's point was not that that "someone" necessarily should be a white man. Describing himself as "a heterogenologist but not a representologist," Meinert was all in favor of allowing diverse groups into clinical trials. But he was deeply concerned about the presumption that there was a scientific need for their representation in large numbers in every case from the outset, so as to be able to conduct statistically significant comparisons.[47] "We should be moving toward unconstrained heterogeneity," wrote Meinert, "not controlled representativeness."[48]

In other words, the statistician critics were by no means opposed to the goals of inclusion and diversity. In fact, Meinert also wrote that, in retrospect, the Physicians' Health Study should have gone ahead and enrolled those female physicians who were available, rather than deciding to exclude all women if there weren't enough of them to provide a definitive answer about aspirin's benefit to women: "We would have been better off with some information on the question than none at all."[49] (In this regard, Meinert was more "inclusionary" in his philosophy than the study's designers, who worried that if they recruited any women at all, then the public would press them for an answer about aspirin's preventive effects for women that they would not feel comfortable providing.[50])

As "heterogenologists" (to borrow Meinert's somewhat fanciful self-description), the biostatisticians in this fight were not among those who felt that trials with homogeneous study populations were scientifically preferable as a rule. At the same time, they made a specifically statistical

argument about the potential dangers of excessive "mining" of trial results for differences by subgroup: the more ways one sliced up the study
population, the more likely one was to erroneously "discover"—purely
by chance—what appeared to be a meaningful difference. (Statisticians
have demonstrated this point by showing that treatment effects in clinical
trials may appear to vary according to subjects' astrological signs.)[51]

In these debates, the Institute of Medicine committee once again
adopted a position that went some distance toward embracing the views
of the critics: promoting inclusion while worrying about "data dredging"
or any blanket requirement of subgroup analysis. With reference to the
NIH Revitalization Act, the committee expressed its concern "that the
policy has gone too far by insisting that each and every clinical trial be designed to ensure sufficient numbers of subjects of both genders to permit
subgroup analyses." Most of the time, there was no reason to anticipate
differences between men and women that would require this approach.
"Person-years of follow-up are person-years of follow-up whether they are
female or male years, *unless* the researchers have plausible hypotheses
about gender differences in response," observed the committee. Only in
those cases where researchers actually did have "convincing hypotheses about qualitative gender-specific differences" should both men and
women be included "in sufficient numbers to test for gender-specific
results."[52]

The Weakness of the Opposition

From the material presented so far in this chapter, it is evident that
opponents of reform not only deployed a wide range of counterframes
but also invoked potent, hot-button terms, such as *political correctness* and
quotas. A few of the more vocal critics had a straightforwardly right-wing
ideological agenda (and there are loose affinities between the opposition
frames and the kinds of arguments that have been deployed elsewhere to
oppose policies such as affirmative action). But other spokespersons are
less easily classifiable in such terms—for example, complaints about the
dangers lurking in inappropriate subgroup analyses reflected mainstream
views in statistics. Moreover, the criticism voiced by opponents spoke
to the concerns of many biomedical researchers as well as some NIH
and FDA officials, and it was endorsed, at least in part, by independent
authorities such as the Institute of Medicine commission. Why, then, did
opposition ultimately prove unsuccessful?

That the counterframes lacked the punch to turn back the tide of
the inclusion-and-difference paradigm in part reflected the strength and

diversity of the reform coalition (even in the absence of a united front). By contrast, vocal critics of reform mostly were isolated. In Meinert's assessment, the biostatisticians and clinical trial experts proved "by and large very passive with regard to this business"—willing to sign a petition, perhaps, but not to do much more. Wittes's analysis was similar: On one side, "there were too many strong political groups that were fighting for this." And on the other side, "I remember trying to get people exercised about it. And there was kind of an 'Eh, it will go away.' "[53]

Furthermore, many researchers simply doubted that the costs associated with the new policies really would prove to be substantial enough to get exercised about—or concluded that these costs were worth it, considering the potential benefits. As Sylvia Smoller, the lead researcher at one Women's Health Initiative site, commented, the fears raised about the inclusionary policy were in a certain sense familiar: "They had the same argument against the [Americans with] Disabilities Act. Right? 'You can't make ramps and you can't make things convenient. It's too expensive.' But you know what, . . . they're doing it. It's a law. And society is functioning. It hasn't broken the bank. . . . So cost is always brought up as an argument. But it's sometimes not valid."[54]

But there is an additional, crucial reason why strong public criticism proved transient and open revolt never materialized. As I describe below, federal health officials within the DHHS played a pivotal role in forestalling any widespread or sustained opposition to the new policies. Rather than attempt to block these reforms, DHHS officials sought to ride the reform wave—but also to divert its flow in directions of their own choosing. These officials embraced the new policies but implemented them in ways that incorporated many of the concerns of the critics.

BOUNDARY WORK AND THE INSTITUTIONALIZING OF REFORM

How did state actors juggle competing demands from advocates and opponents of inclusion and the measurement of differences? The DHHS was in no position, ultimately, to resolve the broader philosophical and practical questions about human differences or about scientific methodology that were posed by the critics and defenders of the standard human: Just how consequential *are* group-specific differences in biomedicine? When must researchers and physicians attend to such differences, and when ought they to assume that "people are people"? What degree of homogeneity or heterogeneity of research subjects is most desirable in clinical research, given the presumed trade-off between controlling variation and ensuring external validity? In this case—where science was under close public scrutiny; where scientific institutions lacked public legitimacy due to perceptions of bias; and where the very terms of discussion, such as *sex*, *gender*, *race*, and *ethnicity*, were controversial and contested, often even at the definitional level—there seemed little possibility of a deep consensus on matters of truth or fact.

What government health officials *could* bring about, however, was something less ambitious but no less important. They could help to engineer the closure of these debates through the elaboration of new, formal procedural standards as well as informal "work-arounds"[55]—ways of doing science that would simultaneously satisfy critics, allow researchers to proceed with their scientific tasks, and defend the jurisdictions of federal health officials, without requiring the resolution of any underlying debates. To bring about closure in this sense, officials had to promote workable policies that could be presented as scientifically based, and they had to defend against the charge of "politicizing" science. In other words, they had to be adept practitioners of what Thomas Gieryn has called "boundary work"—the "rhetorical games of inclusion and exclusion" that reinforce the legitimacy and autonomy of science by designating certain issues as "scientific" and others as "non-scientific."[56]

Perhaps the best example of this process is the NIH's development of guidelines to carry out the mandate of the NIH Revitalization Act. Because of the way that it intruded directly into questions of scientific methodology, the NIH Revitalization Act posed a significant challenge to the autonomy of science and to the discretionary power of NIH officials. However, it is important to note that the legislation was never meant to stand alone as the guide to NIH policy. Congress left to the NIH itself the task of developing formal, published guidelines that would specify in detail the circumstances in which inclusion would be considered appropriate or inappropriate, as well as the manner in which clinical trials should be designed for purposes of subgroup comparisons. These passages in the bill were quite prescriptive in one regard: they insisted that the guidelines drawn up by the NIH could not invoke excessive costs as grounds for sidestepping the inclusionary mandate. In many other respects, however, the legislation gave the NIH a fair amount of leeway in how it translated the law into specific guidelines.[57]

The introduction of this flexibility in the interpretation of the intent of Congress was by no means an accident. Over the previous quarter century, Congress generally had made a point of respecting the autonomy of the NIH. Members of Congress often found opportunities to make its desires and preferences known to NIH administrators, but, as Susan Halebsky Dimock has observed, "Congress has largely steered clear of direct involvement in NIH priority setting by avoiding directives and earmarks in NIH appropriations bills."[58] Even in this case, where Congress clearly pushed the envelope, the staffers who drafted the legislation were careful to work with NIH employees to come up with legislation that would give the agency some wiggle room. Susan Wood, the deputy director of the Congressional Caucus for Women's Issues, recalled that "NIH had a lot of input," though she conceded that "whether or not they felt like they had a lot of input is another question. But they did in terms of trying to get language that they were not upset about, that would not put them in a box." According to Wood, the specific language "went back and forth with NIH," and "we did a couple of different versions."[59] By several accounts, Vivian Pinn, the director of NIH's Office of Research on Women's Health, played an important, if delicate, role in this process: government officials are not permitted to "lobby" Congress, but they are expected to respond to congressional requests for information; and, acting in that latter capacity, Pinn helped steer the legislation in the direction of granting flexibility and discretion to the NIH.

Eventually, many of the concerns raised by researchers and statisticians—both about research methodology and about the threat of the "politicization" of research—were allayed as the NIH went about the business of determining how actually to implement the congressional directive. NIH Deputy Director Wendy Baldwin, a sociologist and the head of NIH's Office of Extramural Research, convened a working group to develop a policy statement that would be "grounded in science."[60] Significantly, the working group not only took advantage of the flexibility afforded the NIH by the wording of the legislation, but also invented new definitions of key terms in order to justify its preferences. As statisticians on the working group expressed it: "Some of the language used in the Act was imprecise and open to different interpretations. The NIH staff has endeavored to interpret and implement the Act in a manner that captures its spirit and intent while fostering the conduct of scientifically and ethically sound clinical research studies."[61]

An important case in point was the requirement that subgroup comparisons be conducted in all "clinical trials." To circumscribe the application of this requirement, the working group effectively redefined "clinical trials": "For the purpose of these guidelines, a 'clinical trial' is a broadly based prospective Phase III clinical investigation, usually involving several hundred or more human subjects, for the purpose of evaluating an experimental intervention in comparison with a standard or control intervention or comparing two or more existing treatments. Often the aim of such investigation is to provide evidence leading to a scientific basis for consideration of a change in health policy or standard of care."[62] The NIH thereby excluded from the definition of "clinical trial" all of the smaller, more preliminary trials, such as the initial Phase 1 trials that test whether a new drug is safe for further study. In so doing, they restricted the imposition of subgroup comparisons to the research most likely to directly inform public health policy—the "effectiveness" trials that would lead to the licensing of a new drug or the revision of a standard of care.[63] While clearly taking some liberties with definitions, the working group arguably was acting in a way that was consistent with legislators' original concerns. Moreover, they were agreeing with the logic expressed by the biostatistician critics about the stages of research—that it was more important to study variation at later stages than at early ones.[64]

Another crucial instance of interpretative work concerned the requirement in the NIH Revitalization Act that when subgroups were compared, a "valid analysis" of differences between men and women, and between ethnic and racial groups, be conducted. "Valid analysis" was an unusual phrase—in fact, it was a deliberately ambiguous one that had emerged out of the conversations between congressional staffers and NIH officials. A subcommittee of the working group, consisting of NIH statisticians, decided that a "valid analysis" of differences did not necessarily mean that subgroups had to be large enough to permit comparisons that would yield statistically significant results—the prospect that the statistician critics had found so alarming because of the enormous sample sizes that would then routinely be required. Rather, "valid analysis" might simply mean an "unbiased assessment"—one that "will, on average, yield the correct estimate of the difference in outcomes between two groups of subjects."[65]

Here again, the NIH statisticians sought a compromise that was, in many ways, consistent with the arguments expressed by critics. Rather than require statistically significant comparisons of outcomes by gender, race, or ethnicity in all cases, the NIH drew an important distinction: only in those specific cases in which "data from prior studies strongly indicate the existence of significant differences of clinical or public health importance in intervention effect among subgroups" are researchers in Phase 3 trials required to design the trials with sufficient sample sizes in each subgroup to be able to answer the research question independently for each subgroup. For example, in a study of a new medication for hypertension, investigators might be compelled to design the trial to determine the efficacy of the medication independently for black research subjects, given existing claims of differences between black people and other racial groups in the effects of antihypertensive drugs. But in all studies where there was no documented evidence of an outcome difference by groups, then a "valid analysis" would suffice—one that reported on any differences discovered, but without requiring, from the outset, that subgroups be recruited in large enough numbers to attain statistically significant results.[66]

These moves on the part of the NIH went along with other reassuring signals sent to clinical researchers. For example, researchers were informed that clinical studies could exclude particular groups as long as a good scientific justification was presented. Moreover, they were told that an individual trial might escape the requirement of diversity if NIH administrators determined that the "overall research portfolio" for that condition or therapy was sufficiently representative of women and minorities.[67] In general, these various interpretations meant that substantial open controversy over the Revitalization Act proved short-lived. Opponents who, perhaps, were unaware of the informal negotiations between the NIH and Congress were cynical about what they saw as the working group's definitional sleight of hand, but they were not displeased with the outcome. As Piantadosi wrote: "The NIH clinical trials community has done a service to us all by making some workable guidelines out of an unreasonable law." Meinert wrote that the working group deserved praise "for trying to rationalize the irrational."[68]

At the end of the day, the NIH's specification of new procedural standards did a reasonably effective job of walling off the "narrowly scientific" problem of study design from "political" claims on all sides—whether of those denouncing past research biases or of those decrying the intrusion into medicine of "political correctness" and "identity politics." Many of the NIH officials generally supported the new policies, but the point is that they now were in a position to promote them as *scientifically* defensible. At the same time, they interpreted the policies in ways that limited the scope of change, thereby defusing critics of the politicization of science while simultaneously maximizing the agency's own autonomy and discretion. While many of those most centrally involved in the process of specifying the new procedures were themselves committed to the goals of inclusion and wanted to see the guidelines succeed, this interest in reform did not preclude the simultaneous pursuit of another institutional goal: keeping the control over disbursement of its funds substantially in the hands of the NIH's own program officers and peer review committees.[69]

Boundary work by NIH officials was one key dimension of the practical tasks undertaken by state agencies to shore up what became the inclusion-and-difference paradigm. In the next chapter, I outline the emergent paradigm and analyze the new standard operating procedures that it prescribes for biomedical research and pharmaceutical drug development.

Then, in the following chapter, I describe the additional "categorical alignment work" performed by DHHS officials to stabilize the paradigm, and I examine the paradigm's distinctive solution to the tension between competing desires—to standardize research practices and to acknowledge human diversity.

CHAPTER SIX

Formalizing the New Regime

Analysts of the politics of women's health research in the United States have treated 1993 as a banner year—understandably so, because that year was marked both by the passage of the NIH Revitalization Act and by the revision of the FDA's previous guideline excluding women from many clinical trials. But it would be a mistake to stop our analysis then. Over the remainder of the decade of the 1990s, the new emphasis on inclusion and difference solidified into what I have termed a biopolitical paradigm—a framework of ideas, standards, and procedures, not always consciously articulated, that specifies how concerns about health, medicine, and the body are made the simultaneous focus of biomedicine and state policy.[1] The structure of this particular biopolitical paradigm—the inclusion-and-difference paradigm—has taken shape through the continued specifica-tion of new federal policies, the creation of new bureaucratic offices, and the extension of its logic to additional social groups. This process of accretion has been relatively ad hoc: it was no one's "master plan." But in the course of these developments the paradigm has acquired inertia and stability. Over time, its guiding assumptions increasingly have been taken for granted—"black boxed," in the vocabulary of science studies.[2] Only by examining events since 1993 can we develop an accurate sense of the transformations in how biomedical research gets performed and understand the implications of these transformations.

The goal of this chapter and the next, therefore, will be to describe the "new regime" that has come into being—or at least, to describe how things are *supposed* to work. (I defer until chapter 8 the important question of how the system actually *has* worked.) In this chapter, then, I trace the steps in the consolidation and institutionalization of the paradigm, includ-ing, first, the creation of additional policies and offices with reference to various underserved groups and, second, the emergence of new standard operating procedures for biomedical research and pharmaceutical drug development.[3]

FROM REFORM AGENDA TO BIOPOLITICAL PARADIGM

In the years since 1993, the inclusion-and-difference paradigm has been extended in at least four ways that I will discuss. First, age categories (particularly pediatric and geriatric life stages) have been understood to be important dimensions of difference for medical purposes and are now recognized in NIH and FDA policies. Second, in response to public pressure, the FDA has taken a number of steps to strengthen its rules and guidelines. Third, inclusion policies of various sorts have spread to other agencies throughout the DHHS, besides the NIH and the FDA. And finally, a series of offices devoted to the health concerns of specific populations have been created within DHHS agencies.

This "thickening" of the paradigm demonstrates a principle familiar to analysts of organizations and of state policymaking: within a given organizational field, efforts to deal with the same set of problems or grapple with the same dimensions of uncertainty often will lead to "homogeneity in structure, culture, and output." People feel increasing pressure to adopt the same organizational solutions that have been taken up elsewhere, resulting in fundamental similarities in organizational structure, or what Paul DiMaggio and Walter Powell have called "institutional isomorphism."[4] Moreover, policies have "feedback effects" or "legacies" that influence the adoption of future policies. As Margaret Weir expresses this notion, "decisions at one point in time can restrict future possibilities by sending policy off onto particular tracks, along which ideas and interests develop and institutions and strategies adapt."[5] Not only do policies provide organizational solutions that others will copy, but, more profoundly, as Frank Dobbins notes, "extant policies shape what is *culturally conceivable*."[6] Thus, the implementation of policies by state actors has considerable implications for future action. Indeed, as Weir and coauthors put it: "Once instituted, social policies in turn reshape the organization of the state itself and affect the goals and alliances of social groups involved in ongoing political struggle."[7]

Not Just Miniature Adults

Although the FDA began requiring drug manufacturers to provide pediatric information in drug product labels and package inserts in 1979, and although reformers began pointing to the underrepresentation of children in medical research at least as far back as the 1980s, additional policies promoting their inclusion in research weren't developed until relatively late in the reform wave. This lag may be due to the generally strong desire to protect children from the risks of participation in biomedical research—that is, in the case of children, the "pendulum swing" away from the protectionism of the 1970s has been somewhat less pronounced.[8] It makes sense, then, that policies focusing on children came only after the first inclusionary policies already were in place to serve as precedent for action.

That children were folded into the inclusion-and-difference paradigm slightly later also may reflect the unusual place that children occupy in relation to "identity politics" in the United States. On one hand, invoking the best interests of children is one of the surest ways to build support for just about any political agenda in a country like the United States, where children are conceptualized as both infinitely precious and infinitely vulnerable.[9] On the other hand, children are not a self-identified political constituency in the United States the way that "women" or "people of color" are, for the simple reason that, most of the time, children themselves are not agents in the political arena. Children don't represent themselves; their interests are always represented by others.

The question of children's inclusion in medical research rose to public visibility, then, only when key representatives began to articulate children's interest. Here, again, AIDS advocacy organizations played an important role. But there was another group that was absolutely crucial to the story: pediatricians. It mattered that children had a medical specialty devoted specifically to their concerns. Moreover, pediatrics is distinctive within medicine in ways that inclined professionals to take an activist posture. As Sydney Halpern has emphasized in her account of the rise of pediatrics, the whole developmental trajectory of this specialty, since its creation in the late nineteenth century, is "grounded in social meliorism and in a tradition of stewardship on the part of the American medical elite": pediatricians very typically have seen themselves as advocates of child welfare; and, over the years, they have responded to, or articulated, a range of social concerns relating to children's needs.[10]

In this case, physicians who were prominent within the American Academy of Pediatrics played a key role as what Howard Becker called "moral entrepreneurs"—crusading professionals seeking reform through new rules.[11] In the mid-1990s, members of the Academy's Council on Pediatric Research, pointing to evidence that showed that the vast majority of medications used by children had never been tested in children, began discussing remedies among themselves—specifically, whether there ought to be legislation that would do for children what the recently adopted policies on inclusion accomplished for women and racial and ethnic minorities. It is likely that this idea would have found a receptive ear in Congress, which was being lobbied on the issue of children's access to medications by AIDS advocacy groups such as the Elizabeth Glaser Pediatric AIDS Foundation.[12] Indeed, reports issued by the House and Senate Appropriations committees informed the NIH in 1996 that Congress was "concerned that inadequate attention and resources are devoted to pediatric research conducted and supported by the National Institutes of Health"; and they "encourage[d] the NIH to establish guidelines to include children in clinical research trials conducted and supported by NIH."[13] Recommendations of this sort—contained in so-called report language from Congress—do not carry the force of law; but government agencies ignore them at their peril, because they often point to areas of concern that Congress will keep pursuing.[14]

At the same time, the views of pediatricians were well represented within the DHHS bureaucracy. Indeed, one FDA official, when asked in a 1991 interview why the agency recently had begun focusing more attention on drug testing in children, responded only half-jokingly: "There's a simple answer to your question: Pediatricians are infiltrating the FDA."[15] In 1994 the agency instituted a rule that required manufacturers of marketed drugs to survey existing data for each of their products to see if enough was known to support adding information on pediatric use to the drug's labeling.[16] Over at the NIH, meanwhile, pediatricians didn't even need to "infiltrate": they had a home at the National Institute of Child Health and Human Development (NICHD), one of the NIH component institutes. Clearly, representatives of the pediatric profession within the DHHS were interested in improving knowledge about the effects of medications on children. At the same time, as DHHS insiders, they often were leery of outside interference from Congress or advocacy groups.

The director of the NICHD, Duane Alexander, was a pediatrician who had spent most of his career working within the agency. Alexander had served on the PHS Task Force on Women's Health, whose 1985 report led to the first guidelines on inclusion; and he had paid close attention to the struggles around inclusion, including the passage of the NIH Revitalization Act in 1993 and the implementation of new NIH guidelines in 1994. Alexander had no intention of ignoring the warning contained in the congressional report language, lest this "nudge," as he put it, be replaced by the "club" of legislation. Moreover, by virtue of his position as director of NICHD, Alexander also was an ad hoc member of the American Academy of Pediatrics' Council on Pediatric Research, which gave him firsthand knowledge of the Academy's interest in passing legislation to enforce the inclusion of children. Thus, Alexander was perfectly situated to pursue his goal—to preempt congressional action through proactive measures on the part of the NIH.[17]

Alexander convinced the leaders of the American Academy of Pediatrics not to "tie our hands" with legislation, but rather to give the NIH a chance to voluntarily institute guidelines on the inclusion of children.[18] To this end, Alexander worked together with Wendy Baldwin, the director of extramural research, and the NIH formally announced its intention to develop such guidelines in January 1997, publishing them in March of the following year. As of October 1998, all investigators applying for NIH funding for research on human subjects are obliged to "provide either a description of the plans to include children and a rationale for selecting or excluding a specific age range of child, or an explanation of the reason(s) for excluding children as participants in the research." NIH study sections (peer review panels) are charged with reviewing proposals to determine whether the stated inclusion or exclusion of children is deemed acceptable or unacceptable.[19]

The guidelines represented an important policy change at the NIH that brought children under the umbrella of the inclusion-and-difference paradigm. But there is no question that preemptive action by Alexander and others at NIH resulted in the adoption of a more flexible policy than Congress might have imposed. The guidelines on children spelled out many possible exemptions from the inclusionary requirement. Moreover, the language on the conduct of subgroup comparison—examining differences within a study between adult and child populations—was considerably less constricting than the corresponding guidelines on women and minorities.

Meanwhile, however, Congress had taken decisive action to address the problem of inadequate data about the effects of medications on children— but by focusing on the FDA and the pharmaceutical industry, rather than on the NIH and the research community. Much as with the NIH Revitalization Act previously, concerned members of Congress were able to tack their proposals onto an existing piece of legislation focusing broadly on the agency. As part of the FDA Modernization Act of 1997, legislators offered a substantial financial incentive in the form of a six-month extension of the life of a patent to a drug company willing to go back and conduct studies of an approved drug in pediatric populations, in order to add pediatric labeling data.[20] Drug companies have a relatively limited period during which their patented drugs can recoup development costs and bring them profits before generic competitors are allowed on the market. The six-month extension of "market exclusivity" was a huge boon to the industry, potentially worth millions of dollars per drug.[21]

Thus, while the inclusion-and-difference paradigm has generally been enforced by confronting researchers and drug companies with "sticks" of varying heft, in this particular case Congress decided to dangle an especially sweet "carrot." Widely considered a success, the policy was granted a renewed lease in 2002, when Congress passed the Best Pharmaceuticals for Children Act, which continued the policy of granting six-month extensions of exclusivity until 2007. This legislation also called on the FDA to pay attention to the racial and ethnic composition of pediatric trials promoted by the policy—an example of the intertwining of concerns about various underrepresented populations singled out by the inclusion-and-difference paradigm.[22]

In 1998 the FDA, with backing from the Clinton White House, took a more aggressive stance and sought to complement the "carrot" with a new "stick." In doing so, the agency ignited a controversy, played out on both ideological and economic grounds, that demonstrates some of the limits of the inclusionary reform wave. The FDA Modernization Act had provided motivation for drug companies to act, but not necessarily right away: companies had little incentive to undertake pediatric studies until their patent protection was about to expire. Nor did the bill do much to encourage studies of drugs whose patents already had expired. Moreover, the FDA was unhappy about the limited response to its 1994 rule requiring companies to assess whether there were sufficient data to add pediatric labeling information for existing drugs. Manufacturers had submitted labeling supplements for only 430 drugs and "biologics" (biological products)—a small fraction of those on the market—and fully half of those labels simply reported that "safety and effectiveness in pediatric patients have not been established."[23] Therefore, the agency issued a "pediatric rule" announcing that the FDA would have the option of compelling manufacturers to conduct studies in pediatric populations—as part of the approval process for a new drug, or, in compelling circumstances, for drugs already on the market—if it seemed that the drug was likely to be beneficial to children.[24]

"Kids deserve the same access to newly developed drugs that their parents get," said DHHS Secretary Donna Shalala, announcing the new FDA policy.[25] The pediatric rule also had the clear support of President Clinton, whose administration was engaged in a number of projects promoting children's health, including a recently passed health insurance program for children.[26] But the pediatric rule provoked an outcry among pharmaceutical companies, and their cause was championed by conservative groups opposed to governmental regulation. In March 2002 the administration of George W. Bush announced that it intended to suspend the rule. Government spokespersons cited a lawsuit brought against the government by three conservative or libertarian organizations (the Association of American Physicians and Surgeons, the Competitive Enterprise Institute, and Consumer Alert), who argued that the FDA had exceeded its statutory authority in issuing the rule. However, the Bush administration quickly retreated from its plan to suspend the rules in the face of protests from pediatricians and members of Congress, including Senator Hillary Clinton.[27]

In October of that year, a federal district court sided with the plaintiffs, determining that the FDA had indeed exceeded its authority.[28] The court ruling in turn ignited a wave of publicity, with broadcaster Peter Jennings noting on ABC News that hundreds of young children die each year from adverse reactions resulting ultimately from "guesswork" in doses.[29] Stepping in to resolve the issue, Congress passed the Pediatric Research Equity Act in July 2003, formally granting the FDA the authority to compel drug companies to test products in children. Although DHHS Secretary Tommy Thompson and FDA Commissioner Mark McClellan issued a press release commending Congress for its action,[30] the controversy does suggest the ongoing contentiousness of more expansive regulations within the inclusion-and-difference paradigm—indeed, their potential vulnerability, especially, perhaps, during a Republican administration.[31]

What about the Elderly?

At the other end of the age spectrum, the elderly also have been incorporated into the set of policies that comprise the inclusion-and-difference paradigm. However, formal attention to inclusion of the elderly has been sparse—surprisingly so, given the size of the elderly population in the United States and its political clout on health policy issues. Perhaps because advocacy organizations such as the AARP have been so heavily focused on cost concerns related to programs such as Medicare, they have not mobilized around questions of inclusion of the elderly in research populations or the study of medical differences between the elderly and other age groups. Neither has Congress appeared to take a strong interest in such matters. Indeed, Douglas Schmucker and Elliot Vesell, in a 1998 article in a pharmacology journal describing the underrepresentation of the elderly in drug trials, lamented that "the elderly have not received attention comparable to that accorded the underrepresentation of women in clinical trials," such as the GAO study and the NIH Revitalization Act.[32]

However, responding in part to concerns expressed by geriatricians and by the NIH's National Institute on Aging, the FDA has passed a few specific policies relating to the elderly. Early in the reform wave, in 1989 the FDA issued a guideline calling upon the pharmaceutical industry to include elderly patients in clinical trials as a general matter of course.[33] Eight years later, in 1997, the agency set forth a rule that requires a "geriatric use" section on all drug labels, providing information on how the medication should be used in patients aged 65 and older. "The medical community has become increasingly aware that prescription drugs can produce effects in elderly patients that are significantly different from those produced in younger patients," the FDA noted in the *Federal Register*. Moreover, while "people over age 65 constitute only 12 percent of the U.S. population, . . . they consume over 30 percent of the prescription drug products sold in this country."[34]

Beefing Up the FDA Policies

Another way in which the commitment to the inclusion-and-difference paradigm has deepened has been in the FDA's implementation of progressively more binding rules that put the burden on drug manufacturers to present data on safety and efficacy broken down by gender, age, and race. The agency called for such information in a 1995 guideline. But the FDA's own investigation subsequently revealed that pharmaceutical companies were providing relevant data only about half the time. Therefore, in 1998 the FDA issued a rule requiring that industry sponsors formally compile safety and efficacy data for "important demographic subgroups, specifically gender, age, and racial subgroups." (FDA rules are binding, while guidelines are not.) Moreover, companies seeking approval of their products would now have to tabulate, in their annual reports, the numbers of subjects enrolled in clinical trials, according to their age group, gender, and race.[35] Thus, the rule emphasized the need both to include groups and to study differences—even if it did not absolutely mandate inclusion or specify the methodology for subgroup comparisons. In that sense, the FDA rules are similar in spirit to their NIH counterparts, while remaining somewhat more flexible.

During the 1990s, AIDS activists continued to press the FDA on these policies. As soon as the 1977 restriction on women's participation in research was lifted in 1993, women from the Lesbian Caucus of ACT UP/New York criticized the change as inadequate; they argued that the new guidelines lacked teeth and did not actually force drug companies to include women.[36] Terry McGovern, the director of the HIV Law Project, the group that had taken the lead in filing the "citizen petition" against the

FDA, also continued to pursue issues of inclusion in drug research. In 1994 she was appointed to the National Task Force on AIDS Drug Development, a commission established by President Clinton that included representatives of government agencies, the pharmaceutical industry, the research community, and activist groups. Along with other AIDS activists, such as Moisés Agosto of the National Minority AIDS Coalition, McGovern used the task force as a forum to press for a much stronger enforcement mechanism at the FDA—actually bringing to a halt any trial that excluded women or people of color from studies of drugs treating life-threatening illnesses.[37]

In 1997 the FDA followed up on this recommendation (at least with regard to gender) and announced its consideration of a "clinical hold" policy: the agency would delay the initiation of a clinical trial, or suspend one in progress, if either men or women were excluded from study of a treatment for a life-threatening condition that affects both genders out of concern of risk to offspring. This clinical hold regulation eventually was implemented, taking effect in July 2000.[38] Not surprisingly, the policy was controversial. According to a reporter for *Nature Medicine*, "many believe that the 'clinical hold' rule will hinder development of the very drugs to which it will be applied—those for life-threatening diseases—because these products normally receive fast-track evaluation."[39] However, to corporate sponsors of new drugs, the threat of a clinical hold communicates in a very powerful way that the FDA is serious about including women in trials for diseases such as HIV infection.

Inclusion Policies Spread through the DHHS

Another demonstration of the gradual institutionalization of the inclusion-and-difference paradigm within DHHS is the spread of various sorts of inclusion policies among its component agencies. For example, the Centers for Disease Control and Prevention (CDC), a large federal health agency with a small clinical research component, implemented policies in 1995 on the inclusion of women and minorities in the research that it sponsors, such as clinical trials of preventive vaccines.[40] In 2003 the Agency for Healthcare Research and Quality (AHRQ), which conducts research on the delivery of health services, announced a new policy "on the inclusion of priority populations in research conducted and supported by the Agency," as well as the "valid analysis" of differences between groups. While not every AHRQ study would need to examine every "priority population," the "overall portfolio" of research would have to include such populations as "inner-city; rural; low income; minority; women; children; elderly; and those with special health care needs, including those who have disabilities, need chronic care, or need end-of-life health care."[41] That same year, the NIH published new guidelines for its conference grant program, calling for conference organizers to "make a concerted effort to achieve appropriate representation of women, racial/ethnic minorities, and persons with disabilities, and other individuals who have been traditionally underrepresented in science, in all NIH sponsored and/or supported scientific meetings."[42] The definitions of the precise groups of concern varied in these policies. But in these instances and elsewhere, DHHS agencies made the commitment to studying group differences a baseline feature of their research efforts.

During the final years of the Clinton administration, the spread of inclusionary policies was both connected to and facilitated by a simultaneous, explicit policy emphasis on the reduction of health disparities related to race and ethnicity. Announced in 1998 during Black History Month, the health disparities initiative was conceived as the health component of Clinton's broad-based "Presidential Initiative on Race," intended to improve racial relations in the United States. "Nowhere are the divisions of race and ethnicity more sharply drawn than in the health of our people," Clinton told the national audience of his Saturday radio address, announcing the $400 million initiative to eliminate the gaps between the health of racial minorities and non-Latino whites by the year 2010. The effort was spearheaded by David Satcher, recently appointed to the dual role of Surgeon General and Assistant Secretary for Health. An African American, Satcher had a strong track record in the area of minority health issues.[43]

As compared to the general tendency within the inclusion-and-difference paradigm to conceive of differences mostly at the biological level, the health disparities initiative was noteworthy for its emphasis on social-structural determinants of health inequalities. While the focus areas were relatively conventional—infant mortality, cancer screening, cardiovascular disease, diabetes, HIV/AIDS, and immunizations—the stated goal was "to identify and address the underlying causes of higher levels of disease and disability in racial and ethnic minority communities." These underlying causes were presumed to include poverty, inadequate access to health care, and environmental hazards.[44] In the conclusion to this book, I will return to the important distinction between a concern with "differences" and a concern with "disparities." However, within the Clinton administration, as a practical matter, the disparities initiative and the various inclusionary policies and programs often overlapped and reinforced once another.

An Office of One's Own

One of the important legacies of the women's health research initiatives of the early 1990s was the creation of specific bureaucratic offices within the DHHS designed to promote women's health. In 1991, a year after the founding of the NIH's Office of Research on Women's Health, an Office on Women's Health was created at a higher level, reporting to the Assistant Secretary for Health; this latter office was charged with coordinating women's health activities across the various PHS agencies. In 1992 President Clinton appointed Susan Blumenthal, a psychiatrist, to head the office and serve as Deputy Assistant Secretary for Women's Health.[45] Other offices devoted to women's health were then created in a number of key DHHS agencies, including the FDA and the CDC. According to a report issued by the Kaiser Family Foundation and National Women's Law Center in 2003, thirteen state governments around the United States also had created women's health offices, whether by legislation, executive order, or administrative action.[46]

A roughly parallel set of federal health offices focus on racial and minority health issues. Indeed, the DHHS Office of Minority Health, headed by the Deputy Assistant Secretary for Minority Health, was established in 1985 (the same year as the publication of the report from the Secretary's Task Force on Black and Minority Health), well preceding the creation of the Office on Women's Health. The CDC founded its Office of the Associate Director for Minority Health in 1988. Within the NIH, the Office of Research on Minority Health (ORMH) was founded at the same time as the Office of Research on Women's Health. Some of the NIH institutes, such as the NHLBI, also have created minority health offices in recent years. Other DHHS agencies fold minority health concerns into the agendas of offices devoted to "special populations," "priority populations," and so on.

Some of these offices are small; others—like the Office on Women's Health, which had more than forty employees by 1999 and had forty-five in 2005—are more substantial. I will review some of the activities of these offices in chapter 8. For the moment, two points are worth making. First, these offices are not merely an outgrowth of the inclusion-and-difference paradigm but also a powerful mechanism for its institutionalization and, sometimes, expansion. This has been evident from the early days of the paradigm, when the NIMH's Office of Special Populations, under Delores Parron, became a locus for activism around issues of research inclusion. Aside from the specific functions performed under their auspices, offices provide a sort of insulated space within the bureaucracy, within which like-minded professionals can advance their agendas.[47] The offices also reflect, and further, the establishment of a limited kind of multiculturalism within the ordinary workings of the executive branch. The ability of the offices to provide a secure home for certain kinds of beliefs and frames is perhaps especially evident in the few cases where Congress has mandated the office, meaning that it cannot be eliminated or de-funded unless Congress changes its mind. Indeed, in recent years, supporters in Congress have pressed, so far without success, for passage of a "Women's Health Office Act," which would permanently authorize offices of women's health throughout DHHS.[48]

Second, the establishment of these offices is a significant indicator of the influence of outside forces on the operations of government. At the FDA, for example, officials whom I interviewed tended to play down the role of Congress and advocacy groups when it came to the passage of guidelines and rules regarding sex, race, and age; they argued that the agency was already on the path to taking action in these areas and would have done so, in the end, even without public scrutiny and pressure. Whether or not this perception is accurate, what is striking is that when it came to the offices, officials were more inclined to attribute them to outside influence from "stakeholders": they acknowledged that the FDA most likely would not have created these offices on their own, absent such pressure.[49]

It may be symptomatic of the perception that the offices are a concession to stakeholders that, in some cases, federal health officials have been loath to see the mandates of these offices expand. For example, in 1999 NIH Director Harold Varmus clashed with Jesse Jackson Jr., a Democratic representative from Illinois, when Jackson and other members of the Congressional Black Caucus sought to elevate the NIH's Office of Research on Minority Health from an office into a "center."[50] (In the NIH organizational hierarchy, centers outrank offices in clout, though both rank below institutes.) The following year Varmus was overruled, as Congress voted to transform the ORMH into the National Center on Minority Health and Health Disparities. President Clinton signed the legislation, claiming it as consistent with his emphasis on the reduction of health disparities by race.[51]

STANDARDIZATION AND FORMALIZATION

In a certain sense, as I have described, the new biomedical paradigm grew out of a revolt against standardization—at least, against the biomedical presumption of a "standard human." But it would be a mistake to imagine that the politics of inclusion have brought about a new world of research free of standardization. Rather, the inclusion-and-difference paradigm is powerfully undergirded by standardization of various kinds, including new ways of standardizing human beings. Standards, as defined by Geof Bowker and Leigh Star, are sets of agreed-upon rules for the production of material or symbolic objects, and they serve as a fundamental and powerful means of organizing everyday life practices.[52] When promulgated by government agencies, standards reflect what Michael Mann terms the "infrastructural" power of the modern state: its capacity to penetrate its territories and coordinate social life.[53] However, standards are often hard to enforce, while those who do find it convenient or necessary to conform to standards may nonetheless resist adopting the values associated with them. Therefore, standards can be thought of as a weaker alternative to either laws or norms, and their use may reveal the limitations as much as the strengths of the organizations that promulgate them.[54]

Standards come in various kinds. Stefan Timmermans and Marc Berg usefully have distinguished procedural standards, which concern the conduct of practices, from other sorts of standards—terminological standards, design standards (which emphasize technical specifications), and performance standards (which focus on outcomes).[55] In the next chapter I discuss the new sorts of terminological standards—the categories of personhood—that correspond to the inclusion-and-difference paradigm. First, though, I want to examine the rise of a new set of procedural standards for biomedical research and pharmaceutical drug development.

The inclusion-and-difference paradigm seeks to reshape the procedural standards of researchers both in academia and in industry through the careful specification, by state officials, of new requirements for experimentation on human beings. Laying out procedures endows the paradigm with stability; as John Kingdon has noted, once policies are built into standard operating procedures, "then inertia sets in, and it becomes difficult to divert the system from its new direction."[56] It follows that the institutionalization of this "new regime" is an example of the extension of bureaucracy—and a demonstration of the not-unfamiliar pattern in the United States by which social reforms that arise out of a democratic impulse have the effect of enhancing the administrative capacities of the state.[57]

New Standard Operating Procedures for Drug Companies

The FDA's data-reporting procedures for pharmaceutical companies are notoriously complex, but before the 1990s there were few requirements with regard to such characteristics of research subjects as race, ethnicity, age, and gender. In the late 1980s, however, the FDA began calling for each "new drug application" to "give the number, age range, and sex distribution of subjects" as part of a table showing all studies conducted on the drug being considered for licensing.[58] More recently, in response to a request from Congress made in 2002, the FDA has begun developing a database into which these figures from individual clinical trials can be entered. With the aggregate demographic information from the database, the agency will be in a better position to report its inclusion statistics.[59]

In addition to providing figures on clinical trial participants, pharmaceutical companies are required to give specific information by "subset" for any differences in response to a drug revealed by the clinical trials. The "subsets of interest," the FDA noted, might well vary with the drug and condition being studied, but usually would include sex, race, age, and size, along with such diverse potential factors as the severity of the disease, whether patients suffer from other ("concomitant") illnesses, the patients' histories of therapy with other medications for the condition, and smoking and alcohol use. The subsets that pharmaceutical companies are specifically requested to tabulate, however, are the so-called major ones of age, sex, and race. The list of adverse events experienced by patients in the trials must also indicate patients' age, sex, race, and weight.[60] After a drug has been marketed, the agency also has special procedures for reporting adverse reactions to the FDA. Since 1993, these "MedWatch" forms have collected data on the age, sex, and weight of patients suffering adverse reactions, while "race" and "pregnancy" are listed as possible examples for data entry under "other relevant history."[61]

Interestingly, the FDA does not require formal statistical analysis of differences between subsets. As described in the preceding chapter, the NIH Revitalization Act forced the NIH to call for subgroup comparisons in its funded research, and NIH officials have gone to some creative lengths to specify precisely when such comparisons are really needed. The FDA, by contrast, is under no such injunction. Therefore, FDA guidelines simply instruct pharmaceutical companies that "the examination of subsets need not routinely involve formal statistical analysis." Companies should be on the lookout for obvious differences—what the FDA calls "differences of clinically meaningful size." But pharmaceutical company statisticians need not pursue "minor differences" that lack real-world medical significance.[62]

Formalization at the NIH

Academic biomedical researchers are most likely to encounter the inclusion-and-difference paradigm when applying for NIH funds to conduct clinical studies. As a consequence of the NIH Revitalization Act, the standard grant application form PHS 398 was revised to include a "Targeted/Planned Enrollment Table" on which investigators must enter their study recruitment targets by "sex/gender" and by race and ethnicity (see fig. 1). If the proposal is then funded, the investigator also is required to submit annual reports on accrual of subjects, demonstrating that the actual demographics of the study are consistent with the inclusion plan that was proposed originally.[63] The NIH then aggregates these figures in a database and uses the information to prepare reports for Congress, as mandated by the NIH Revitalization Act.

If investigators do not intend to include both women and men, a range of racial and ethnic groups, and children as well as adults in a proposed study, then they must explain the rationale for exclusion as part of their grant application text.[64] Justifications for exclusion are sometimes obvious—no one expects to see women in a study of prostate cancer, for example. In other cases, however, researchers have to marshal their knowledge of the field in order to make a compelling case for exemption. For example, an applicant might argue that because an ongoing research study is already examining children with a given medical condition, then it is acceptable to design a new study that focuses strictly on adults.

When received by the NIH, all applications are coded by peer review panels (called "study sections") with three codes, indicating whether women, minorities, and children are included and whether the inclusion or exclusion is considered acceptable or unacceptable (see fig. 2). Reviewers also are instructed to create headings in their written critiques labeled "Inclusion of Women" and "Inclusion of Minorities" and comment specifically on the inclusion plans. In addition, if the applicant is proposing a large, Phase 3 clinical trial, then reviewers are expected to comment on whether the investigator is planning to conduct subgroup analysis (either a full-fledged analysis capable of showing statistical significance, in those cases where prior evidence suggests that results may vary by sex/gender, race, ethnicity, or age; or a simpler "valid analysis" of differences, in those cases where there is no reason to expect variation by subgroup). In theory, the reviewer's consideration of the inclusion plan and the analysis plan is supposed to be factored into the "priority score" assigned to the application—that is, it affects the determination of the overall scientific merit of the proposal and, hence, its fundability relative to the pool of applications.[65]

If a proposal coded as "U" (for an "unacceptable" inclusion plan) is otherwise deemed worthy of NIH funding, then a "bar-to-funding" is imposed on the proposal until the issue of inclusion has been satisfacto-

FIG. 1 NIH GRANT PROPOSAL INCLUSION TARGETS

Targeted/Planned Enrollment Table			
This report format should NOT be used for data collection from study participants.			
Study Title: _____			
Total Planned Enrollment: _____			
TARGETED/PLANNED ENROLLMENT: Number of Subjects			
		Sex/Gender	
Ethnic Category	Females	Males	Total
Hispanic or Latino			
Not Hispanic or Latino			
Ethnic Category: Total of All Subjects*			
Racial Category			
American Indian/Alaska Native			
Asian			
Native Hawaiian or Other Pacific Islander			
Black or African American			
White			
Racial Categories: Total of All Subjects*			
*The "Ethnic Category: Total of All Subjects" must be equal to the "Racial Categories: Total of All Subjects."			

Source: http://grants1.nih.gov/grants/funding/phs398/phs398.html.

rily addressed. As Eugene Hayunga, who worked for the NIH's Office of Research on Women's Health (ORWH) expressed it, "That 'U' is a very powerful administrative tool," because when it is assigned, then "everything stops."[66] At that point, the NIH program officer has the discretion to propose a range of potential solutions. The program officer may require the applicant to include a certain demographic group, for example, or he or she may recommend that the applicant work in collaboration with another investigator located in another geographic region that has a higher representation of a racial or ethnic minority group.[67]

After the passage of the NIH Revitalization Act, the NIH promoted awareness about the new emphasis on inclusion through extensive education about these requirements. First, employees of the ORWH conducted a two-hour training with more than one thousand NIH employees with responsibilities in areas such as grant management and proposal review. As Hayunga recalled, "We had to make sure that everyone at NIH understands what the requirement is and knows what the standard is"—especially given previous congressional criticism of NIH's failure to publicize the earlier policy on inclusion. NIH employees who received

FIG. 2 NIH REVIEW PANEL CODES

GENDER CODE

First character = G

Second character:

　1 = Both genders

　2 = Only women

　3 = Only men

　4 = Gender unknown

Third character:

　A = Scientifically acceptable

　U = Scientifically unacceptable

MINORITY CODE

First character = M

Second character:

　1 = Minority and nonminority

　2 = Only minority

　3 = Only nonminority

　4 = Minority representation unknown

Third character:

　A = Scientifically acceptable

　U = Scientifically unacceptable

CHILDREN CODE

First character = C

Second character:

　1 = Children and adults

　2 = Only children

　3 = No children included

　4 = Representation of children is unknown

Third character:

　A = Scientifically acceptable

　U = Scientifically unacceptable

Source: "NIH Instructions to Reviewers for Evaluating Research Involving *Human Subjects* in Grant and Cooperative Agreement Applications" (National Institutes of Health, Bethesda, MD, April 25, 2001).

this training then had the responsibility of explaining the requirements to applicants and peer reviewers.[68] The ORWH also published and distributed several thousand copies of an "outreach notebook" intended to explain the policy to researchers around the country.

The NIH's Office for Protection from Research Risks (OPRR) advertised the new policy in its educational workshops with IRBs charged with reviewing research protocols at academic centers, hospitals, and

other research sites around the country.[69] The fact that IRBs have become attentive to issues of inclusion when reviewing research protocols
is highly significant for the broader diffusion of this new emphasis, because IRBs must approve nearly all academic research on human subjects. Typically, each IRB requires investigators to conform to a standard
set of instructions when writing a research protocol—whether or not
the investigator intends to seek government funding. Thus, nearly every academic researcher doing research involving human participants is
likely to be confronted with questions about whether he or she intends
to include women, minorities, and children in the research. This near-
universalization of the inclusionary injunction extends well beyond the
biomedical arena. In fact, in order to conduct interviews to write this
book, I was obliged to submit a research protocol to my university's IRB
for the social and behavioral sciences, which instructed me as follows:

> **Inclusion of women and minorities** must be addressed in all research
> protocols. For example, what is the study population and how/where will
> subjects be recruited? What percentages of women and minorities make
> up the demographic area under study and what percentage will be in your
> study? If inclusion of women or minorities is inappropriate, the scientific
> rationale must be explained and justified.[70]

Given the topic of my research, it was not hard for me to assure the IRB
that I would indeed be interviewing a substantial number of women and
minorities. But these practices demonstrate the considerable reach of the
inclusion-and-difference paradigm, at least in a general form.[71]

Standardizing Persons

The development of new standard operating procedures is a story about
the diverse kinds of work that make it possible to institutionalize new
ways of doing things. The inclusion-and-difference paradigm depends on
the creative employment, especially by federal health officials, of techniques to formalize abstract goals, convert them into practical targets, and
measure and assess the outcomes. The requisite work of formalization,
standardization, and quantification is often largely invisible to outsiders,
but it is no less significant for being hard to observe.

However, in this chapter my account has focused on research procedures, and I have not had much to say yet about the form of standardization that was the original target of reformers: the standardization of
the human subject as a research object. What has become of the much-

maligned "standard human," and who or what has taken his place? In fact, the new procedural standards are closely linked to another kind of standardization—the formalizing of the categories used to classify human subpopulations for research purposes. In this regard, one of the most important functions of the new biopolitical paradigm is also one of the most abstract: to specify a new mode of standardizing the human. Understanding this development is the goal of the next chapter.

CHAPTER SEVEN

From the Standard Human to Niche Standardization

With the rise of new, scientific conceptions of medical practice and medical research in the twentieth century came increased pressure to stabilize and standardize a scientific working object for experimental purposes—a "human subject" whose body could yield generalizable scientific knowledge.[1] However, advocates of the inclusion-and-difference paradigm repudiated the notion that humanity could be standardized at the level of the species—that is, they rejected the presumption that biomedical knowledge could be derived from the study of, or be broadly applicable to, the "standard human." At the same time, these skeptics of universalism did not veer fully to the opposite extreme of embracing total particularity. Though they frequently invoked the rhetoric of "individualized therapy," their response in fact was *not* to insist on the medical uniqueness of each individual. Rather, advocates proposed that the working units of biomedical knowledge-making could be groups: women, children, the elderly, Asian Americans, and so on.

The inclusion-and-difference paradigm therefore enshrines what might be termed *niche standardization*: a general way of transforming human populations into standardized objects available for scientific scrutiny, political administration, marketing, or other purposes that eschews both universalism and individualism and instead standardizes at the level of the social group—one standard for men, another for women; one standard for blacks, another for whites, another for Asians; one standard for children, another for adults; and so on. Instead of a standard human, niche standardization proposes an intersecting set of standard subtypes.

This chapter begins by sketching the general logic of niche standardization and then considers its specific application to the case of clinical research in the United States in recent years. I analyze why certain ways of disaggregating and categorizing humanity have flourished within the inclusion-and-difference paradigm while others have been deemed inappropriate or undesirable. Then, I examine the mechanisms by which this new way of categorizing people gets "operationalized," or put into practice, especially by federal health agencies that rely on the "symbolic power" of the state; and I pay particular attention to the extraordinary difficulties that sometimes arise when research subjects must be sorted into categorical boxes, particularly according to their race and ethnicity. Finally, I emphasize the significance of the nation-state and state agencies to the success of biomedical categorization by considering an example of a less successful attempt to standardize pharmaceutical drug development and regulation at the transnational level.

NEITHER THE UNIVERSAL NOR THE PARTICULAR

Though it is not hard to think of examples of niche standardization, the phenomenon mostly has fallen below the radar screen of social science. Many analysts of state bureaucratic practices have emphasized the tendency of modern states to homogenize populations—what Max Weber called the "leveling of the governed," or what James Scott described as the creation of "standardized citizens" who were conceived of as "uniform in their needs and even interchangeable."[2] Alternatively, analysts of practices of governing have considered the contrary tendency to administer through individuation. These analysts have emphasized how states have controlled populations through technologies of identification such as passports, fingerprints, and biometrics, which seek to precisely distinguish one citizen from another; or how states make use of the practices, emphasized by Foucault and his followers, of surveillance and comparison of persons against norms.[3] Some scholars, such as Philip Corrigan and Derek Sayer, have emphasized both dimensions: the universalistic ideology of state formation on one hand and the individualizing practices of state administration on the other.[4] However, what all these discussions share is the presumption of a polar opposition between leveling and individuation or between universalism and particularism. This binary focus diverts attention from niche standardization: the biopolitical management (and redefinition) of population subgroups via a specification of standards at the "intermediate" level of the categorical group.

At the most general level, niche standardization offers different opportunities to different actors in society. For state bureaucrats, it can serve as a way of segmenting the population in order to provide differential benefits to recognized political constituencies. (Affirmative action policies constitute an important example.) For corporations (including pharmaceutical companies), niche standardization can undergird niche marketing practices, in which products are tailored not to a mass market but to distinct social groups, or "demographics."[5] For political organizers, niche standardization specifies the basic units of identity politics. Moreover, insofar as niche standardization challenges a model of politics that presumes that all citizens are homogeneous, it is also consistent with the political vision put forward by critics of universalistic conceptions of citizenship such as the political theorist Iris Marion Young. In a world in which differences matter, Young argues, the goal of equality is best served not by the pretense that all citizens are alike but rather by the development of appropriate mechanisms for group representation.[6]

Niche standardization has become so much a part of the cultural logic of societies like the United States that it can be found at work not only in obvious places, such as marketing and opinion polling, but in all sorts of unlikely locales. Consider, for example, the crash-test dummy, used by automobile manufacturers and safety experts to predict the outcomes on human life of car crashes. How should the crash-test dummy be designed? By constructing a composite of many sorts of automobile drivers and passengers, one might seek to develop the single, perfect crash-test dummy that comes closest to representing the effects of collisions on the average person—the "standard dummy." Alternatively, those who doubt the utility of the standard dummy to model the real-world car-crash experiences of distinct individuals might favor the development of fully individualized dummies—but of course, it would be thoroughly impractical to expect companies to repeat their tests using millions of different dummies. The compromise proved to be niche standardization: the production of a few standard types of dummies, male, female, child, and infant.[7] Another interesting case concerns attempts to map the size of the "average American body." The first such survey since the Second World War was completed in 2004 under the sponsorship of clothing and textile companies, the Army, the Navy, and several universities. After measuring ten thousand adults using a "light-pulsing 3-D scanner," the investigators "redefined" the average American, who not only had grown heavier in recent decades, but also could best be comprehended as a series of subtypes. The average American was either a male or a female and either white, black, Hispanic, or "other"; and he or she belonged to one of six discrete age groups. Thus, the survey presented forty-eight standard subtypes, each with average chest, waist, hips, and collar measurements.[8] In these examples and others, the trick is to determine which particular ways of differing matter for the problem at hand—typically, sex, age, and race—and then to institutionalize that typology as the standard.

Those who see a global movement toward valorization of the individual as the basic social unit might question the significance of niche standardization. For example, David Frank and John Meyer, in their analysis of the trend in recent decades toward the global recognition of "the individual as the main element of reality and thus primary repository of legitimate roles and identities," have described identity-group formation as temporary "exceptions" that develop "at the frontiers of individualization."[9] The United States has long been recognized as a society that valorizes individualism,[10] and there is in fact some evidence one might point to of individualism triumphing over niche standardization—for example, in the recent efforts by multiracial citizens to resist the requirement that they assume a group identity by "checking a box" on forms, surveys, and censuses.[11] Still, given the extraordinary salience of standardized group identities in diverse arenas of political and economic life in the United States (and elsewhere), it seems a bit misleading to describe these as simple exceptions.[12]

Within the world of modern biomedicine as well, niche standardization also has been overlooked because of the presumption of a fundamental tension between the universal and the individual. A familiar and continuing debate in biomedicine juxtaposes two ways of conceiving the patient. On one hand, modern scientific medicine is associated with universal, homogeneous, standardized approaches to patient care—often preached under the rubric of a movement called evidence-based medicine, which prescribes treatment protocols that are well supported by research. On the other hand, when treating individual patients, physicians frequently reject these standardized formulas (which they sometimes dismiss as "cookbook medicine") in favor of more particularistic approaches that depend less on data than on experience and seasoned judgment—the "art," as opposed to the "science," of medicine.[13] New scientific developments like pharmacogenomics that aim eventually at so-called personalized medicine through access to the patient's genetic profile represent a different individualizing approach, one that would be particularistic but also scientific.[14] But if these are the usual polar alternatives, then, again, the inclusion-and-difference paradigm suggests an interesting intermediate solution, targeted at the "middle level" of the collective actor: medicine that is not "personalized" but, rather, group specific.

Once again, the Human Genome Diversity Project offers a parallel example. In reaction against the abstract universalism of the Human Genome Project, which sought to construct a single map of "the human genome," a group of reformers from within the genetics establishment proposed an auxiliary program, the Human Genome Diversity Project. However, the goal of the Diversity Project was not to insist, as critics of mainstream genomics such as Michael Flower and Deborah Heath have done, that "we are each *singular variants* of 'the' human genome."[15] Rather than attempt to substitute radical individuality in place of the standard human, the Diversity Project organizers intended to roam the globe sampling the genomes of deliberately selected, supposedly "isolated" populations in order to compile a warehouse of these distinct genetic types. That is, the project would use a predetermined classification of human subtypes in order to construct a series of group-specific genetic standards.[16] These group-based standard types are then an instance of niche standardization.

Interestingly, proponents of niche standardization in medicine often adopt a language of individualism but then develop policies that are aimed at social groups. For example, an article by FDA officials published in *Science* in 1995 observed: "Since the early 1980s, [the FDA] has been interested in the individualization of therapy, that is, determining whether and how treatment should be modified for various demographic groups within the population."[17] This slippage between referencing individuals and groups is a common feature of discourse surrounding the inclusion-and-difference paradigm; it endows the paradigm with legitimacy by associating it with individualism, one of the cherished values of U.S. political culture.

The Logics of Classification

What determines how the human species will be disaggregated into subunits? Who decides which categories will rule? Clearly, in different situations, different logics come into play. Sometimes the "groups" designated by bureaucrats or experts are inventions that do not interpellate any preexisting, self-defined collective actor. For example, a policy may be specified to apply to a statistical risk group, such as "young men aged 25 to 34."[18] Or a class-action lawsuit may effectively create a category of people who share a particular life circumstance, such as "all female employees of Wal-Mart." Or a geneticist may propose that all those individuals who share an allele or genetic marker constitute a group insofar as they have a particular genetic risk in common. In each of these cases, what is noteworthy is that the category has little real-world significance prior to or apart from its creation by some authority in a given situation.

While it is possible that the category may eventually *become* a meaningful social identity—for example, that individuals who share a genetic marker may come to see themselves as part of a group and may organize around that "biosocial" category[19]—the point is that the emergence of the social identity is, in these situations, mostly an aftereffect of expert labeling.

The case described here, though, is interestingly different. In the inclusion-and-difference paradigm, the subdividing of humanity has made convenient use of preexisting, familiar, and everyday understandings of salient group difference. To put it another way, in the policies and practices of the inclusion-and-difference paradigm, niche standardization has leaned on categorical alignment—the merging of social categories from different worlds, such as medicine, social movements, and state administration. Here, the groups designated both by state and biomedical authorities correspond roughly with mobilized collective identities, or with what Michèle Lamont and Virág Molnár call the "phenomenology of group classification": how ordinary individuals "think of themselves as equivalent and similar to . . . others [and] how they 'perform' their differences and similarities."[20] In such cases, bureaucratic and scientific classifications come to be treated as functionally equivalent both to one another and to the categories of everyday life.

It is very much worth noting that dividing humanity by categorical identities was only one of several conceivable way of organizing an attention to difference in biomedicine. For example, there are many biomedical risks that are more directly associated with *practices* or *behaviors* than with identities. Whether one smokes, how much one exercises, and what sort of food one eats are choices that all have significant health consequences. Might it not make scientific sense, at least in some medical studies, to make sure that research populations include both smokers and nonsmokers and to measure differences in outcomes between the two groups?[21] Other ways of categorizing are less intuitive but may make sense in particular circumstances. For example, a cardiologist reported in 1994 that people shorter than five feet tall have a seven percent higher risk of dying from a heart attack than patients who are over six feet—apparently because of differences in the diameters of their arteries.[22] Perhaps, then, clinical trials of heart medications ought to be certain to include subjects of varying heights and to compare results between shorter and taller participants. Or what about classifying people by hair color—given the finding reported in 2002 that redheads experience more pain and need more anesthesia during surgery?[23]

Still other, more complex risk measures might also be invoked as a way to subdivide research populations. For example, in 2001 the FDA licensed a drug called Xigris to treat severe sepsis. In a study that led to licensing, the drug appeared much less effective for patients whose APACHE II scores (a statistical measure intended to predict the likelihood of recovery on the part of a patient in the intensive care unit) fell below a certain threshold. Thus, the FDA-approved labeling for the drug restricted claims about its efficacy to patients with higher APACHE II scores.[24] Clearly the division of patients according to APACHE II test scores reflects a substantially different logic than one that classifies them according to social identities such as age, race, ethnicity, sex, or gender.

Thus, the choice of categories for niche standardization was highly consequential. In part, these were simply the categories of political mobilization: for example, organizations such as the Congressional Caucus for Women's Issues and the Society for the Advancement of Women's Health Research took shape in relation to the political category "women." In part, the singling out of groupings determined by sex, gender, race, ethnicity, and age reflects the everyday apparent naturalness of these ways of differing in U.S. society: when we look around us, we tend almost inevitably to categorize people in these terms, and it may be hard for some to imagine an alternative. But in addition, the obviousness of these categories is a testament to their entrenchment within public health discourses and statistics in the United States, and their present-day use is a legacy of their previous use. In particular, sex or gender, race, and ethnicity have been treated as relevant health indicators in the United States for more than a century, in large measure, as Nancy Krieger has explained, because they are typically (though by no means always properly) treated as self-evident, immutable, and easily recordable characteristics of individuals.[25]

The point is not just that differences seen as natural or obvious are adopted for use by medical and public health authorities. Reciprocally, those authorities, through various public activities aimed at specific groups (including health promotion campaigns, reports of research findings, and targeted recruitment for participation in research) help to constitute various publics or social identities—they shape the meanings of those groups through the circulation of health discourses about them.[26] Thus, the incorporation of categories within the inclusion-and-difference paradigm is potentially quite consequential for their broader social meanings. In particular, reformers did not simply *presume* the biomedical significance of categories: through their actions, they *reinforced* this perception. In chapters 10 and 11, I will argue that one of the problematic consequences of the new paradigm is precisely that it reshapes how we think about sex, gender, race, and ethnicity—specifically, that it encourages the tendency to imagine these ways of differing as grounded strictly in our biological make-up. So, on one hand, biomedical institutions borrow the categories and groupings of everyday life, but on the other hand, the categories are infused with new meanings through that borrowing, and they are handed back to us in transformed character. Of course, this is nothing new. For several centuries in the modern West, the meanings of categories such as gender, race, and ethnicity have evolved regularly out of the complex dialectical interplay between expert labelers and the claims about selfhood of those being labeled.[27]

An additional example of the subtle shifts in the meaning of identities and categories lies in the construction of rough equivalences among the various forms of difference that are recognized within the inclusion-and-difference paradigm. That is, from the standpoint of DHHS policies and procedures, sex/gender, race/ethnicity, and age are all treated as formally equivalent modes of difference to be "handled" administratively in similar ways. Because of contingent factors relevant to their histories, the policies and standards that make up the inclusion-and-difference paradigm do vary somewhat from one type of difference to another. (For example, the NIH does not compile statistics on the age distribution of subjects in its research portfolio, for the simple reason that Congress never required it to do so.) There are also some differences between agencies in the definitions of terms. (For example, the NIH considers anyone under the age of 21 to be a "child" for research purposes, while at the FDA the definition is 16 or younger.) Nevertheless, in a more overarching sense, the paradigm tends to "flatten" differences—to conceptualize sex/gender, race/ethnicity, and age as ways of differing that are all analogous or commensurate from a policy standpoint.[28] Formally, the policies also tend to treat sex/gender, race/ethnicity, and age as discrete characteristics of individuals, rather than as complexly intersecting relational properties of groups.[29] Hence, out of different differences, the policies of the inclusion-and-difference paradigm have created a sort of generalized difference. This flattening may facilitate bureaucratic administration, but it also may problematically presume equivalences and analogies across very different sorts of categorizing systems.

Which Categories, Which Identities?

What permits particular social identities to achieve recognition within systems of niche standardization such as the inclusion-and-difference paradigm? Why do other identities fail to "qualify"? In general, I would argue that the inclusion-and-difference paradigm is well disposed to recognize categorical identities when the identity is already socially salient, when the representative group is highly mobilized, when the group lays claim to a form of difference that is already authorized by state classifications, and when proponents are able to convincingly deploy frames that link justice arguments to biological difference claims. Conversely, the likelihood of recognition of a way of differing is reduced when the group is not well mobilized; when it articulates demands in relation to a form of social difference that is not already institutionalized in state policies; and when its frames do not resonate with the public or policymakers, perhaps because of the difficulty of advancing a biological difference argument.

We gain further insight into the logic of the inclusion-and-difference paradigm by considering examples of well-known social identities associated with types of difference or inequality that have *not* been recognized, or fully recognized, within it. I should clarify that here I take up the question of the group's "suitability" in the abstract. In chapter 12, I examine other cases (especially that of sexual identity) in which strong attempts actually have been made to fold the group or category into the policies of the inclusion-and-difference paradigm. Those cases will demonstrate additional factors that help determine who becomes a "special population"—whether the group is able to present itself as analogous to others already included and whether it is able to leverage that similarity and attract allies from within the existing policy environment.

In thinking of cases not included, perhaps the most important one to consider is that of social class. Health researchers universally acknowledge the correlation between poverty and poor health outcomes, and in other countries, such as the United Kingdom, the use of measures of socioeconomic status are routine. But in the United States—despite the best efforts of the NIH's Office of Behavioral and Social Sciences Research to call attention to these issues—the poor or working class are only sometimes treated as a "special population," and one rarely hears calls for greater inclusion of people of different social classes within study populations or encounters worries about the dangers of extrapolating findings from the rich to the poor or vice versa. (However, the Clinton administration's emphasis on health disparities did place social class issues under consideration to a much greater degree than in the preceding recent decades or in those years since.) Yet it is plausible to imagine that social-class differences may significantly affect the generalizability of medical findings.

For example, Marcia Angell, formerly the editor-in-chief of the *New England Journal of Medicine*, has insisted that class is "*numero uno* as the determinant of good health," something that "swamps every other difference," and pointed to the controversial Physicians' Health Study as an interesting case: everyone zeroed in on the exclusion of women from the study, while no one mentioned that its focus on a highly affluent group—physicians—made the sample extremely unrepresentative of the U.S. population in quite a different way.[30] Similarly, Janet Wittes, one of the strong critics of the NIH Revitalization Act, has suggested that while extrapolation across racial groups is rarely a concern, extrapolation from upper-middle-class research subjects to the poor may be highly problematic—not because of biological differences between the well-off and the poor, but because of social factors that can affect the response to medication, such as nutrition.[31] And Otis Brawley, another who voiced concerns about how the NIH Revitalization Act conceptualized racial differences, has proposed that poor whites are the "forgotten minority" who are not being included in representative numbers within studies of diseases such as prostate cancer.[32]

Yet despite these sentiments and findings, there has been no formal attempt to incorporate social class within the policies mandating inclusion of groups within clinical studies and the testing of differences across categories. In this case, so-called American exceptionalism (the reduced political salience of class in the United States) and the relative absence of collective actors mobilized around class categories in the domain of health policy likely help to explain the failure to incorporate class in the paradigm, even when the government has some history of programs and policies that target poverty in the domain of health (for example, Medicaid). Here again, the lesser degree of biologization of class in the United States in recent decades may mean that the biological-differences frame appears less relevant to researchers or policymakers in this case. Moreover, there is relatively little history in the United States of the public collection of medical statistics by social class, and class is taken by medical researchers and epidemiologists to be much harder to operationalize and measure than race or gender.[33] It is not hard to see, then, why proponents of legislation such as the NIH Revitalization Act did not promote such goals as subgroup analysis by social-class background.

Yet the absence of class from the formal policies and offices of the inclusion-and-difference paradigm matters greatly for how health and research issues are conceptualized in the United States. Indeed, if social class were incorporated as a standard classifier, the political effects might be significant: because social class is not seen as a biological category, to call attention to differential health outcomes by class is to call attention to the effects of social inequality on health. By contrast, differential health outcomes by race or sex—while perhaps in fact produced by social inequality—may often be framed as a simple consequence of biological difference. As this example clearly suggests, classification systems have important consequences through what they omit as well as through what they include.[34]

Other negative cases are revealing as well. For example, religion is not treated as a categorical variable by the DHHS. Although there are examples of health risks that accrue unequally to certain religious groups (such as a greater risk by Ashkenazi Jewish women of inheriting the genetic mutations known as BRCA that are associated with breast cancer), in most discussions such epidemiological differences are subsumed under the category of ethnicity. At least in the present-day United States, religion, per se, is not typically associated with biological differences, so that frame would not be likely to resonate, even if there were a strong advocacy group putting it forward. (Indeed, in the case of Ashkenazi Jews, mobilization mostly has worked the other way: because of the historical legacy of Nazism, Jewish organizations have been fearful or ambivalent about embracing any association between Jewishness, disease, and bodily difference.[35]) In addition, religious identification often is considered a private matter in the United States, one that government should not take into account.

Another intriguing example concerns the politics of size, an issue of relevance as obesity increasingly becomes a topic of great concern within federal health agencies. On one hand, as Abigail Saguy and Kevin Riley have described, "fat acceptance" activists who promote the philosophy of "health at any size" epitomize what I have termed an antistandardization movement that resists the notion of there being a single "standard human." In that sense, their activism resembles that of other proponents of the inclusion-and-difference paradigm. On the other hand, many of these activists are ambivalent about the medicalization of obesity and would reject the idea that being large is inherently medically problematic.[36] Thus, they might be disinclined to cooperate in a coalition calling for inclusion of people of different weights within research populations. The absence of a committed advocacy group promoting weight as a relevant research variable helps to explain why weight is not a formal dimension of the inclusion-and-difference paradigm.

Yet another telling case that sheds light on the classificatory logic of the inclusion-and-difference paradigm is the formal emergence as a mobilized identity of what used to be the "unmarked category": men. As George Lundberg, the former editor of the *Journal of the American Medical Association*, observed, "Male gender is a ticket to death earlier than women";[37] and medical experts as well as social scientists have been paying increasing attention to understanding this brute fact as well as the dynamics that result in poor health outcomes for men. In 2003 the *American Journal of Public Health* published a special issue on men's health, while the American Medical Association formally "encourages research and medical education to address the reasons that men have shorter life spans, to develop ways to engage men in their health care and to develop methods to improve access to care."[38]

Much of the recent attention to men's health focuses on problematic aspects of masculinity—for example, men's greater propensity to engage in risky behaviors, or a cavalier attitude about health that translates into a disinclination to seek medical attention.[39] By contrast, political attempts to promote a concern with men's health within DHHS are more emblematic of the politics of antifeminist backlash. The Web site of the men's health advocacy group Men's Health America characterizes the growing inclusion of women in NIH-funded clinical trials in the wake of the NIH Revitalization Act as a "setback" for men: "Any way you look at it—sex-specific budget allocations, declining male participation in NIH studies, or comparative risk of death—over the past decade, men's health has been shortchanged by medical research."[40] Consistent with the concern that men are now underrepresented, and on the heels of increasing interest in specific men's health issues such as prostate cancer, several conservative male members of Congress have introduced legislation to create an Office of Men's Health within the DHHS.[41] According to a June 2000 press release from Randy "Duke" Cunningham, a Republican from California, announcing his introduction of such legislation in the House, "men have a higher death rate than women do for each of the ten leading causes of death in this country."[42] Strom Thurmond, the Republican Senator from South Carolina, introduced a companion bill in the Senate. The legislation has yet to garner much enthusiasm. (Interestingly, however, the 2001 version of the bill was endorsed by the National Medical Association, the African American physicians group.[43])

Thus, the case of men's health provides an example where political mobilization exists (though mostly at elite levels[44]), where the biological-differences frame resonates, and where the form of difference (gender) is well institutionalized—but where the collective identity (men) cannot very plausibly be presented as the victim of injustice. Of course, an even more striking example than men's health would be "white people's health"—something that does not exist as a mainstream political project, although white people (or Caucasians) are claimed to be at higher risk for certain diseases and conditions.[45] In these limiting cases, we see the importance not just of making scientific arguments about difference but of tying them effectively to claims about the pursuit of social justice.

OPERATIONALIZING RACIAL AND ETHNIC CATEGORIES

In facilitating categorical alignment and shoring up niche standardization, DHHS employees have played a critical and defining role. This is not surprising: as the social theorist Pierre Bourdieu argued, modern states have tremendous power to shape the ways in which social reality is perceived: "Through classification systems (especially according to sex and age) inscribed in law, [and] through bureaucratic procedures . . . , the state molds *mental structures* and imposes common principles of vision and division."[46] For example, as John Skrentny has shown in an analysis of a comparable case (the development of affirmative action policies in the United States), government agencies and committees played an important role in creating the list of "official minorities" that would be deemed appropriate candidates for affirmative action.[47] Similarly, in the case of the inclusion-and-difference paradigm, state actors have endowed the policies with a vital measure of stability. They have accomplished this not just by brokering agreement between proponents and opponents of reform, as described in chapter 5, but also through their work in operationalizing the categories—defining, more or less precisely, terms such as age, race, and ethnicity for policy purposes. This is no trivial accomplishment; the success of the paradigm presupposes the ability to take characteristics of personhood—one's race, one's gender, and so on—and convert them into discrete measurable "variables" within biomedical experiments.

The clearest and most interesting example of this operationalizing work is also the one that is the most vexing in practice: defining race and ethnicity for purposes of ensuring compliance with the new inclusionary policies. A substantial body of scholarship has demonstrated that, in the domains of medicine and public health, classifications of individuals by race and ethnicity are subjective and often arbitrary. At a 1993 workshop sponsored by federal health agencies on the "Uses of Race and Ethnicity in Public Health Surveillance," expert participants agreed that "concepts of race and ethnicity are not well defined or consistently measured among Federal agencies."[48] Indeed, CDC epidemiologists noted that the challenges involved in collecting usable data on race and ethnicity included variability in the use of terms, misclassification, and undercounting.[49] As Robert Hahn has observed, one symptom of the unreliability of categorization by race and ethnicity in health documentation is that the same individual "may be assigned a different race at birth, during the course of life, and at death."[50] Of course, the difficulties in assigning individuals to particular races and ethnicities on forms, certificates, and documents in the domain of health ultimately reflect the precariousness of such classification in the society more generally. Precise definitions of these categories are impossible to provide, the boundaries separating them are gray, the practices of classification change as the society evolves, and people's willingness to adopt racial and ethnic identifiers may reflect the desirability of group-specific benefits provided by state agencies.[51]

The success of the inclusion-and-difference paradigm, therefore, has depended in part on the ability of federal health bureaucracies to impose some workable means of assigning racial and ethnic identifiers to individuals participating as human subjects. In doing so, DHHS practice has been shaped by "policy legacies": officials have imported standards and classifications from other domains, including other government agencies that have dealt with issues of inclusion and affirmative action.[52] For example, in its 1994 guidelines implementing the new provisions of the NIH Revitalization Act, the NIH invoked "Statistical Policy Directive No. 15" of the Office of Management and Budget (OMB), entitled "Race and Ethnic Standards for Federal Statistics and Administrative Reporting." Published in 1977, Directive No. 15 specified the racial and ethnic categories used in the U.S. census. It identified four racial and ethnic minority group categories—"American Indian or Alaskan Native," "Asian or Pacific Islander," "Black, not of Hispanic Origin," and "Hispanic"—along with one majority group category, "White, not of Hispanic Origin."[53] As Michael Omi has observed, although Directive No. 15 was "originally conceived solely for the use of federal agencies, [it became] the de facto standard for state and local agencies, the private and nonprofit sectors, and the research community." It is thus a striking historical example of how "state definitions of race have inordinately shaped the discourse of race in the United States."[54] Indeed, Dvora Yanow has described how the U.S. government uses official racial and ethnic categories for counts of "AIDS cases; birth defects; cancer; cataract surgery; drownings; firearm accidents; hysterectomies; bubonic plague; smoking habits; [and] suicides."[55]

The Politics of the Census

This way of operationalizing race and ethnicity provided the initial basis for the coding scheme used by the NIH in determining researchers' compliance with the NIH Revitalization Act. Researchers are expected to use the OMB categories—more precisely, they are expected to require their research participants to self-classify according to these categories. Like many standards, this one facilitates various kinds of work practices through the enforcement of consistency. In its own words, "NIH has chosen to continue the use of these definitions because they allow comparisons to many national data bases, especially national health data bases."[56] It is important to say, however, that census categories are determined in response to particular sets of political needs and pressures, and they have changed with regular frequency since the initiation of the U.S. census in 1790. In 1890, for example, the U.S. census included racial categories such as "quadroon" and "octoroon" to designate people who were one-quarter and one-eighth (or less) black.[57] A growing body of sociological and historical scholarship based on work conducted in several countries has demonstrated that census-taking is not a neutral act of counting or measuring but is in fact an active way of organizing the state and society. More specifically, as Melissa Nobles and David Theo Goldberg both have described, the census functions as a powerful technology of racialization: it crystallizes particular understandings of race and ethnicity, embeds those understandings within a host of government programs, and diffuses them throughout the society—thereby "bringing into being the racial reality that census officials presume is already there, waiting to be counted."[58] That these classifications and meanings matter is widely perceived. In 1993, when Congress held hearings on proposed revisions to the census categories, a host of groups lobbied for the inclusion or reclassification of their identities on the census forms, in large part because the census results may guarantee a seat at the table of what one analyst called "a smorgasbord of set-asides and entitlements and affirmative-action programs" administered by the federal government.[59]

Indeed, debates about racial and ethnic categories on the U.S. census that played out in the 1990s resulted in significant changes to the census in the year 2000—changes that then had to be taken into account by the NIH and other DHHS agencies. In response to diverse political pressures, the OMB revised its list of categories in 1997 to treat "ethnicity" (now described as "Hispanic or Latino," and "Not Hispanic or Latino") as independent from "race" (slightly redefined as "American Indian or Alaska Native," "Asian," "Black or African American," "Native Hawaiian or Other Pacific Islander," and "White"). That is, each individual would be expected to answer two questions, one about their ethnicity and the other about their race. Furthermore, the OMB was caught in the crossfire between the emergence of a noisy new movement on behalf of multiracialism, which called for a new multiracial category on the census, and opponents of such a change who feared the dilution of minority-group clout if their absolute numbers appeared to decline. The compromise was that no new category of "multiracial" would be created, but that individuals would be permitted to describe themselves on the census using more than one of the racial terms if desired.[60]

The NIH switched to this new scheme in 2000.[61] On the eve of this change, NIH officials such as Vivian Pinn, director of the Office of Research on Women's Health, worried that "having people pick multiple categories of racial origin [is] going to be impossible for our tracking."[62] And responses to the 2000 census provide ample indication of why DHHS agencies might encounter practical difficulties in getting research participants categorized according to the logic of the new guidelines. In the 2000 census, not only did 6.8 million Americans select more than one racial category to describe themselves, but also nearly half of all those who chose "Hispanic or Latino" as their ethnicity declined to identify themselves with *any* of the five approved racial categories.[63] Nevertheless, like other federal agencies, the NIH has embraced the new OMB categories and has made pragmatic adjustments to accommodate them. In 2003 the FDA announced that it, too, was proposing to formally adopt the OMB categories as "a standardized approach for collecting race and ethnicity information in clinical trials conducted in the United States and abroad for certain FDA regulated products"; the agency translated this intention into a formal "guidance" for industry in 2005.[64]

Using census terms for biomedical purposes is a premier example of what I have called categorical alignment, demonstrating its pragmatic uses as well as its limitations. By virtue of simply adopting categories already employed elsewhere in state administration, the DHHS has been able to finesse the question of the precise correspondence between political and scientific classifications. Although the NIH, like the OMB, describes the ethnic and racial categories as "socio-political constructs," there is an inevitable tendency to naturalize them. And although the fine print of grant instructions tells researchers that they may also use any additional or more specific subpopulation descriptors that they deem relevant to their study and report those numbers in an attachment, these are the categories that are counted and which, therefore, effectively "count." Given that few clinical researchers themselves hold clear understandings of just what race "really is" (in my own interviews with biomedical researchers studying racial differences in health, I found that researchers consistently were unable to articulate clear definitions of "race") reliance on an official list of categories proves convenient for just about everyone.

But the work of force-fitting bodies to labels can become quite messy. This is perhaps especially evident in the growing number of cases where researchers or pharmaceutical companies make use of human subjects from countries outside of the United States. On one hand, NIH investigators are encouraged to collect identifying data from their participants in ways that allow participants to use meaningful, indigenous identifying terms. On the other hand, investigators nonetheless must take these culturally specific responses and "aggregate" them into the sanctioned OMB categories.[65] Exactly how this aggregating work is to be performed is not explained in NIH guidelines—or rather, the question itself is hidden behind a haze of bureaucratic reporting procedures:

> [T]he investigator can report on any racial/ethnic subpopulations by listing this information in an attachment to the required table. . . . When completing the tables, investigators should asterisk and footnote the table indicating that data includes foreign participants. If the aggregated data only includes foreign participants, the investigator should provide information in one table with an asterisk and footnote.
>
> However, if the study includes both domestic and foreign participants, we suggest the investigator complete two separate tables—one for domestic data and one for foreign data, with an asterisk and footnote accompanying the table with foreign data.[66]

The instructions speak volumes about the complexities of making a standardized classification system function "on the ground." Regardless of whether participants identify as Yoruba or Thai or "simply" use conventional U.S. racial and ethnic descriptors, the question that becomes submerged beneath the level of policy debate is why the OMB classification system, with all of its particularistic history reflecting political pressures from mobilized groups, makes *biomedical* sense. "With our present state of knowledge, this is perhaps the best way to start framing the question, using those categories," commented Eugene Hayunga, a staff member in the Office of Research on Women's Health responsible for tracking inclusion. "We might learn from this, five, ten years in the future, that maybe we should frame the questions a little bit differently."[67] In essence, federal officials, along with many researchers and policymakers, pragmatically "act as if"—they proceed on the assumption that the identity categories of everyday life and bureaucratic politics can be successfully marshaled in the service of biomedicine, even when they understand the limitations of this assumption. Of course, if the point were to study the health consequences of social processes that the census categories more obviously track—such as racial discrimination—then the use of these categories might indeed make biomedical sense. Almost always, however, the research questions have to do with biological processes for which the relevance of the census categories is simply assumed.

Transnational Alignment Work?

For the most part, categorical alignment work is socially invisible when it is successful. The seams begin to show, however, when the stitching is especially rough—as in the example above concerning the incorporation of foreigners into U.S. research populations. But even then policies can be successful, provided that some authority is in a position to enforce the categorical scheme—and this is precisely the case with the DHHS, which is able to bring the symbolic power of the state to bear in operationalizing the classifications of the inclusion-and-difference paradigm.

The striking power of the state to impose human classification schemes can be seen clearly through a brief comparison with a less successful project, an attempt to align categories at the transnational level for purposes of pharmaceutical drug development and regulation. At this level we can observe striking tensions. On one hand, multinational pharmaceutical companies seek global markets for their products, and they have a financial investment in the belief that people are everywhere enough alike that a drug found safe and efficacious in one population can be expected to have similar effects in all populations. On the other hand, regulatory agencies and researchers have long been concerned that data from clinical trials performed in one country cannot credibly be extrapolated to another country. Indeed, at least until relatively recently, the presumption in many countries, notably including Japan, was that foreign data simply could not be trusted for these purposes.[68] The boundaries of legitimate generalizability across borders have been drawn in diverse and sometimes rather stark ways. At a conference in 1993, one expert on the acceptability of foreign clinical data recalled being told by a regulator in the United Kingdom twenty years previously "that English data was very good, Scottish reasonable, Welsh data was acceptable, and that US data was not very helpful for an English population."[69]

What happens to the "category problem" as we move to the transnational level? What are the relevant dimensions of difference? How can these categories be standardized such that trust can be managed across national borders? These problems were taken up by the International Conference on Harmonisation of Technical Requirements for Registration of Pharmaceuticals for Human Use (ICH). A transnational body created in 1990 with no formal governmental authority, the ICH has the goal of "harmonizing," or standardizing, the registration of pharmaceutical products in three regions: the European Union, Japan, and the United States. The six sponsors of the ICH are the three governmental regulatory agencies (the European Commission, the Japanese Ministry of Health and Welfare, and the U.S. Food and Drug Administration) and the three trade associations representing the pharmaceutical industries of these regions.[70] In effect, the work of the ICH constitutes a countertrend to the concern with the limits of extrapolation described in this book— an attempt to generalize widely across human populations. But in order to advance this mission, the ICH members had to confront the issue of ethnic differences.

In February 1998 the ICH adopted a final draft of a document called "Ethnic Factors in the Acceptability of Foreign Clinical Data," intended "to facilitate the registration of drugs and biologics among ICH regions by recommending a framework for evaluating the impact of ethnic factors on a drug's effect." A few months later, the FDA published the document in the *Federal Register* as a guidance representing the agency's current thinking on the topic. In essence, the goal of the document is to reduce the likelihood that additional clinical trials must be conducted before introducing a drug into a region where it has not previously been studied. The practical innovation proposed by the ICH is something called a "bridging study"—a supplemental study performed in the new region that is designed to provide just enough additional data about the drug's effects on people in the new region to warrant its licensing there, without the expense or time investment of full-scale clinical studies.[71]

The ICH's document on "ethnic factors" describes a bewildering array of kinds of differences that might be found between nations and that might complicate the process of accepting that data generated in one place might be transportable to another—and all of these differences are called "ethnic." That is, "ethnicity" is here taken as a catch-all term to refer to nation-specific or region-specific variation in such matters as lean body mass, organ function, genetic polymorphisms, diet, medical practice, exposure to pollution and sunshine, use of alcohol and tobacco, compliance with prescribed medication regimens, and practices in clinical trial design and conduct, among other things.[72] What work, then, does this document do? On one hand, its practical impact lies in the specific mechanism of the bridging study, which may provide a way for locally generated knowledge about human response to medications to travel comfortably across national borders.[73] On the other hand, the document obscures rather than clarifies what kinds of social groupings count as "ethnic."

The point is that the ICH, as a weak supranational body, lacks the definitional authority often possessed by nation-states: it lacks what Bourdieu would call the symbolic power to impose systems of social classification that will be accepted as both legitimate and obvious. Given time, the ICH's overall work may end up encouraging the spread of some aspects of the inclusion-and-difference paradigm across national borders—a point I return to in chapter 12. However, at the global level, there is simply no consensus about which ways of chopping up humanity into distinct groups are relevant to the domain of biomedicine, and it is unlikely that an organization such as the ICH could impose such a consensus by fiat. Thus, in the domain of biomedicine, categorical alignment and niche standardization continue to depend crucially on the nation-state—no matter how much biomedical research and pharmaceutical drug development have become transnational industries subject to the pressures of globalization.[74]

CHAPTER EIGHT

Counts and Consequences: Monitoring Compliance

If the beliefs and practices associated with "inclusion and difference" constitute a new biopolitical paradigm, then for whom does this paradigm actually matter? Previous chapters of this book have described the creation and the institutionalization of the paradigm. The remainder of the book assesses its real-world *consequences*—for a variety of distinct actors and audiences. I begin with an emphasis on the groups most immediately affected by the guidelines and policies: the researchers and drug companies expected to comply with new directives and the federal health agencies charged with the practical task of monitoring, policing, and documenting that compliance. The inclusion-and-difference paradigm has rescripted the everyday work practices of both of these social actors, as well as the choreography of the dance that locks them together.[1]

Studying compliance with regulations as a social interaction immediately calls attention to the inevitable gap between the rhetoric and reality of social change. The preceding two chapters described the formal apparatus of a "new regime" of biomedical inclusion, complete with regulations, procedural standards, and techniques for classifying and standardizing human groups—at least, they described how things are supposed to work. But to what degree *do* medical researchers or pharmaceutical company sponsors comply with its provisions? To what extent is the paradigm enforced, whether by state officials, Congress, IRBs, or anyone else? More importantly still, how much have the new policies and procedures brought about meaningful, substantive outcomes? These questions matter for those who care about health, equity, and the politics of gender, race, ethnicity, and age. They matter, as well, for those who seek to understand the more general tendencies of institutional change.

This chapter begins by examining the DHHS perspective on the implementation of the policies and practices that make up the inclusion-and-difference paradigm. I then contrast the views of DHHS employees with those of two groups—on one hand, critics of the policies, who remain unconvinced of their merit; and on the other hand, proponents of reform who see the changes to date as insufficient. Using sociological perspectives that are relevant to thinking about compliance, I consider the capacity of these reforms to bring about significant changes as well as the clear limits placed on that potential.

Finally, to extend my consideration of the practical effects of the new paradigm for biomedical work and pharmaceutical drug development, I briefly examine several additional signs of its consequences. These include various reverberations or spillover effects that are less directly measurable by state officials charged with counting up the numbers of different sorts of persons enrolled in medical research. I consider the activities of new offices within DHHS, the rise of new single-group research studies, changes in medical education and in the policies of medical journals, and the practice of niche marketing by pharmaceutical companies.

POLICIES IN PRACTICE

NIH Perspectives

NIH officials concerned with extramural research or with women's health research were quick to embrace the new policies as successful. Writing of them in the journal *Applied Clinical Trials* in 1996, staff of the NIH's Office of Research on Women's Health (ORWH) observed that opinion within the research community continued to be divided, but they suggested that criticism and skepticism were misplaced. Though opponents of the NIH Revitalization Act had predicted a slew of difficulties with its implementation, after more than a year under the policies, it was demonstrably evident "that the new requirements have not brought clinical research to a screeching halt."[2] Nor had the policy "bankrupted" clinical research— the specter raised by opponents of the NIH Revitalization Act.

Arguing that the inclusionary policies had been implemented successfully, the ORWH authors, Eugene Hayunga and the office's director, Vivian Pinn, also presented statistics demonstrating that compliance with inclusion policies quickly had become high. For example, of more than five thousand proposals for experimentation with human subjects that were reviewed at the NIH's January 1995 review meeting, 92 percent met the standard as submitted. Awards were made to 1,187 of the proposals,

96 percent of which had met the standard as submitted. Only twenty-two of the awards received a "bar-to-funding" based on inadequate gender inclusion, and only forty-three were barred based on minority inclusion. The majority of these bars were lifted once investigators supplied additional information about their inclusion plans. A small minority of studies required a modification of the study design in order for the bar to be removed. ORWH staff also sat in on some of the initial review group meetings and "found that reviewers were knowledgeable about the inclusion policy and were following NIH instructions."[3]

By 2000, more than 95 percent of NIH applications met the formal criteria for inclusion of women and minorities as submitted.[4] Similarly, although precise figures on the inclusion of children are not kept, Duane Alexander, director of the National Institute of Child Health and Human Development (NICHD) at the NIH, reported after the first two rounds of reviews under the guidelines (which went into effect in 1998) that "a very, very small percentage" of applications were not in compliance. This reflected an important change in practice, since a review of a sample of proposals from the previous year had indicated that about 15 to 20 percent of applications either were inappropriately excluding children or, at minimum, constituted "missed opportunities" to include them.[5]

My own research, conducted in 2003, corroborated the claims of NIH officials that in recent years there are relatively few wholesale exclusions of social groups from biomedical research, with the exception of pregnant or nursing women. My research assistant examined all Phase 3 trials reported in the NIH's online database of clinical trials, ClinicalTrials.gov. Whether sponsored by industry or by the NIH, very few such trials had blanket eligibility restrictions by gender, with the exception of studies of sex-specific conditions. (However, a large proportion of trials excluded women who are pregnant or nursing, and only one trial in the database specifically indicated that pregnant women could participate.) Of 231 Phase 3 trials sponsored by industry, only 6 were restricted to men, and only 11 to women. Of 369 trials sponsored by the NIH, only 3 were all-male, and only 15 were all-female. In addition, only three trials in the database restricted participation to specific ethnic groups. (One such trial was studying Japanese subjects, another African Americans, and a third was comparing African Americans to Caucasian Americans.)[6]

NIH officials also described the evolution of productive relationships with investigators wondering how to bring their proposals into compliance. Wendy Baldwin, the director of extramural research, noted that researchers sometimes reacted with surprise when faced with the implications of inclusion, but that practical remedies typically were not that hard to devise: "People [would] come back and say, 'I'm going to have to translate my questionnaire. I'm going to have to hire a Spanish-speaking nurse.' And our reaction was, 'Yes. Yes, that does seem to be the solution, very good, you have found the solution. Congratulations.'"[7] Evidence also suggests that NIH-funded researchers, whether happy about the requirements or not, have adjusted their practice to conform to the guidelines. In interviews with epidemiologists, Janet Shim found in 2002 that nowadays "race is almost ritualistically included in [epidemiological] research. . . . One researcher refers to the inclusion of race as just something that everyone has to do—that is, a practice that once may have come with explicit justifications, but that is now so taken-for-granted that epidemiologists perceive it as a standard operating procedure . . . with which they must comply."[8]

For the NIH, the proof of the pudding is in the actual statistics on inclusion. However, these are not equally available for every group. In the case of children, for example, because the NIH instituted its policy so as to preempt congressional action, the agency is under no legal obligation to collect or aggregate data on the numbers included in studies—and therefore doesn't do so.[9] While NIH officials describe having a good general sense that applicants are complying with the policy on including children, they cannot report any specific numbers on how many children or adults are now being studied.

With regard to women and racial and ethnic minorities, NIH record-keeping is considerably more extensive. Thanks to the implementation of a tracking system based on the entry of data from investigators' annual updates, a Tracking/Inclusion Committee has been able to prepare annual reports on the inclusion of women and minorities, as required by the NIH Revitalization Act. In its first "snapshot," presented in January 1997, the NIH reported that 52 percent of more than one million total human subjects represented in ongoing clinical research were women (45 percent were men, 3 percent "unknown").[10] Data from subsequent years suggest a trend toward higher inclusion of women. Of all extramural studies funded in fiscal year 2000, women represented 61.3 percent of subjects. Phase 3 trials—the large trials with clear public health implications—were even more likely to include women.[11]

Data for the year 2000 also showed that at least some racial minority groups were being represented in numbers consistent with their share of the U.S. population. Non-Hispanic whites were 62.4 percent of those studied; Asians and Pacific Islanders, 11.4 percent; non-Hispanic blacks, 11.3 percent; Hispanics, 7.9 percent; and American Indians and Alaskan Natives, 0.9 percent (with 6.1 percent classified as "other/unknown" in terms of race/ethnicity). However, minority inclusion varied significantly by NIH institute, especially for Phase 3 trials. For example, 93.4 percent of those in Phase 3 trials sponsored by the National Institute on Aging trials were white.[12]

More recent NIH data on race and ethnicity are harder to interpret, because of the introduction of new census categories along with the "check more than one box" option in 2000. As late as 2004, some investigators were still using old forms with racial and ethnic categories dating from 1977, while others were using the newer forms with the 2000 census categories. In their tracking report, NIH officials did their best to provide numbers in a series of rather confusing tables. Perhaps the clearest statement that can be made is that minorities overall were estimated to constitute 36 percent of extramural and intramural research participants in 2004, as well as 27 percent of those in Phase 3 trials.[13]

An important question is whether members of specific groups are now being represented in numbers that reflect how much they suffer from particular diseases or conditions. For example, a study by a group of researchers called the HIV Cost and Services Utilization Study Consortium, published in the *New England Journal of Medicine* in 2002, examined rates of participation in AIDS research trials. The burden of AIDS on communities of color was indicated by the fact that nationwide, slightly less than half of all adults receiving care for HIV infection were white—yet 62 percent of the adults participating in trials were white. Patients who were black, who had not completed high school, who had private insurance through an HMO, and whose doctor's offices were located more than eight miles from a major clinical trial center, were all far less likely to be participating in a trial.[14] An accompanying editorial in the journal suggested that "investigators have a narrow view of the sort of person who makes a good participant in an HIV-related clinical trial: a white, college-educated, employed, housed, homosexual man."[15]

Some recent studies also raise serious questions about the progress in improving research on heart disease in women, a focal point of concern during the debates in the early 1990s. David Harris and Pamela Douglas, writing in the *New England Journal of Medicine* in 2000, examined all cardiovascular disease trials funded by the National Heart, Lung, and Blood Institute (or its predecessors) from 1965 through 1998. The news was in some respects good: not only was the overall enrollment rate for women 54 percent, but also the percentage of participants who were female increased significantly over time. However, fully half the women were enrolled in just two all-women trials, the Women's Health Study (on the preventive effects of aspirin) and the gigantic Women's Health

Initiative. Excluding single-sex studies, the percentage of women overall dropped to 38 percent. Moreover, the percentage of participants who were female showed *no* statistically significant increase since 1965, once single-sex studies were removed from the analysis. Given this finding, the investigators concluded that, apart from single-sex trials, "federal mandates with regard to the sex composition of study cohorts" (i.e., the NIH Revitalization Act) had not had any effect on increasing women's participation in cardiovascular research.[16]

FDA Perspectives

Though the FDA has been under pressure to promote inclusion and the study of difference, the agency has not had to confront any directive as overtly prescriptive as the NIH Revitalization Act. One analyst, Karen Baird, has argued that, precisely as a result, the FDA has been slower than the NIH in promoting meaningful reform.[17] This is a particularly significant issue given that growth in the pharmaceutical and biotech fields in recent years has caused private-sector clinical research to surge ahead of publicly funded efforts: by 2003, the total dollar amount of industry-sponsored clinical research was three times the amount provided to clinical researchers by the NIH.[18] Yet even as medical research increasingly passes through the FDA, the agency's capacity to monitor industry has lagged in recent years, leading to much criticism of the agency's overall performance in protecting the public from risk.[19]

FDA officials do report generally good compliance by drug companies with the various policies on inclusion that they have implemented. Of course, in the case of the pediatric exclusivity provision, companies find it greatly to their financial advantage to perform studies on children: "We just have to fight them off now," commented Robert Temple, the associate director for medical policy at the Center for Drug Evaluation Research (CDER, the FDA's center responsible for approval of drugs). Moreover, as Duane Alexander noted, studies in children were simply becoming routine for new drugs coming onto the market: "Companies are not going to risk even being slowed down by the FDA, by the FDA raising questions about their study in kids, they are just doing them."[20] The chair of the American Academy of Pediatrics's Committee on Drugs called the amount of progress "absolutely astounding" and suggested that "we are entering what could be the golden age for kids and pharmaceuticals."[21] Some complained that the pediatric exclusivity provision was a gigantic windfall for pharmaceutical companies, placing them in a position to recoup billions of dollars in profits for an investment of perhaps $100,000.

Other argued, however, that even if, as the FDA predicted, the provision ended up costing consumers $13.9 billion over twenty years (because of the higher amounts they will have to pay for brand-name drugs rather than generics), this was a reasonable price for better knowledge about the effects of drugs on the bodies and minds of children.[22]

In 2001, in its first report to Congress as mandated by the pediatric exclusivity legislation, the FDA observed that the extension of patent protection "has done more to generate clinical studies and useful prescribing information for the pediatric population than any other regulatory or legislative process to date." The agency described receiving 191 proposals from pharmaceutical companies to conduct pediatric studies. In less than three years, fifty-eight such studies had been conducted, resulting in the granting of the six-month patent protection to twenty-five drugs treating conditions ranging from fever to allergies to epilepsy to HIV. Twelve drugs, including Motrin, Advil, and Zantac, had received labeling changes—in some cases simply extending the age range, but in a few cases adding information about the proper dosages by age.[23] Since 2001 the upward trend in response to the pediatric exclusivity provision has continued steadily. In late 2005 the FDA joined with a number of children's advocacy groups to publicly celebrate reaching a milestone: the one hundredth drug to have new information for children included in its labeling since 1997.[24]

At the same time, the FDA's report to Congress noted that the inducements didn't extend to drugs no longer under patent protection.[25] This was the problem for which the FDA's controversial "pediatric rule" and the subsequent Pediatric Research Equity Act (passed by Congress in 2003) were devised as solutions.[26] Although the Pediatric Research Equity Act granted the FDA the authority to compel drug companies to test products in children, critics have complained that loopholes in the legislation have undercut its effectiveness by allowing drug companies to delay conducting studies in children. Moreover, the legislation contains a "sunset clause" that may result in the expiration of the new enforcement measures in 2007.[27]

With regard to the elderly, FDA initiatives have been modest (while the NIH has been even less inclined to issue policies). So it is perhaps not surprising that a number of studies published between 1998 and 2002 concluded that the elderly continue to be substantially underrepresented in biomedical research and pharmaceutical drug development. For example, an article published in the *Journal of the American Medical Association* (*JAMA*) in 2001 reported that the percentage of all trials studying acute coronary syndromes that had explicit age cutoffs (most commonly, 75 years of age) declined during the 1990s, after climbing sharply in the previous decade. However, "even among . . . trials published in the period 1996 through 2000, more than half still failed to enroll at least 1 patient aged 75 years or older." In short, while greater consciousness about the importance of studying the elderly had meant a removal of formal barriers, it had not translated into a successful recruitment of this population into clinical trials.[28] To remedy this problem, some have called for new legislation "requiring the FDA to issue regulatory standards to mandate an appropriate proportion of older persons in clinical trials and directing the NIH to establish formal guidelines for the inclusion of older people in NIH-funded clinical research."[29]

In the case of women's participation in drug trials, the removal of the FDA's 1977 restriction certainly had changed the picture. But it was not always clear that a removal of a ban on women's participation necessarily had translated into active recruitment of women for drug trials, as FDA staff themselves observed in a presentation at an international AIDS conference in 1996.[30] As late as 2001, an article in a pharmaceutical industry trade publication noted the continuing fears on the part of drug developers of liability in the case of harm to a fetus or to an infant being breast-fed. In theory, the article noted, women were now supposed to be able to participate in trials provided they were using birth control. However, "some investigators, uncertain of what constitutes an 'acceptable' control method and fearful of patient noncompliance, simply refuse to enroll female patients of childbearing age in their trials."[31]

Only recently having been pressured by Congress to maintain and compile demographic information, the FDA has little information available about compliance with its guidelines and rules. However, two internal investigations suggested considerable room for improvement in the areas of gender and racial inclusion and attention to differences. The first study, performed by the FDA's Office of Special Health Issues, went back over the internal reviews conducted by the FDA's medical officers to determine the extent to which women had participated in clinical trials for 185 new drugs approved by the FDA from 1995 through 1999. For about a quarter of the 500,000 individuals who participated in clinical trials for these drugs, sex could not be determined from the FDA's records. But for the remaining three-quarters, women and men were nearly equally represented—though less so in the cases of antiviral and cardiovascular drugs, two of the areas of greatest concern in the push to remove the restriction on the participation of women in drug trials. However, the research also found that in a quarter of the cases, medical officers failed to comment on whether any gender analysis had been performed. And while gender differences were noted for 32 of the 185 products, a review of the approved product labeling revealed that in 6 of these cases the labeling failed to indicate the gender differences that had been reported to the FDA.[32]

A comparable study examined racial and ethnic inclusion for the same 185 new drugs approved by the FDA from 1995 though 1999. In this case, however, the medical officers' reports left it impossible to determine the race or ethnicity of nearly half the participants in the clinical trials that led to licensing. In those cases where race or ethnicity could be established, fully 88 percent of participants were white. Relatively few product labels "contained statements about whether the effect of race was known." The study's understated conclusion was that "attention to race by CDER medical officer reviews is variable."[33]

My own analysis of the labeling for drugs approved by the FDA in one sample year (1998) likewise suggests that relatively few analyses of differences across groups were being performed or reported. Of 142 drugs not intended for use strictly in a specific population, only nineteen labels indicated that male/female differences were studied (and such differences were found in four of the nineteen cases). Only twelve labels reported that racial or ethnic differences were studied (with differences found in two of them); only seven reported the study of pediatric differences (which were found in three); and only five reported studying differences between geriatric patients and adults at a younger age (with differences found in four of the five).[34]

The Skeptics

As my discussion in chapter 5 of the NIH's implementation of the NIH Revitalization Act also suggested, DHHS agencies have been forced to walk a careful balancing act—promoting the new policies and standards while being responsive both to investigators' concerns and to broadsides from outright opponents of the inclusion-and-difference paradigm. Certainly the agencies have faced no shortage of criticism. As early as 1995, two researchers from Oregon complained in a biomedical journal about the feedback that one of them had received on a recent grant application: "A profound weakness of the proposed study," the researcher was told by the peer reviewers convened by the NIH, "is the low percentage of minority subjects expected to be in the study. . . . The findings of this study will have limited external validity." Noting that there was no evidence to indicate that ethnic differences would limit the generalizability of their study, the authors commented: "Experiences like these will have a chilling effect on clinical research in areas of the country with small minority populations."[35]

Over the years, many researchers have focused their criticism on NIH "bean counting." They have suggested that the formal requirements not only are bureaucratic impositions but also come at the expense of substantive attention to underlying issues of clinical importance. Thus, while Janet Shim noted the perception among epidemiologists that race must be included as a variable, she also observed a good measure of cynicism and resentment about the "ritualistic" character of that inclusion. Shim quoted one female epidemiologist (pseudonymously identified as "Karen") who complained: "What's happening with the mandate—that you have to check the little boxes [to show] that you include everyone—[is that] people comply." But "checking the boxes," Karen suggested, may do little to encourage the appropriate studies, which might in fact be studies specifically of women or minority ethnic groups. Calling the policy "a huge mistake," Karen also saw it as "a waste of research dollars."[36] Karen's comments joined together a critique of misguided priorities with a repudiation of the notion that methodologies imposed from above by the bureaucrats function better to advance research on ethnic or gender differences than studies designed by the experts themselves.

NIH officials confronted such challenges directly in 2003 at a conference sponsored by the ORWH called "Science Meets Reality: Recruitment and Retention of Women in Clinical Studies and the Critical Role of Relevance."[37] While most of the discussion at the conference presumed or demonstrated the virtues of the inclusion-and-difference paradigm, critics were also in evidence. Steven Piantadosi, one of the early opponents of the subgroup comparison requirement, introduced himself as a "heretic" and proceeded to declare that "the foundations of subset mandates, particularly those for sex and race representation in clinical trials, have a political rather than a scientific origin."[38] Lewis Kuller, chair of the epidemiology department at the University of Pittsburgh Graduate School of Public Health, was even more unequivocal in his judgment: "The NIH approach to include minorities and women in every study is one of our biggest mistakes," he commented. In place of a representational model of "bean counting," which Kuller called "nonsense" and "an embarrassment," he proposed: "We should increase the number of women and minorities, but in a more focused manner." Kuller's position, like Karen's cited above, is that more studies of specific groups made more sense than inclusion of members of all groups within all studies. In that sense, the new procedures were missing the point: "Requiring a percentage of women and minorities is a rationalization for the failure of public health and preventive medicine," he maintained. When Vivian Pinn, director of the ORWH, insisted that NIH guidelines are designed to be flexible precisely to prevent irrational outcomes, other participants complained, in contrast, that the new policies had rigidified into a de facto quota system. If you want to get past NIH scrutiny, Kuller suggested, "it'll be a cold day in hell when you don't include women and minorities."[39]

Dissatisfied Reformers

While critics consider the inclusionary policies an inappropriate imposition, many proponents of reform, by contrast, complain that the new approaches don't go far enough, and they point to inadequacies in design and implementation. First, advocates of inclusion describe inconsistent levels of knowledge about, and attention to, the rules and varying degrees of commitment to their enforcement. Spero Manson, head of the division of the American Indian and Alaskan Native Program and the Department of Psychiatry at the University of Colorado Health Sciences Center, commented in 1999: "Serving on a variety of review committees, I am impressed that there remains significant variability in the understanding and application of those criteria. I think its getting better, but it's still got a ways to go.[40]

One individual who worked at the NIH in the late 1990s described his disappointment sitting in on review meetings and seeing people "going through their little checklist on the review"—certifying inclusion without looking closely at the applicant's proposed recruitment plan: "And I, of course, would be there [with] a full copy of the application in my hands, and I am like, are they reading the same thing I'm reading?" That same person complained of the disinclination on the part of DHHS officials at the time to use enforcement mechanisms at their disposal. He did recall hearing of "one project officer who got fed up with an investigator who said she was going to do a certain kind of thing in recruiting . . . and she never did it. So that for the next year, and to her credit, this one lonely staffer said, 'Cut her budget!'" However, when the investigator then complained about the budget cut to the division director, the project officer "had to fight her division director to sustain it."[41]

One of the NIH component institutes, the National Institute of Mental Health, adopted a policy in 2005 that potentially could add teeth to its enforcement of recruitment diversity. The new policy obliges researchers to specify recruitment "milestones" in advance, with attention given "to recruitment plans for women and men, members of racial and ethnic minority groups, and to children." If actual recruiting ever falls "significantly below the milestones," then the investigator must correct the deficiency; ultimately, the agency reserves the right to "consider suspending, terminating or withholding support and in some instances, may choose to negotiate a phase-out of the award."[42]

FDA officials also have enforcement mechanisms at their disposal, such as the clinical hold procedure, but rarely, if ever, invoke them. Karen Weiss, the director of the Division of Clinical Trial Design and Analysis at the FDA's Center for Biologicals Evaluation and Research (CBER, which is responsible for "biologics") reported in early 2003 that she never had imposed a clinical hold for inadequate inclusion of women,[43] while Robert Temple suggested there had been few, if any, clinical holds at CDER. To be sure, a clinical hold is a measure of last resort, and FDA reviewers might find ways of making sure that companies get the message before things reached that stage. As Temple described the process, "You'd talk to the company" and convince them to make changes, rather than formally invoke the hold procedure.[44]

In a perfect world, commitment by investigators themselves would obviate the need for careful scrutiny by review panels or DHHS employees. But, in Spero Manson's view, while some researchers are doing an excellent job with inclusion, "the vast majority of investigators are less thoughtful, less critical, less committed to understanding the importance of the inclusion of ethnic minorities in research."[45] Others suggested that investigators who won grants on the basis of intentions to recruit people of color or the elderly for their studies may then encounter difficulties recruiting the proposed population and consequently "revert" to a whiter and younger population. "It's just reality, that's what ends up happening, and they don't go the extra lengths that it takes to make sure that the recruitment processes and strategies are effective," said Anna Nápoles-Springer, who studies elderly African Americans and Latinos at the University of California, San Francisco.[46] Some researchers also described to me the pernicious practice, on the part of white male senior investigators, of bringing on board junior researchers who are people of color, largely with the intent of legitimating the study. Manson, for example, reported being "absolutely convinced . . . that many young ethnic minority scientists are in fact invited to participate in the efforts of senior investigators largely as an attempt to increase the attractiveness and potential fundability of research proposals. [But] once those proposals are funded, it is often the case that those investigators receive little or, even more likely, no follow-up inclusion" in the design and conduct of the research.[47]

A final concern raised by those who think the new policies have not gone far enough is one that affects not only investigators, drug companies, and DHHS agencies but also medical and scientific journals: the issue of analyses of differences between subgroups. A range of critics have presented convincing evidence that, at least in its earliest years, the inclusion-and-difference paradigm has done much more to promote "inclusion" than it has to ensure the study of "difference." While various populations (women, in particular) are being included in greater numbers, either the subgroup analyses are not performed or the results are not being reported and published. Thus, the premise that underrepresentation matters because results cannot necessarily be generalized is not actually translating into a careful study of when or where generalizations break down—let alone an investigation of the underlying causes or mechanisms that bring about medical differences between human groups.

This was the implication of the FDA's internal reviews, cited above, which noted that, in a substantial proportion of new drug applications, FDA medical officers failed to comment on whether subgroup differences had been studied. But outside assessments were harsher than those produced by the agency itself. In 2001 four senators (Tom Harkin, Jim Jeffords, Barbara Mikulski, and Olympia Snowe) and one member of the House of Representatives (Henry Waxman) asked the General Accounting Office to conduct a follow-up to its 1992 study of the inclusion of women in drug trials. The GAO investigators reviewed the new drug applications submitted to the FDA from August 1998 through December 2000 and approved by the agency. In its report, the GAO concluded that pharmaceutical companies frequently were failing to present data on gender as required by the 1998 regulations. In particular, about a third of the time, the new drug applications failed to present safety and outcome data by sex. That is, although women were being included, no indication was given of whether there were differences between men and women in response to the new drug. The "FDA has not effectively overseen the presentation and analysis of data related to sex differences in drug development," the report concluded, recommending that the agency introduce new management procedures and devise a means to track data on the inclusion of women.[48]

Another GAO report, presented earlier that year, had studied drugs taken off the market in recent years and had determined that women were more likely than men to have reported adverse effects, even in cases where men and women were prescribed the drug in equal numbers. These results appeared to underscore the importance of subgroup analyses.[49] Advocates of women's health seized on these various findings to promote the goal of improved analysis of subgroup differences. "If you don't analyze the sex differences, it doesn't make any difference to enroll women," commented Denise Faustman, a physician on the Harvard Medical School faculty.[50]

The previous year, the GAO had conducted a similar follow-up study of NIH efforts with regard to women's health, also at the request of members of Congress. While praising the NIH for making progress in including women and for establishing the database on research participants, the GAO found that "NIH has made less progress in implementing the requirement that certain clinical trials be designed and carried out to permit valid analysis by sex, which could reveal whether interventions affect women and men differently." Their recommendation—that NIH staff focus more attention on implementing the "valid analysis" requirement—not only attracted attention in the mass media but also was trumpeted by groups such as the Society for Women's Health Research (SWHR). "It's important to have women in clinical trials," Phyllis Greenberger, the director of the SWHR told a reporter for *Science* magazine, "but not for the hell of it. The point is to do the gender analysis."[51]

Soon after the GAO report came out, SWHR representatives met with Ruth Kirschstein (formerly the acting director of the ORWH when it was first established, but then the acting director of the NIH after Bernadine Healy's departure) to discuss how to improve compliance with the goal of conducting subgroup comparisons.[52] The following year, the NIH issued revised guidelines that spelled out the requirements more forcefully. In cases where either a "valid analysis" of differences or a statistically significant analysis of differences is warranted, investigators must present a research plan showing how they will test for those differences, both when applying to the NIH and when submitting their protocols to their IRB for approval. All grants that are funded will be awarded with the condition that results from any promised subgroup analyses be reported to the agency in the investigators' progress reports. Finally, investigators are strongly encouraged to report the results of their subgroup analyses in the publications resulting from NIH funding.[53]

This latter point—the publication of subgroup analysis results—also reflected pressure from women's health activists. In their advocacy work, SWHR staff emphasized not only the GAO findings, but also an analysis, by SWHR staff in conjunction with a statistician, that was published nearly simultaneously in its own *Journal of Women's Health and Gender-Based Medicine*. Regina Vidaver and coauthors examined all original articles derived from NIH-funded studies that were published in four medical journals (the *New England Journal of Medicine*, *JAMA*, the *Journal of the National Cancer Institute*, and *Circulation*) in 1993, 1995, 1997, and 1998.

The authors reported that between two-thirds and three-fourths of the studies that were not single-sex "made no mention of either a presence or absence of effects due to the sex of the subjects." Moreover, there was no statistically significant increase over time in the reporting of gender comparisons—though one would expect to see such an increase if compliance with the 1994 guidelines was growing over the 1990s.[54]

Though it had not yet appeared in print, the article by Vidaver and coauthors was mentioned by the GAO report as presenting evidence that corroborated its own critique.[55] However, as Vivian Pinn pointed out in an editorial in *USA Today*, scientific articles published from 1993 to 1998 may simply be too recent to reflect changes from a policy that began affecting funded research only in fiscal year 1995, given how long it takes to organize and conduct clinical research and write up the results.[56] In retrospect, Pinn may have been unduly pessimistic: later that year, Vidaver and coauthors ran a correction (which, unlike the original article, attracted little, if any, media attention), in which they presented revised figures for many of their numerical calculations. Notably, the authors now concluded that there indeed *was* a statistically significant increase in reporting of sex/gender analysis in the sample over the time period studied.[57]

Pinn also emphasized the limits of NIH enforcement capabilities in the world of publishing: "NIH does not dictate the editorial policies of scientific journals."[58] Moreover, the authors themselves, who conducted telephone interviews with some of the investigators who had not indicated whether gender analyses had been performed, found a variety of legitimate reasons in many cases. Some researchers had tested for differences between men and women and, not finding any, had not seen any purpose in reporting a null outcome. Others had indeed found differences by sex and had chosen to report them in a separate article devoted specifically to the topic.[59] The SWHR has lobbied major medical journals, hoping to convince them to require reporting of subgroup analyses as a standard procedure, even when no differences are found.[60] And an effort spearheaded in part by Delores Parron at the National Institute of Mental Health already had resulted in an agreement by a number of journals that publish work on children and adolescents not to accept articles that fail to spell out both gender and ethnic breakdowns and subgroup analysis findings.[61] However, there is little reason to expect that journals will adopt a blanket policy in this regard, given the lack of unanimity in the scientific community about the need to conduct subgroup comparisons routinely. As Marcia Angell rather forcefully expressed it in 1999, when she was executive editor of the *New England Journal of Medicine*: "We are not going to say . . . we will not publish a study unless you have enough women, Hispanic Americans, Presbyterians, to permit a separate analysis. We are not going to say that."[62]

But in specific areas of concern, such as studies of heart disease in women, the issue of subgroup analysis is not going away. A report presented in 2003 by the Agency for Healthcare Research and Quality, a DHHS agency, found that of 272 systematic reviews and 55 randomized trials on heart disease published from 1985 to 2001, "only 32 systematic reviews and 25 randomized trials contained evidence on the key question in women." Despite the fact that substantial numbers of women and minorities were included in these studies, "most authors . . . that we identified did not perform subgroup analyses in women or ethnic minorities."[63]

Formalism, Substance, and the Meaning of Successful Reform

The continuing, heated debate between the DHHS agencies, the skeptics of the new policies, and their not-yet-satisfied promoters revolves, in part, around different ways of "doing the math" when monitoring outcomes. Clearly, by some measures, things have changed, while by other measures they haven't; and it is difficult to make sense of these competing analyses or to draw firm conclusions from numbers alone.[64] At a deeper level, this review of perceptions of compliance with new NIH and FDA guidelines suggests the unsettled character of reform and the continued contention over the basic assumptions that underlie the inclusion-and-difference paradigm. Critics denounce the procedures as empty rituals and bureaucratic impositions, while proponents of these changes point to the gap between intention and reality and complain that genuine social change has stalled. Caught in the crossfire are the officials responsible for instituting and monitoring the new policies, who mostly claim success in their efforts. These officials also have gone to great lengths to take positive steps to make the policies succeed, for example by seeking to educate investigators about how they might better recruit members of underrepresented groups for their studies.[65]

As evident in the review of the debate over the inclusionary policies, perhaps the most serious problem with their implementation is the substantial degree to which the inclusion-and-difference paradigm really has become a matter of following "rules for rules' sake." Even if we acknowledge some measure of flexibility on the part of monitors within DHHS, and even if we take with a grain of salt investigators' complaints about "bean counting," it is hard to escape the perception that at least part of what researchers and pharmaceutical companies are being asked to do is go through the motions of compliance—to provide a quantitative documentation of their inclusionary efforts, so that federal health agencies can feed the numbers into their databases and generate reports to satisfy external critics. Many perceive the requirements essentially as one more "hoop" through which they are expected to leap on the way to receiving NIH funding or FDA approval. And some suggest, with no small measure of cynicism, that at least some DHHS officials view the matter in much the same terms. Thus, some researchers describe having encountered considerable variation in attitudes toward the formal bureaucratic monitoring even on the part of NIH officials across the different institutes, ranging from those officials who take the issues very seriously in meetings with scientific investigators to others who communicate to the peer reviewers who evaluate grant proposals that, in effect, "this is bullshit, but we have to do it."[66]

Whenever abstract political goals are translated into concrete numerical targets, there is always the risk that "formal rationality" will swamp "substantive rationality"—that is, the emphasis on systematization and measurement will become more salient than the achievement of the original policy objectives. In such cases, procedural standards become ends in themselves, rather than means to an end.[67] The dilemma may well be inescapable: those seeking demonstrable changes want to see "hard numbers," but the fetishizing of counts and percentages obscures the real issues at stake—in this case, issues of justice, equity, and fairness, as well as medical efficacy. Thus, on one hand, critics of the policies (such as the epidemiologists cited above) complain that a prescriptive, "bean-counting" approach fails to address in a creative fashion the actual research needs of underrepresented groups. And on the other hand, dissatisfied proponents of the policies complain that mere technical compliance with the inclusionary requirements is not sufficient to bring about meaningful changes in research design, publication patterns, and other aspects of biomedical knowledge production. Despite their differences, both sets of interlocutors seem to perceive the width of the gap between the imposition of formally rational systems and the achievement of substantively rational outcomes.

However, in considering the meaning of so-called bean counting, two qualifications are necessary. First, as Lauren Edelman has pointed out in a study of a different domain (that of corporate affirmative action policies), organizations often respond to external pressure by creating formal structures (offices, positions, rules, programs, and procedures) precisely "to create visible symbols of compliance" that they can show off. But to say that compliance is "symbolic" is not to say it is "merely" symbolic. Even if the organization appears to prize formalism over substance, the outcome may still be one of meaningful social change.[68]

Second, if this consideration of the impact of formal rationality paints a somewhat negative picture of the reform effort, it is important to temper this criticism through analysis of the often complicated relationship between formal and informal procedures. In principle, the inclusion-and-difference paradigm is enforced through a whole series of procedures and policies that are laid out in an increasingly detailed fashion in DHHS documents. However, as James Scott has observed, "formal order . . . is always and to some considerable degree parasitic on informal processes, which the formal scheme does not recognize, without which it could not exist, and which it alone cannot create or maintain." Susan Leigh Star has made a similar point in describing the relation, within the lives of organizations, between formal representations on one hand, and "ad hoc strategies, work-arounds, and local knowledge" on the other.[69]

This complex relation between formalism and informality is well demonstrated by the creative ways that both researchers and NIH program officers sometimes find to "fudge" the inclusionary mandates. An example mentioned previously is pertinent: sometimes an individual clinical trial is exempted from the requirement of diversity if NIH administrators determine that the "overall research portfolio" for the condition or therapy under investigation is sufficiently representative of women and minorities.[70] Such solutions are neither surprising nor necessarily inappropriate. To the contrary, Star's analysis suggests that no organization could function without some set of ad hoc mechanisms of this sort. In this regard, defenders of the inclusionary policies such as Pinn are right to point to their flexibility in practice as a guarantor of their legitimacy. Indeed, as the discussion in chapter 5 of the "valid analysis" requirement demonstrated, careful negotiations between NIH insiders and Congress led to the institutionalizing of flexibility from the get-go, even in the language of the NIH Revitalization Act itself, and certainly in the writing of guidelines to implement it.

A very literal defender of the inclusion-and-difference paradigm might complain that ad hoc exemptions, ambiguous definitions, and work-arounds vitiate the policies, while a critic of the paradigm might suggest that such practices lay bare the extent of official hypocrisy. But such evaluations beg the question of what, ultimately, the new rules and standards are meant to accomplish. The point here is that policies can have multiple effects. For example, Claude Lenfant, the director of the National Heart, Lung, and Blood Institute, acknowledged the possibility that "maybe we are using the wrong tool to solve the problem," but went on to credit the inclusionary policies for raising "societal awareness" about outcome differences by sex and race.[71] Similarly, some researchers suggested to me that forcing investigators at least to *think about* inclusion is one of the key practical benefits of the new policies. James Jackson, a psychologist who studies elderly African Americans, commented about critics of the new policies: "I think people have really missed the thrust of the argument. The purpose of the stipulations was to force researchers to think about women and minorities. . . . In the guidelines, it clearly states you don't have to include women and minorities in your studies. You just have to lay out the rationale as to why you didn't."[72] Someone like Jackson presumably would be relatively untroubled by informal mechanisms and work-arounds, to the extent that they left standing this goal of promoting a new conscientiousness or reflexivity among biomedical researchers.

REVERBERATIONS

My analysis has suggested the real but limited success of the institution-alization of reform, and it helps explain why both proponents and critics remain dissatisfied. But for purposes of evaluating the inclusion-and-difference paradigm, my emphasis so far has been in some respects a nar-row one. Arguably, the substantive effects of the inclusion-and-difference paradigm extend beyond the so-called bean counts—the numbers of re-search subjects included or subgroup analyses performed. Therefore, in the remainder of this chapter, I briefly consider some additional signs of the consequences of the inclusion-and-difference paradigm for biomed-ical researchers and pharmaceutical companies. Where have the new policies made a difference, and what sort of difference have they made? I identify four specific domains: the work of the new DHHS offices; the new, large research studies that have emphasized populations considered to have been underrepresented previously; the "spillover" effects of the inclusion-and-difference paradigm on other biomedical institutions such as medical schools and medical journals; and the rise of niche marketing by pharmaceutical companies focused on women's health or minority health.

Offices and Their Projects

One topic worthy of more attention than I can devote to it here is the im-pact of the various offices that have been created within DHHS agencies to promote research on so-called special populations. These offices are

involved in considerably more than monitoring compliance with guidelines: they cofund research projects, organize conferences and workshops,
and generally seek to articulate a research agenda. The ORWH has been
exemplary in this regard. The ORWH has taken primary responsibility for
collecting statistics on inclusion of both women and minorities—a role
that appears to reflect the concerns of its energetic director, Vivian Pinn,
who is an African American woman with a longstanding commitment
to the health needs of communities of color. But in addition to promoting inclusion of diverse groups of women in NIH-funded research,
the office also has sought greater amounts of research on diseases that
are more prevalent in women and has worked to increase the number
of female scientists pursuing biomedical careers. The ORWH cofunds
research studies with other NIH agencies and provides "supplements" to
funded NIH grants.[73] For example, in 2003 the ORWH distributed funds
to support research on topics as diverse as outcomes of hysterectomies,
vaccines for human papillomavirus, the effect of a plant-based diet in
breast cancer recurrence, macular degeneration in older women, alcohol
effects in postmenopausal women, lower back pain, gender differences
in drug abuse, cognitive therapy for irritable bowel syndrome, and relax-
ation therapy for Alzheimer's caregivers.[74] Moreover, the office has been
involved in strategizing a broader national agenda for advancing women's
health research.

The ORWH's counterpart, the Office of Research on Minority Health,
played a similar role until 2000, when it became the National Center
on Minority Health and Health Disparities and thereby gained enhanced
importance within the NIH.[75] Other significant research innovations consistent with the inclusion-and-difference paradigm are located within
existing NIH institutes. For example, the NICHD runs the Pediatric
Pharmacology Research Unit program, a national network of academic
research sites funded to conduct studies on the effects of medications
on children.[76] There seems little question that these various offices and
programs encourage biomedical research projects that otherwise would
be much less likely to be performed.

Group-Specific Research Studies

The rhetoric of the inclusion-and-difference paradigm has emphasized a
diversification of subject populations, as if the ideal study would be one
that included representatives of every social group, all in the same clinical
trial. In practice, however, a consistent emphasis of those concerned with
the health of disadvantaged groups has been to promote new, group-

specific research studies—where every participant belongs to a single social group. Studies such as SWAN (Study of Women's Health Across the Nation), the Black Women's Health Study, AASK (the African American Study of Kidney Disease and Hypertension), AAASPS (the African-American Antiplatelet Stroke Prevention Study), and Strong Heart (on cardiovascular disease in American Indians) have focused exclusively on women or selected racial or ethnic minority groups. In the process, these studies have set recruitment records. For example, the Black Women's Health Study, assessing risk factors for a variety of diseases and funded by the National Cancer Institute, is the largest epidemiological study of African American women ever conducted.[77]

Without question the most striking example of a single-group study is the Women's Health Initiative, the largest disease prevention study ever conducted in the United States. Funded by the National Heart, Lung, and Blood Institute with the collaboration of the ORWH, the Women's Health Initiative included both an observational study of 93,000 women and a randomized clinical trial of 68,000 women, recruited from forty centers around the United States, to test the effects of diet on cancer and heart disease, hormone replacement therapy on heart disease, and calcium and vitamin D on hip fractures.[78] Ten of the forty centers were specially charged with the goal of "overrecruiting" racial minorities, with the result that "18.5 percent of the women in the trial are of African American, Hispanic, Asian American/Pacific, or Native American extraction."[79] At the time of its initiation, the entire study was expected to cost as much as $625 million.[80]

The headline-making findings from the Women's Health Initiative on the unexpected health risks associated with hormone replacement therapy testify to the potential benefits of studies of this massive scope conducted in specific populations. In 2000 Congress also allocated funding for the NIH to plan a very large, national longitudinal study of children's health and development. The study is intended to enroll one hundred thousand children and track their health from before birth until age 21.[81]

Spillover Effects

The impact of the inclusion-and-difference paradigm also can be observed in its more diffuse ripple effects on other biomedical institutions. For example, its inclusionary goals are broadly consistent with new emphases within medical school curricula on women's health and minority health (or on the development of "cultural competence"[82])—emphases promoted by advocates within DHHS agencies, among other places. Progress is especially evident in the arena of women's health. In 1992 Congress requested the DHHS to survey medical schools to determine the degree to which women's health issues were represented in the curriculum. A survey sent to all U.S and Canadian medical schools in 1994 found that only 12 percent of them integrated women's health across the clinical disciplines.[83] Over the course of the decade, however, the amount of change appeared to be noteworthy. In 2003 the SWHR surveyed 125 U.S. medical schools and found that, of 68 schools that returned the survey, 44 percent offered a women's health curriculum and another 18 percent had plans to develop one.[84] To be sure, some complained that curricular emphases on various "special populations" tended to get stuck in at the end of the semester and sometimes received short shrift.[85] Still, these curricular emphases constituted important changes from the not-so-distant past. As a New York Times article expressed it in 1997, commenting on a "quiet revolution" in medical school curricula: "Much has changed in medical training since the days when anatomy professors ordered students to discard the breasts from female cadavers."[86]

Another arena in which spillover effects can be observed is in biomedical publication policies and patterns. The 1997 version of the "Uniform Requirements for Manuscripts Submitted to Biomedical Journals"—endorsed by all the major U.S.-based journals—instructs authors to "identify the age, sex, and other important characteristics" of the research subjects.[87] At the same time, publishing on women's health issues in particular has accelerated. It was only in 1991 that the Index Medicus of the National Library of Medicine first introduced "women's health" as an index entry.[88] Yet in 2000, when JAMA devoted a special issue of the journal to the topic of women's health, the editors reported having received 238 manuscript submissions for the issue—one of the highest responses ever to a specific call for papers. "The articles in this issue . . . suggest that women's health research has entered the mainstream," said the editor, Catherine DeAngelis, and the deputy editor, Margaret Winkler, observing that such research was now "dealing with many of the same issues that mainstream medicine seeks to avert, [such as] cardiovascular disease, dementia, [and] osteoporosis."[89] Notably, with DeAngelis's appointment the previous year, both JAMA and the New England Journal of Medicine—the two top medical journals in the United States—were at that point under the direction of women. Six years later, JAMA devoted another theme issue to the topic of women's health, this time receiving 412 manuscript submissions—an all-time record for the journal.[90]

In a third example of "spillover," the American Medical Association has endorsed a series of "inclusionary" policies. These policies promote "the need to include both genders in studies which involve the health of society at large," further study of gender disparities in health, and the removal of gender bias in medical treatment decisions.[91] In 2000 the AMA also recommended "that all medical/scientific journal editors require, where appropriate, a sex-based analysis of data, even if such comparisons are negative."[92] These new emphases paralleled an impressive trend toward gender parity in medical practice at the entry level, with medical school classes now nearly 50 percent female. By contrast, in terms of race and ethnicity, the profession continues to be heavily white. As a percentage of medical school graduates, blacks increased from 5.3 percent in 1992 to 6.9 percent in 2003, and Hispanics went from 5.5 percent to 6.0 percent.[93]

Pharmaceutical Profits and Niche Marketing

A more complex case of the downstream impact of the inclusion-and-difference paradigm concerns the pharmaceutical industry and its marketing practices. "Wall Street investors, the pharmaceutical and hospital industries and Madison Avenue marketers all agree: Women's health care has become one of the hottest fields in medicine and marketing," declared the *Washington Post* in 1997 on its business page, singling out the political agitation by the Congressional Caucus for Women's Issues as one of the forces that had propelled corporate interest. The *Post* article cited a number of indicators of this surge, including the decision by ten new companies developing products aimed at women's health to go public in the previous year alone and the determination by the investment banking firm Smith, Barney Inc. that "investor interest in women's health companies had grown enough to warrant devoting an investment analyst to the subject."[94] Two years later, the *New York Times* agreed that "pharmaceutical makers have discovered women in a big way," noting that, according to analysts, pharmaceutical companies had devoted a fifth of their total research budgets in 1998 (about $12 billion) to developing products for women.[95] In 1999 Jonca Bull, acting deputy director of the FDA's Office of Women's Health, also described the increased trend in pharmaceutical company interest in women. Bull pointed to "the proliferation of offices of women's health in the larger pharmaceutical companies," as well as "the proliferation of pages of ads in women's magazines."[96] (Bull didn't mention the ways in which some of these companies benefited from the "revolving door" between industry and government: her predecessor at the Office of Women's Health, Ruth Merkatz, went from the FDA to Pfizer's offices in New York City to direct its women's health research activities there.)

Whereas in the 1980s "women's health" products focused almost exclusively on reproductive health issues, by the 1990s pharmaceutical companies had expanded their interests to include both diseases specific to women and general conditions, such as heart disease and cancer, that may affect women and men differently. A report issued in 2001 by PhRMA, the pharmaceutical industry lobbying group, quoted Dr. Freda Lewis-Hall, a leading figure in industry-based women's health research and the director of the Lilly Center for Women's Health in Indianapolis: "It's not just maternal and child health anymore—it's broader and deeper. . . . And pharmaceutical companies are doing gender-based research, looking at both the sameness and the differences between men and women."[97]

A similar, though less pronounced, tendency toward niche marketing is also observable in the recent relation of pharmaceutical companies to racial and ethnic minority groups. Michael Montoya has described the emergence of "multicultural pharmaceutical marketing conferences," at which exhibitors are attentive to strategies for creating "brand allegiance" for their products on the part of distinct ethnic groups.[98] One recent conference featured panels on topics such as "Zeroing In on Special Market Segments to Accelerate Your Multicultural Growth Strategies."[99]

To analysts of broader trends in the development of modern capitalism, these moves on the part of the pharmaceutical industry will not seem at all unusual. If the existence of a single "standard human" is the presumption of Fordism (the old-fashioned system of producing mass commodities as predictably invariant as the Model T, to be sold to a universal consumer), then what I have called niche standardization is consistent with post-Fordist production (the niche marketing of diverse products to well-defined subgroups).[100] Many commentators have noted the inroads that niche marketing practices have made into biomedicine generally. As Adele Clarke and coauthors have argued, the rejection of one-size-fits-all medical solutions and the substitution of niche-marketed drugs, devices, and technologies is a defining characteristic of present-day biomedical practice—but one that, all too often, transforms social identities into market niches through the commodification of difference.[101] Indeed, while just about any sort of group can be construed as a potential consumer niche, there are special implications when niche marketing leans on identity politics. For social critics such as Naomi Klein, the cooptation of identity politics by niche marketing reflects a transition from a homogenizing cultural imperialism (the "Coca-Colonization" of the world) to a thin multiculturalism—a "market Masala" exemplified by the so-called diversity of the ethnic food court.[102]

The point is not that women and members of racial and ethnic minority groups don't potentially gain from industry attention. Indeed, PhRMA has emphasized the extraordinary potential benefits of this "women's health revolution," publicizing the fact that drug companies have hundreds of drugs in the pipeline for diseases primarily affecting women.[103] But to what degree are pharmaceutical companies just "cashing in" on the political mobilization on behalf of women's health research? An advertisement by Pfizer that appeared in the mass media in 1999 seemed to epitomize the corporate capture of a political reform movement. In the ad, a raised fist inside a blood pressure cuff appeared with the caption "Women's Rights: We're empowering women to take charge of their total health."

Several pharmaceutical company practices raise troublesome questions about the reverberations of reform and its real beneficiaries. One example is the "rebranding" of existing products solely to attract women's dollars—as Nathan Greenslit has described in the case of Eli Lilly and Co.'s Sarafem. The pill is chemically identical to Lilly's well-known drug Prozac but produced in a special pink-and-purple version for sale to women suffering premenstrual dysphoria disorder.[104] Does the availability of Sarafem constitute a victory for women's health?

A second and equally striking example is the interest of the pharmaceutical industry in invoking ethnic differences in response to medications as a way to resist pressure to cut the enormous costs of prescription drugs in the United States. While the U.S. Congress has sought to promote the substitution of generic drugs for more expensive, name-brand drugs, PhRMA has adopted the "one size does not fit all" slogan for its own purposes. Citing differences in responses to medications, the lobbying group argues against the universal use of a single drug for any given condition with the claim that specific subgroups that respond differently, such as racial minorities, require access to a range of therapeutic options and not just a single generic drug.[105] Similarly, the National Pharmaceutical Council, another trade association, has argued against "cost containment tactics" such as restrictive formularies, therapeutic substitution, and mandatory generics, all of which presume "that related medicines having the same general effect are almost identical in their actions and are therefore interchangeable." Here, sensitivity to ethnic minorities and what the Council's president and chief executive officer calls "an acknowledgment and celebration of cultural diversity" are marshaled in the service of a political campaign against attempts to rein in drug expenditures.[106]

A third example equally suggests the potentially opportunistic use of "difference findings" for financial gain. In a drug regulatory environment that is newly sensitive to arguments about group differences, some pharmaceutical companies unable to establish the efficacy of their products in all humans have, when possible, sought FDA approval to market their products only for use in a designated subgroup. In 2002 two drugs treating irritable bowel syndrome (Zelnorm, a drug made by Novartis, and Lotronex, made by GlaxoSmithKline) became the first drugs ever approved by the FDA for use only in women for a condition that affects both sexes. The drugs' advantages over a placebo in a mixed-sex population could not be demonstrated with statistical significance.[107] BiDil, a drug that treats heart failure, in 2005 became the first drug ever approved for use only in African Americans. Here again, the drug initially had failed in tests with a diverse population, but analysis of racial subsets had suggested a reduced mortality for African Americans. A subsequent trial with 1,050 African Americans, conducted by the manufacturer, NitroMed, with the support of the Association of Black Cardiologists, appeared to bear out the claim of benefit.[108]

In the cases of these three drugs, niche marketing might be viewed as the happy outcome of a proper attention to subgroup analysis: arguably, in the absence of such analyses, drugs with real efficacy for certain subpopulations might have been tossed out as useless, and a real opportunity to help those groups would have been lost.[109] At the same time, the "racializing" and "gendering" of drugs raises quite troublesome questions that I will address in chapters 10 and 11—questions about what some have denounced as "racial profiling" in medicine, a critique that might be extended to "sex profiling" as well.[110] More generally, these and the other examples of the affinity between niche standardization and niche marketing demonstrate how reforms advanced under the banner of identity politics can end up promoting the commercialization of those identities in the service of profit-making.

Intended and Unintended Consequences

The analysis in this chapter has suggested that the inclusionary reforms in biomedical policy have had measurable effects of various sorts. Most immediately, they have affected the responsibilities of federal agencies charged with ensuring and measuring compliance. But they also have brought about change in everyday biomedical work practices; ensured at least some attention to questions of inclusion on the part of researchers, IRBs, drug company scientists, federal regulators, peer reviewers, and journal editors; and encouraged important new research studies focused on populations such as women, children, and racial and ethnic minorities. Moreover, they have had reverberations elsewhere in the world of biomedicine through the varied work of the new offices, the promotion of key single-group studies, the boost they provide to niche marketing, and other spillover effects. Some of these influences are precisely what reformers had in mind; other consequences are somewhat less intended.

In the chapters that follow, I continue the process of assessing the effects of reform. I begin by considering, in the next chapter, one of the most powerful effects of the paradigm on researchers and pharmaceutical companies involved in conducting clinical studies. For these actors, the new policies create substantial pressures to find innovative approaches to a thorny practical problem: how to locate members of underrepresented groups and convince them to enroll in clinical studies.

CHAPTER NINE

The Science of Recruitmentology and the Politics of Trust

One concrete arena of scientific work is being reinvented in light of the new imperatives of inclusion: the on-the-ground practices of finding and recruiting research subjects to participate in biomedical studies. To comply with new requirements and expectations, academic investigators and drug companies, first and foremost, have to find members of various groups—women, children, the elderly, and racial and ethnic minorities— and get them into their studies. Partly as a result, recruitment, once considered merely a chore, is now emerging as an applied science, one that presupposes and generates knowledge about the characteristics of medically underserved communities. New understandings of the medical significance of race, gender, and community are being generated in the crucible of this practical and intellectual work, where concerns about biological difference intersect with new conceptualizations of culture, history, and power.

This chapter tracks the consequences for biomedical research of the new emphasis on the practicalities of recruiting participants. I begin by briefly considering some of the new challenges that underlie recruitment and retention in light of the inclusionary requirements. Then, I analyze how, in the United States, the increased pressure to enroll participants has helped bring into being a new science—one that hasn't named itself, but that might be called "recruitmentology." Practitioners of recruitmentology seek to produce and disseminate knowledge about how to recruit and retain successfully—particularly, how to understand and reach out to so-called hard-to-recruit populations. Increasingly, recruitmentologists are developing an empirical body of studies scientifically evaluating the efficacy of various social, cultural, psychological, technological, and economic means of convincing people (again, especially members of hard-to-recruit populations) that they want to become, and remain, human subjects. That is, whereas the science of clinical trials evaluates the efficacy of therapies or regimens, the auxiliary science of recruitmentology evaluates the efficacy of techniques necessary to get bodies into a trial in the first place and to keep them there throughout the life of the experiment.

The risk is that recruitmentology threatens to substitute a methodological formalism for a substantive concern with the reasons why certain populations may be hard to recruit in the first place. Inevitably, to be effective, recruitmentology must address collective memories of racism and abuse of research subjects, and it must respond in meaningful ways to the highly charged politics of trust and mistrust that characterize relations between researchers and many of the communities from which they hope to recruit, particularly communities of color. I consider the practical solutions to the problem of trust that some recruitmentologists have devised, including new models of participatory research that emphasize a more politicized understanding of race relations. Finally, I examine the increasingly transnational character of biomedical research and the ways in which globalization intensifies the dilemmas surrounding recruitment and retention while heightening the risks of biomedical exploitation of a racialized global underclass.

THE BODY HUNT

Especially with the growth of clinical research, one of the most daunting tasks to confront researchers is the practical challenge of finding appropriate individuals to participate in clinical trials. Recruiting (or "enrolling," or "accruing") research subjects is a *sine qua non* for biomedical investigators in both academic and commercial settings, who simply cannot perform the experiments that are their bread and butter unless they can convince living, breathing human beings to become research material and to offer up their bodies to medical manipulation and scrutiny.[1] Similarly, the retention of participants during the months or years over which a clinical trial may continue (and the willingness of those participants, along the way, to comply with or adhere to all the conditions of the experimental protocol) is critical for generating scientifically valid conclusions.[2] Research teams need to do more than make a good first impression on research subjects, as important as that may be: they need to do the hard work of maintaining a long-term relationship.

For those concerned about reversing health disparities—or, perhaps more immediately, complying with the formal requirements of new policies mandating the inclusion of underrepresented groups in biomedical research—the practicalities of recruitment and retention are truly "where the rubber meets the road." The opening sentence of a 2003 article on the recruitment of African Americans and Latinos for research on lung cancer observes: "The National Institutes of Health 1993 Revitalization Act mandates inclusion of minority groups in clinical research to address their historical underrepresentation."[3] The authors' arguments about recruitment techniques essentially follow from that premise. While not every researcher is as explicit about it, certainly the laws and policies that comprise the inclusion-and-difference paradigm are a consistent point of reference in the burgeoning scientific literature on recruitment, and they are never too far from consciousness. Multiple rationales underlie the interest in figuring out how to recruit women, racial and ethnic minorities, children, the elderly, and other groups effectively, including the goals of reversing past practices of underrepresentation, eliminating health disparities, and responding to distinctive health needs of specific medical constituencies. But clearly at least part of the boom in interest in the mechanics of recruiting subjects reflects a practical concern with satisfying requirements imposed by Congress, the NIH, and the FDA: academic researchers and pharmaceutical companies are under pressure not only to come up with the bodies, but to come up with the *right mix* of bodies.

Employees at DHHS offices charged with promoting inclusive practices, including the NIH's Office of Research on Women's Health among others, have sought to help researchers with this task. They have devoted considerable attention to the issues of recruitment and retention, holding conferences on the topic and publishing and distributing how-to books.[4] Moreover, the DHHS has created and funded a number of specialized academic research networks in the hopes of better promoting outreach to various demographic groups, including the Resource Centers for Minority Aging Research, the Pediatric Pharmacology Research Units, and the National Centers of Excellence in Women's Health. But no one underestimates the difficulties inherent in recruitment and retention or believes that magical solutions are to be found.

That accomplishing these goals can be quite a challenge points to an important irony at the heart of the inclusion-and-difference paradigm. Much of the rhetoric of reformers in the 1980s and 1990s about the unwarranted exclusion of various groups from biomedical research seemed almost to paint an image of a mass of medical have-nots pounding on the walls of research institutions, demanding to be let into the experimental domain. But, in fact, only sometimes does the supply of willing bodies exceed research demand. In the late 1980s and early 1990s, for example, in the absence of approved therapies to fight HIV, people with AIDS and HIV infection often clamored for entry into clinical trials, insisting, in the process, on their right to serve as "guinea pigs."[5] Inspired by their example, others have pressed for greater availability of public information about ongoing clinical trials—a mandate endorsed by Congress in the FDA Modernization Act of 1997, which requires the DHHS to maintain a publicly accessible database of all clinical trials "in a form that can be readily understood by members of the public."[6] But even if an increasing number of highly motivated, potential research subjects find their own way to clinical trials, much more typically—and especially in the many cases where experimenters seek out healthy volunteers rather than sufferers in need of cures—those responsible for the orchestration of large clinical trials find themselves engaged in a vexing and time-consuming body hunt.

All scientists at times have difficulty obtaining research materials; all scientists confront recalcitrant materials that may not behave as the researcher would like or would expect, and they may exert considerable energy in getting those objects to perform properly so that the experiment may proceed.[7] But research materials that "talk back"—or that can "vote with their feet"—present scientists with unique challenges. Here, human subjects emerge as "subjects" in both senses of the word—at times subject to the will of the experimenter, at times endowed with subjectivity, agency, and a capacity to pursue their own interests.[8] Therefore, in their engagement with potential participants, clinical researchers must grant recognition to an "other," and must grapple with ethics, commitment, and responsibility.

Thus, along with the many other hats that biomedical researchers already wear—as grant writers, administrators, and public advocates—they now don new ones as marketers and persuaders.[9] However, chasing after human subjects—and perhaps particularly subjects who come from ethnically diverse backgrounds—is a costly endeavor. It demands dedicated staff time not only on the part of researchers, but also from nurses functioning as clinical trial coordinators and other personnel hired specifically to assist with outreach and recruitment efforts.[10] Producing and disseminating publicity and recruiting materials adds to the expense—altogether, more than $500 million is spent on mass media promotion annually[11]—as does the screening of potential research participants. One article published in 2001 about an estrogen replacement and atherosclerosis trial estimated the average cost of recruiting and screening each participant to be $2,500.[12] In addition, delays associated with recruiting subjects can add significantly to the cost of a study. In 2001 it was estimated that 57 percent of clinical trials ran a month or more late in recruiting.[13] Such delays may reduce the time remaining for reaping a profit before patent protections expire.[14]

But where some see a challenge, others perceive a business opportunity: as more and more aspects of clinical trials get outsourced to private companies, recruitment is sometimes being turned over to for-profit consultants who specialize in managing this task on behalf of drug companies and who maintain extensive databases of potential participants, cross-referenced by demographic and medical characteristics.[15] Between 1992 and 2001, the number of study participants recruited by private companies grew from 7 million to 20 million.[16] Insiders refer to this development as the professionalization of recruitment, and they note the increasing reliance on "metrics-driven recruitment practice."[17] In 2005 a small contract research organization named Anaclim, a minority-owned business based in Indianapolis, became the first such business launched specifically to recruit minority participants for clinical trials.[18]

New expectations about the social identities of the research participants—that some numbers of them should belong to a specified sex, race, ethnicity, or age group—add to the expense of recruiting. But at the same time, new financial incentives intensify the challenges by generating competitive pressures. For example, the extension of "exclusivity" (the period of exclusive marketing rights) offered to drug companies that test products in children has set off what Robert Temple of the FDA's Center for Drug Evaluation and Research has characterized as a recruiting "frenzy," with companies competing for the available supply of child subjects. A *Wall Street Journal* article in 2002 quoted Temple's ironic comment: "If you have a hypertensive kid, hold on to him. He'll be in hot demand."[19]

Indeed, at least some experts have worried that researchers might now be *overly* motivated to recruit groups such as women and minorities, with potentially pernicious results. For example, some have voiced concerns that the requirements associated with the inclusion-and-difference paradigm will promote research by those who simply have not taken the time to learn about the communities they hope to study and that such efforts are likely to fail. Barbara Howard, the principal investigator of a Women's Health Initiative (WHI) site in the Washington, D.C., area that was quite successful in enrolling minorities, complained about how the new policies mandating inclusion "resulted in a flood of researchers . . . who thought this [studying minorities] was a way to get money"—researchers who then found themselves "falling flat" because they had no idea how to recruit the subjects they claimed to want to study.[20] A related concern, expressed by Otis Brawley, an oncology researcher and the former head of the National Cancer Institute's Office of Special Populations Research, had more to do with the abridgement of rights to informed consent in the face of new demands to recruit racial and ethnic minorities. Brawley speculated about the tremendous pressure confronting a hypothetical "Dr. John Smith" to enroll people of color: "If this woman in his office is white, he gives her all the pros and cons of going into the trial. . . . But the black woman or the Hispanic woman, they get a very hard sell because he's got to produce, and if he doesn't produce he loses his grant."[21]

Few investigators or DHHS officials whom I interviewed felt that this practice of the hard sell was especially common, and many of them suggested that either careful scrutiny by IRBs or resistance on the part of potential trial participants would militate against it. One might then rephrase the issue to suggest that investigators potentially face several cross-cutting pressures simultaneously. At the same time as they may confront the imperative to show recruitment results, they also must satisfy IRBs that they are not exploiting "vulnerable populations," and they must respond to deep suspicions about participating in biomedical research that are prevalent within many racial and ethnic minority communities. Thus, ironically, the diverse kinds of people that academic researchers and pharmaceutical companies operating in the United States now are expected to enroll in their studies include some, such as children, whom IRB members are most vigilant in protecting from risk, and others, such as African Americans, who may be highly distrustful of the medical research enterprise and little interested in placing their bodies and their lives in the hands of scientists. In such circumstances, those seeking to carry out clinical trials truly find themselves in a quandary.

Incentives, Altruism, and the New Duties of Citizenship

The question of how a hard-to-recruit participant might be induced to participate in a clinical trial quickly provokes another one: What might that person conceivably get out of it? In treatment trials that enroll patients suffering from a condition, the main incentive may simply be access to therapies. In addition, participants and observers frequently cite the draw of free health care, including special medical attention and state-of-the art monitoring, as more than sufficient inducements, particularly in a society such as the United States that lacks national health insurance.[22] For prevention studies and others that enroll healthy volunteers, as I will discuss, altruistic motivations are widespread and not to be ignored, and investigators routinely seek to nurture and reward them. Yet for a growing number of studies of all sorts, the most typical quid pro quo is a simple offer of cash. For example, in her study of private-sector clinical trials in the U.S. Southwest, Jill Fisher found that Phase 1 trials—typically enrolling healthy patients for an initial study of safety and efficacy—are especially likely to be populated by the indigent, some of whom become "serial participants," enrolling in one experiment after another.[23]

It has long been recognized that investigators walk a fine line between suitable payment and unethical inducement.[24] Yet the amplified concern with these issues in recent years is not surprising. On one hand, it reflects a growing sense within biomedicine and pharmacotherapy that human bodies and body parts are now commodities whose "biovalue" fetches a price.[25] On the other hand, it is an obvious accompaniment of the recruitment pressures that stem from the new policies associated with the inclusion-and-difference paradigm. In an essay published in the *New England Journal of Medicine* in 1999 entitled "What's the Price of a Research Subject?" two authors affiliated with the NIH, Neal Dickert and Christine Grady, observed: "The frequency of payment may also increase in response to requirements for greater inclusion of women, minorities, and children in research studies."[26]

Indeed, now that children are in high demand as companies seek to extend the period of patent exclusivity, a good deal of commentary has focused on the particular issue of paying the families of child participants—in some cases $1,000 or more, according to a story in *U.S News and World Report*.[27] (In other cases the incentives are aimed even more narrowly at the children themselves, as in the provision of gift certificates for toy stores.[28]) Sometimes the offer of a substantial monetary incentive seems calibrated to compensate for unacceptable risk—for example, a study sponsored by the Environmental Protection Agency in 2005 on the effects of pesticides on infants and babies in Duval County, Florida, was canceled in the face of scathing media and congressional criticism. According to the *New York Times*, "a recruiting flier for the program . . . offered $970, a free camcorder, a bib and a T-shirt to parents whose infants or babies were exposed to pesticides if the parents completed the two-year study."[29] To be sure, most pediatric studies target children who have medical conditions, often serious ones, and the studies present the theoretical possibility of direct medical benefit. Still, "there's something worrisome about parents getting money to enroll their kids in a study that has, at the least, discomfort, and, at the worst, risk," a professor of pediatrics and medical ethics at the University of Wisconsin told the *New York Times*, adding that the recent "explosion" of drug testing in children had intensified the problem.[30] In 2004 the Institute of Medicine took up the issue, suggesting that IRBs and research institutions adopt formal policies governing payments to parents of participating children.[31]

The practice of obtaining informed consent is supposed to do much of the work of ensuring that participants in research know what they are getting themselves into, before they accept any sort of inducement or compensation. Yet many critics have noted the limitations of this formal procedure (both in its conception and in its execution), suggesting, among other things, that consent is rarely all that "informed."[32] One investigator at a WHI site acknowledged frankly that "virtually no one, I think, other than somebody with a professional education, can understand the consent forms that we ended up using, [though] we did our darnedest to explain it to them."[33] At the same time, the recent emphasis on recruitment of diverse social groups has raised new questions about what consent means and who provides it, and this has posed new complications for investigators. Researchers studying Native Americans, for example, may be required to obtain not only consent from individual research subjects, but also permission from an IRB representing the tribe—a sort of collective consent.[34] The case of children's participation provides a different example of complexity: pediatric researchers whom I interviewed all agreed that it was generally inadvisable to proceed with enrollment unless both the child and his or her guardians were comfortable with the protocol. "You don't force studies on children, they have to want to participate, otherwise you don't do it," commented one researcher.[35] And conversely, according to another, if a fifteen-year-old wants to participate in a study but the parents are opposed, then "I generally say no way, because if we don't have a full team support you are generally asking for a problem."[36]

While the issue of inducements and incentives has attracted considerable attention, at the same time no one doubts the potency of altruistic motives on the part of participants in clinical research. When altruism prevails, biovalue is given away for free, in a striking example of the promotion of social ties through what Marcel Mauss once termed the "gift relationship."[37] The Women's Health Initiative is a case in point. In this enormous project that enrolled 93,000 women in an observational study and 68,000 women in a randomized clinical trial, researchers studied the effects of various measures to prevent heart disease, cancer, and hip fractures. Many of the WHI investigators whom I interviewed made special mention of the impressively altruistic inclinations of the older female participants, whose values resonated favorably with the study's official slogan: "Be Part of the Answer." More to the point, the WHI, like other studies, specifically sought to cultivate and nurture such altruistic behaviors and to promote them as aspects of responsible biomedical citizenship. That is, whereas early proponents of the inclusion-and-difference paradigm invoked ideas of citizenship to demand that researchers attend to the health research needs of disadvantaged groups, investigators seeking to recruit subjects have counterposed such citizenship *rights* with citizenship *duties*: the good citizen is one who volunteers on behalf of his or her community.

These instances of altruism are of a particular kind. Often when we speak of altruism we imagine an expressed commitment to society or humanity in the abstract. For example, in the medical arena, the gift of blood has often been seen as a prime means by which an individual can affirm his or her solidarity with the social whole.[38] By contrast, here as throughout the inclusion-and-difference paradigm, the social unit that is invoked is larger than the individual but smaller than the nation; potential participants are encouraged to make the sacrifice of enrolling in studies for the benefit of "their daughters and granddaughters" or, in other cases, for their racial or ethnic community.[39] WHI promotional materials sought precisely to invoke group allegiance while interpellating specific social identities. "If we don't do this, who will?" asked one advertisement, featuring the photo of a black woman.[40]

Uncertainty and the Rise of Recruitmentology

How exactly do researchers go about recruiting subjects for large clinical trials? The manifold methods testify to the absence of any single dominant strategy. Depending in part on whether the trial is a prevention study or a test of a therapy, whether it seeks to study healthy volunteers or ill people, and whether it addresses a common condition or a rare one—but also depending on the local culture of research or individual researchers' idiosyncratic judgments about how best to proceed—subjects might be recruited through their primary care physicians; in hospitals or clinics; through newspaper, radio, and television advertising; through public notices, billboards, or signs posted on public transportation; through flyers, brochures, or doorknob literature packets; through listings in searchable online databases; through direct mail, random-digit-dialing, or "cold calling"; through celebrity campaigns; or by means of various forms of community outreach at places such as health fairs, churches, and nursing homes.[41]

Overall, interviews with investigators involved in large clinical studies of women, minorities, children, and the elderly revealed few consistent opinions about the efficacy of the various recruitment methods. Some researchers praised community outreach events for the kind of trust they can engender,[42] while others spoke with a bit of resignation of having to embark on "dog-and-pony shows."[43] Some swore by direct mail and have spent upward of $100,000 on it in a single study-year, while others pursuing similar studies called it next to useless.

Given the uncertainty over effective techniques in a high-stakes environment, it is not surprising that researchers increasingly are interested in obtaining reliable, generalizable answers to the question of how best to enroll. Hence, a steady stream of journal articles—typically, spin-off articles from large, collaborative research projects, essentially framed as "lessons learned" from a given study—has reported on experiences with diverse recruitment strategies. These publications, along with conferences, workshops, and reports, all have provided assistance to researchers hoping to nail down the right approaches. While some of the advice—for example, "that the study leaders develop an eye-catching logo and use colors and catch phrases consistently throughout all publications"[44]—has a generic quality to it and is borrowed from the worlds of marketing and advertising, other lessons are more context-specific and reflect attempts to situate clinical research projects within their social milieus.

Success stories play an important function within this body of literature, not only in suggesting specific approaches, but also in presenting concrete evidence that recruitment of "special populations" is a doable task. Studies such as the African-American Antiplatelet Stroke Prevention Study (AAASPS), the Dietary Approaches to Stop Hypertension Collaborative Research Group (DASH), and the Strong Heart study are frequently pointed to as positive examples of recruitment of racial and ethnic minority group members. The WHI, which specifically designated ten of its forty centers around the United States as "minority centers" charged with the goal of overrecruiting minorities, has been lauded for achieving an ethnic representation that is not far from that of the U.S. population as a whole.[45]

Alongside this advice literature—what might be called "soft" recruitmentology—a more rigorous, "hard" recruitmentology also has taken shape that attempts a scientific analysis. "For many researchers recruitment is not always guided by empirically tested rules, but instead occurs in a 'hit or miss' fashion," complained Virginia Nacif de Brey and Virginia González, explaining the motivation behind one example of this genre, a comparative study of the efficacy of methods used to recruit Hispanics in the Bay Area.[46] Sometimes "hard" recruitmentologists attempt to synthesize and summarize the insights from multiple studies, along the lines of a meta-analysis. Others go a step further by setting out formally to compare different recruitment strategies, for example by building a prospective experimental design into a planned clinical trial or into a feasibility study conducted prior to undertaking a trial.[47]

Recruitmentology reflects an explicit attempt to transform the art of recruiting into a science. But at the same time, the rise of recruitmentology reminds us that even as biomedicine becomes increasingly scientific in so many respects—rationalizing its treatment algorithms, employing more sophisticated technologies, and turning its attention to the molecular and genetic levels—it also remains a "human science" in Foucault's terms, one that concerns itself with monitoring the bodies and souls of individuals.[48] Not just in the clinical encounter, but in increasingly varied settings "from bench to bedside," biomedical experts do their work by coordinating or coercing the activities of laypeople—something they cannot accomplish unless they have an understanding of how people function in society. Indeed, in the case of trial recruitment and retention, the hybrid character of biomedicine as both a natural and a human science is being reinforced by a knowledge infusion from the social sciences. As clinicians come to realize that they need to know something about cultures, communities, groups, networks, and individual psyches in order to carry out their experiments while meeting inclusionary mandates, they import concepts and frameworks from sociology, anthropology, psychology, and economics. Social scientific knowledge—in both its formal and folk variants—is deployed to help research teams advertise trials effectively, find appropriate subjects, forge alliances with the communities that subjects come from, and ensure their continued participation. In the process, the teams that conduct clinical trials generate cognitive maps of what both the biological world and the social world look like—they "co-produce" natural and social order.[49]

Recruitmentology studies take several forms. One subgenre of the literature seeks to determine the barriers that keep individuals from volunteering. Sometimes recruitmentologists use formal methods, such as surveys, to acquire a clearer sense of the motivations for participation or the reasons for refusal, while other have used focus groups to gauge attitudes toward research in specific communities.[50] A second type of study engages in various sorts of analysis of, or introduces knowledge about, the cultures of specific groups that are targeted for recruitment. For example, some researchers have pointed to the kinds of confidentiality issues that may affect potential participants living in rural areas or small towns.[51] Others have invoked the language of endangerment often used in reference to black males to characterize young African American males as "an endangered research species."[52] Still other recruitmentology studies—

very much of the "hard," quantitative variety—adopt the economists' language of cost-benefit analysis. Such studies have compared the costs of different recruitment strategies to what they term the "yield" (the ratio of enrolled participants to the total who had to be screened in order to find them).[53]

POWER AND COMMUNITY

Trust and Mistrust

Economic, psychological, anthropological, and sociological ways of knowing the "other" increasingly are seen as pivotal for conducting clinical research in biomedicine: diverse epistemologies of the social are being yoked to the study of biological disease processes and pharmaceutical treatments through the new emphasis on recruitmentology. The benefits of this research seem obvious, but the formalization of recruitmentological research does raise a question: Is there a risk that the ever more elaborate studies of how to find and hold onto various kinds of research subjects may end up encouraging researchers to misconceive of the problem fundamentally as a technical one, to be solved through ingenuity and the appropriate mix of tactics? As with other dimensions of the inclusion-and-difference paradigm discussed in previous chapters, it could be that methodological formalism will come to stand in for a substantive concern with profound and sometimes intractable issues, which here include trust, citizenship, collective memory, and the power relations between researchers and their research participants.

The point is that the history of abuses of patients by researchers is well preserved in the collective memories of many social groups. For example, because of the notoriety of the Study of Untreated Syphilis in the Negro Male (more commonly known as the Tuskegee Syphilis Study, discussed in chapter 2), the question of trust in biomedical research is interwoven in complicated ways with the politics of racial justice in the United States. Investigators conducting research with African Americans routinely report confronting suspicions of being used as "guinea pigs" like in the Tuskegee study.[54] Indeed, a whole branch of recruitmentological scholarship has examined the social-psychological impact of Tuskegee.[55] In one survey mailed to residents of Detroit, about half of the African American respondents reported that they had less trust in medical researchers as a result of Tuskegee, compared to only 17 percent of the white respondents.[56]

At the same time, experts on African American health issues have consistently emphasized that mistrust of medical research long predated Tuskegee—as much as that study has come to epitomize such attitudes. According to the historian Vanessa Gamble, it is a mistake to place "emphasis on a single historical event to explain deeply entrenched and complex attitudes within the Black community."[57] As Giselle Corbie-Smith and coauthors noted, mistrust among African Americans "may be rooted in experiences extending back to slavery and continuing to the present day."[58] At a community forum, Eliseo Pérez-Stable cited examples from the historical record that are commonly invoked, including the use of slaves for medical experimentation in the antebellum South; the use of black cadavers for dissection purposes in the nineteenth century; legends about "night doctors" in the postbellum period, who were hired to kidnap blacks in the South for medical experiments; and more recent concerns about genocide, that link Tuskegee together with forced sterilization, the HIV/AIDS epidemic, and drugs in black neighborhoods.[59] Corbie-Smith recalled that issues as diverse as the use of Agent Orange in Vietnam and the claim that the CIA had deliberately promoted the sale of crack cocaine in black neighborhoods surfaced in discussions with African American groups about their attitudes toward biomedicine.[60] According to Julia Scott, the director of the National Black Women's Health Project, "It's not just history. And people try to say, 'Well, that was done, that is over, that wasn't me.' But there are current medical, everyday medical and scientific practices that reinforce [that] we still are seen as guinea pigs . . . that people will take a risk with."[61]

It is also important to observe that African Americans are not the only group to confront medical researchers with profound mistrust. As Gina Moreno-John and coauthors have noted, for a number of racial and ethnic minority groups in the United States, mistrust of research "is rooted in a general mistrust of mainstream society," while the possibility of exploitative or unethical treatment remains a serious one.[62] According to the authors:

Unfortunately, detrimental research outcomes continue to occur. For example, in Los Angeles in 1989, African American and Latino infants received the experimental Edmonston-Zagreb vaccine from the Centers for Disease Control and Prevention to study whether it could prevent measles in infants. Their parents were not informed that it was not licensed in the United States and had potentially lethal effects. . . . Recently, members of one Native tribe were ostracized after their reservation was identified in a study on syphilis, and another received adverse credit ratings by lenders after they were identified in a study on alcoholism. . . . The confidentiality of these participants was violated despite requests by tribal leaders that researchers not identify the tribes. . . . Ethnic minorities have participated in studies where researchers did not obtain informed consent, changed the protocol without consulting participants, withheld information, or did not follow-up as planned, resulting in a lack of trust.[63]

Thus, while "Tuskegee" often functions as a placeholder in discussions of resistance to participation in clinical research on the part of communities of color, the problem of mistrust cannot really be addressed without considering a much broader set of historical and political issues affecting a range of racial and minority groups in the United States.

An important dimension of the problem of overcoming such distrust concerns attitudes toward research among primary-care physicians serving racial and ethnic minority communities. As Mary-Rose Mueller has described more generally, practicing physicians often function as crucial mediators between patients and clinical researchers, passing on information about ongoing trials and influencing the decisions of patients about whether to enroll.[64] On one hand, a patient may be willing to place greater trust in a personal physician than in some unknown researcher; on the other hand, physicians may be particularly inclined to refer patients to trials when they know and trust the investigators conducting them. Mueller cited the comments of one of the physicians in her study: "I know [the principal investigator] very well and I trust him. I know he's not going to let my patient get into any trouble."[65] Thus, trust is critical at both linkage points in the chain connecting patients to researchers via the intermediary of physicians. The apparatus of the randomized clinical trial might properly be seen as a "technology of trust," and adequate trust relationships may be as central a component to its proper functioning as correct statistical methods.[66] To acknowledge this point is to assert that recruitmentology must indeed go beyond the formal analysis of yields and motivations to imagine the construction of new models of trust relationships.

The Politics of Participation

An important subset of recruitmentological work has proposed that deficits of trust need to be met with sincere and concerted trust-building measures. At the most basic level, these include working through community gatekeepers, such as clergy and politicians, and employing bilingual or multilingual staff when working with linguistically diverse communities. Some also recommend what might be called "identity matching" (that is, making sure that at least the front-line employees for the study, if not the principal investigators, are members of the group being studied), though, in fact, recruitmentology studies do not always confirm the efficacy of this practice.[67] For research in African American communities, the NIH also has touted the virtues of alliances between researchers in universities with predominantly white faculties and those situated in historically black institutions.[68] Clinical researchers also have been advised to think more about the duration of their commitment: Do researchers disappear after the trial is over—what Victoria Cargill, a panelist at a conference on recruitment, characterized as "drive-by research"[69]—or do they make a concerted effort to bring the lessons and benefits of the research back to the community?

On one hand, there can be little doubt that the perceived need to promote trust as an avenue to recruitment of subjects has sometimes given rise to cynical half-measures. One young physician told me about being invited to be a co-investigator on a study directed by a prominent researcher, only to conclude eventually that what the senior investigator really sought was a "black face" to display at community forums for purposes of reassuring potential participants.[70] Another troubling anecdote was related at a conference by Aníbal Sosa of the Latino Health Institute in Boston. When a researcher sought his help in recruiting Latinos for a study, Sosa asked him, "What's the study about? What's the study design?" According to Sosa, the researcher replied, "I don't have time to get into all that. I just need your help arranging a meeting with your people." To which Sosa replied, "Well, I need to know a bit more, before I put you in touch with 'my people.'"[71]

On the other hand, much of the literature on trust-building explicitly challenges such approaches by connecting the issue of trust directly to that of transforming the power imbalance between the researcher and the community under study. One extended discussion of the implementation of trust-building measures, by Gina Moreno-John and coauthors, is based on the work of three of the Resource Centers for Minority Aging Research funded by the NIH (one at the University of North Carolina, one at the University of Colorado Health Sciences Center, and one at the University of California, San Francisco). The authors described strategies such as collaborating closely with community leaders, including members of community-based organizations on advisory boards, providing technical assistance in grant writing and event planning to those community-based organizations, attending community events, and maintaining contact with communities after research ended.[72] Perhaps most significantly, the authors advocated a "participatory approach to research" involving "a reciprocal relationship, with a mutually beneficial exchange of expertise and resources."[73] Along these lines, other recruitmentologists have called for adopting "participatory action research," a model of scholarly investigation that seeks to abolish the power imbalance between experts and laypeople by promoting "community ownership" of research, based on community-driven determinations of research priorities.[74]

In practice, participatory research can mean many different things, and exhortations of the virtues of community participation at times simply beg the crucial definitional questions: What constitutes a community? Who gets called upon to serve as a community's representative?[75] Nor does participatory research always equalize power between researchers and communities. At times, the rubric of participatory research may simply offer investigators another tactic to get the "bodies" that they seek for the research they already have determined to conduct. However, various reports suggest the potential benefits of these sorts of participatory approaches for successful recruitment and retention. For example, at a conference on the topic, Barbara Howard described a study on Genetics of Coronary Disease in Alaskan Natives, being conducted in fifteen remote Alaskan villages—places with "no street signs." To recruit the 1,200 participants, researchers sought "continuous community input," including consultation with tribal leaders, involvement of community recruiters, and the presence of American Indian physicians as investigators and on the steering committee.[76] More generally, participatory styles of research presume a certain amount of deference to the authority of community leaders. As Ilena Norton and Spero Manson have described in the case of work with American Indians, this may mean a willingness on the part of investigators to accept suggestions with regard to "study questions, implementation, presentation of the results, and publications." And the authors warn: "Investigators who object to the review of results by non-scholars are unlikely to be allowed by tribal governments to undertake their research."[77]

Recruiting Gone Global

As this chapter has suggested, scholarship in the "recruitmentology" vein ranges from the most technical considerations of strategy and tactics to the most overtly political analyses of power and inequality in a historical context. However, nearly all of this work makes an assumption that is increasingly less likely to hold true—that the participants to be recruited by U.S.-based researchers or pharmaceutical companies are themselves located within the borders of the United States. Beginning in 1987, the

FDA has allowed pharmaceutical companies to file applications for drug approvals based solely on data obtained abroad, and the percentage of patients being studied in foreign countries has climbed rapidly since then.[78] An FDA study of the approval of "new molecular entities" between 1995 and 1999 found that up to 35 percent of the trials included foreign sites, translating into about 1,140 foreign clinical trials per year.[79] Contract research organizations (CROs, one of several kinds of private consulting companies to which drug companies increasingly outsource their recruitment) are especially inclined to move their operations offshore. In addition, many university-based researchers with federal funding from the NIH, such as academics involved in tests of AIDS vaccines and therapies, are conducting research in foreign settings, often in collaboration with local investigators.

It should be clear that the foreign locales in question here are not usually places like England, Germany, or France. They are countries like India, Uganda, Thailand, China, and Indonesia—places where the costs of conducting research are much reduced and where patients have the experimental virtue of being "pharmacologically naive" (that is, lacking previous exposure to treatment). As Adriana Petryna has described, " 'Treatment saturation' is making Americans increasingly unusable from a drug-testing standpoint, as our pharmaceuticalized bodies produce too many drug-drug interactions, providing less and less capacity to show drug effectiveness and making test results less statistically valid."[80] Less wealthy countries not only provide unexposed bodies; in addition, as David Rothman has pointed out, they offer the "advantage" of a comparative absence of "effective review boards, or, for that matter, highly inquisitive and demanding patients."[81] Web sites for CROs advertise their specialized capacities to deliver research subjects in particular regions of the world. For example, a company called LatinTrials, featuring research in Mexico, Argentina, Brazil, Uruguay, and Chile, asks "Why Latin America?" and provides a range of attractive answers: "strong enrollment rates," "good patient compliance and retention," and "availability of treatment-naive patients."[82]

Recently, much attention has focused on India—described by the *Financial Times* in 2003 as "A Test-Bed for Western Drug Companies"— where the world's largest CRO, the U.S.-based company Quintiles, began operation in 1997 and where as many as a dozen such companies were operating by 2003. Along with offering "an enormous pool" of treatment-naive patients, India can provide well-trained, English-speaking researchers, nurses, and staff "at less than a third of Western wages." According to the *Financial Times*, "some executives believe India could become as prominent in pharmaceuticals as it is in information technology."[83] However, as an editorial in the *New England Journal of Medicine* observed (under the title "A New Colonialism?"), the scramble to take advantage of the growing financial opportunities in India has led to a range of "ethically dubious" practices, including side-stepping informed consent.[84]

India is a country with extraordinary health needs, where millions die of parasites and tropical diseases. But only a tiny fraction of the drugs tested there are intended to treat such conditions, and, in any case, "the sponsors do not guarantee that new drugs tested in India will be made available there at affordable prices."[85] Certainly some transnational medical research, for example on the efficacy of AIDS vaccines, may someday directly benefit the countries in which the research is being conducted. For the most part, however, rich Western countries will be reaping the benefits of the substantial and growing corpus of research now being conducted on the bodies of the global poor.

Clearly, the globalization of clinical research has significant implications for the story told in this chapter (and, indeed, for this book as a whole).[86] A growing subset of recruitmentological work has emphasized the importance of trust and respect toward, and a genuinely participatory role for, the people and communities under study, as a prerequisite of successful recruitment as well as ethical treatment. But the outsourcing of research seems potentially to obviate these concerns, both ethical and practical. Will the primary solution to the dilemmas of recruitment and retention prove to be simple exploitation of vulnerability on a global level—and the neocolonialist extraction of biovalue from a racialized "other"? If so, then all of the programmatic statements and recruitmentological research supporting such worthy goals as trust enhancement, community empowerment, and participatory research will simply be for naught.

In considering likely trajectories, several matters appear significant. One obvious issue concerns ideas about the meanings of difference, with the reliance on foreign settings and non-Western bodies prompting renewed concerns about the generalizability of data: Will it prove possible to apply the results of such research to U.S. patients? For example, at a meeting of the FDA's Antiviral Drugs Advisory Committee in 1999 that considered international studies of drugs to prevent vertical transmission of HIV (that is, transmission from mother to fetus or newborn), at least one member worried that the "use of study populations that would differ from the U.S. in many ways, might make it difficult to extrapolate the results to American patients and clinical practice."[87] For the most part, however, despite the considerable attention to group difference in medical testing in recent years at both the rhetorical and the policy levels, as well as the vocal warnings about inappropriate extrapolations, little concern has been expressed about the use of people of color from the global South as experimental stand-ins for the consumers of pharmaceutical products in wealthy nations. Such opportunism with regard to the problem of generalizability seems to hark back to past moments in the history of medical research discussed in chapter 2, where humans typically became research subjects as a consequence of highly unequal power relations and where this "availability" of subjects trumped all other concerns, whether scientific or ethical, about who to include as subjects. Indeed, the new global research environment, often characterized by the conjunction of strong financial incentives and weak regulatory structures, seems especially likely to produce such "availability."

However, the globalization of research has also, at moments, prompted close attention to ethical and political questions as well as vigorous public discussion. Indeed, the implications of global inequality for medical research ignited a fiery controversy in 1997 that proved to be one of the most divisive bioethical debates in recent years—coincidentally, also focused on NIH-funded studies of antiviral drugs to interrupt vertical transmission of HIV. In the United States, the drug AZT already had been shown quite effective in stopping transmission as much as three-quarters of the time, but the course of treatment was too expensive for most African countries to afford. Therefore, researchers sought to test cheaper alternatives, such as reduced doses or courses of administration of various antiviral drugs. The catch was that most of these studies were designed to demonstrate the efficacy of the less expensive therapy via comparison with a control group receiving a placebo. Whistle-blowing critics vehemently insisted that all participants in U.S.-funded clinical trials were entitled to the present-day standard of care, regardless of where the trial took place.[88] Indeed, for Marcia Angell, executive editor of the prestigious *New England Journal of Medicine*, the withholding of any therapy from the control group when known therapies existed suggested that "we have not come very far from Tuskegee at all."[89] This incendiary analogy was strenuously rejected by the NIH, which funded the research, as well as by the local research collaborators in African nations. Debate about the case and similar studies effectively split the bioethics establishment and led to a formal reconsideration of ethical standards.[90] Much attention was devoted to this episode, and a good deal of ink was spilled in discussing the appropriate response.[91] But it remains unclear whether such cases will prompt a more extensive consideration of the human and social costs and benefits of the new global production of biomedical knowledge and commodities.

Conflict surrounding the globalization of research points to the boundaries of my analysis, which has emphasized how a biopolitical framework that is still largely particular to the United States and is policed by its federal agencies has sparked new ways of apprehending identities and differences.[92] Within the bounds of that framework, the theory and practice of recruitmentology have promoted new fusions of biological and cultural knowledge about the medically "other," and policies mandating their inclusion and the measurement of cross-group differences have inclined many researchers to think anew about the characteristics of medically disadvantaged groups. This epistemic work is closely intertwined with a series of concurrent debates—about the new genetics, about health disparities, about racial profiling in medicine, and so on—though, again, in ways that often reflect the particularities of the United States. How these developments will articulate with transnational research practices, or with the global politics of health inequality, is much more difficult to discern.

The Remaking of Race and Gender

The increased pressures to recruit human subjects and the rise of a new applied science of "recruitmentology" are by no means purely a consequence of the inclusion-and-difference paradigm; they reflect the intensification, corporatization, and globalization of clinical research in recent years. However, the mandate to diversify subject populations has shaped these endeavors in significant ways. Now that attention to inclusion and difference is institutionalized, clinical researchers and pharmaceutical companies cannot escape the demand to think seriously about who to recruit and how to enroll them. In this way, the everyday, hands-on work of clinical research becomes linked to the broad-scale operation of a biopolitical framework for administering and classifying bodies and populations.

One important consequence of recruitmentology is that those engaged in it develop and promote new understandings of social groups—their characteristics and their histories. In effect, new meanings of identities such as "race" and "gender" emerge from the practical work of recruitment and the science of recruitmentology. Yet this is only one way in which the inclusion-and-difference paradigm remakes the meanings of race, ethnicity, sex, and gender. In the next two chapters, I address this latter topic specifically. While this chapter and the previous one have focused on the practical consequences of the inclusion-and-difference paradigm for biomedical insiders, the next two chapters detail the broader social consequences, particularly for racial and ethnic minorities and for women. In these chapters, I develop a critique of how the inclusion-and-difference paradigm promotes a problematic reliance on "racial profiling" and "sex profiling" in modern medicine—practices that may not be to the betterment of those they are intended to help.

CHAPTER TEN

To Profile or Not to Profile: What Difference Does Race Make?

How different is different? When assessing medical knowledge and determining medical treatment, just how important is it to take into account a person's sex, race, ethnicity, age, sexuality, or other dimension of identity? Which differences really matter? When and why? These questions are pivotal for this book, and they merit renewed scrutiny here, now that the story of the inclusion-and-difference paradigm has been told. My historical account emphasized how ideas about medical difference, when yoked together with claims about justice and citizenship, helped inspire new biomedical policies and priorities since the 1980s. But in turn, the new inclusionary requirements, coupled with growing attention to health disparities along with the rise of "recruitmentology," have intensified the tendency to take difference into account and have spawned an impressive quantity of "difference findings" from biomedical research. Thus, the argument that medical knowledge travels poorly across categories of persons—that there are limits to generalizability—is more firmly entrenched now than at the dawn of the inclusion-and-difference paradigm, in large measure because of practices and tendencies that the paradigm has promoted.

At the same time, open controversy has erupted in recent years over whether knowledge of at least one aspect of a person's identity—his or her race—should guide medical diagnosis and treatment. Should the well-informed physician take into account the patient's race or ethnicity when deciding which medication to prescribe? Not only in the pages of medical and scientific journals, but also in the popular press, commentators have fiercely debated the merits of "racial profiling" for medical purposes—a controversy that joins divergent interpretations of scientific findings to varied understandings both of good practice and of racial justice. The

FDA's licensing for sale in 2005 of the first "race-based medicine"—the drug BiDil, approved to treat heart failure only in African American patients—cast a spotlight on this controversy while cranking up the volume on claims and counterclaims. Some have embraced race-based "niche marketing" of pharmaceuticals and other types of racial profiling in medicine as a victory worth savoring in a long struggle to bring medical attention to the excluded and the underserved. Others have accepted it more reluctantly as a short-lived holding pattern—a way station on the path toward the fully individualized therapy that purportedly will be the offspring of the mapping of the human genome. However, critics of medical profiling by race have argued that its use reflects a truncated understanding of the biological and social production of bodily difference, which may not only harm human health but also inappropriately reinforce ideas about the reality of essential differences between groups. From the standpoint of critics—among whom I number myself—health inequalities by race are an enormous social problem deserving sustained attention, but focusing on biological differences is *not* the way to address them.

This chapter will present some of the recent racial and ethnic "difference findings" and reconstruct the debates. The goal is to make sense of new ways of understanding human beings, their bodies, and their medical needs that are consistent with, and have been propelled by, the inclusion-and-difference paradigm. Because I agree with the critiques of racial profiling, my goal will be to make a case for the potential hazards—though also to consider the potential benefits—that follow from the emphasis on human biological difference in medicine, as well as from the understanding of group identities in biological terms. My efforts in this regard have been aided and influenced significantly by the recent outpouring of academic work by scholars in the field of science studies and elsewhere, writing on the nexus of race, genetics, and medicine.[1] Therefore, my intent will not be to recount every detail of their careful analyses—for example, about the implications of recent work in genetics for the understanding of race. Rather, I will summarize the overall relevance of this body of work for the questions at stake here, as well as situate the concerns raised by these other scholars in relation to the recent historical and political changes that I have charted in this book.

In addition, I will argue that we gain some analytical mileage by doing something that these others haven't done: formally juxtaposing recent uses of racial difference in medicine (the topic of this chapter) with simultaneous emphases on differences of other sorts, particularly sex or gender (the following chapter).[2] To the degree that sex and race pose divergent implications for biopolitics, then differences across types of difference matter—which suggests that the tendency of the policies of the inclusion-and-difference paradigm to treat all forms of difference in a standardized way may be problematic. But I also will argue that the contrast in some respects has been overstated. The case of "sex profiling" bears some important affinities with racial profiling in terms of the risks it may pose, and we learn something by considering the two examples side-by-side.

THE NEW RACE DEBATES

The controversy over the virtues or dangers of racial profiling in medicine reflects the new policy environment that I have described in previous chapters: the imposition of requirements for the inclusion of racial and ethnic minorities as research subjects, as well as the emphasis on addressing health disparities by race. At the same time, the controversy has arisen out of the convergence of three streams of public and expert discussion: disagreement in the health arena about the reliability and meaning of schemes of racial classification, perceptions about the booming production of racial "difference findings" in medicine, and recent debates in the field of population genetics about the meaning of race. I will briefly review these three topics, before moving on explicitly to the profiling debate.

The Debate over Racial Classification in Medicine and Public Health

During the 1990s—at the same time as the passage of the NIH Revitalization Act and other policies that required the racial classification of biomedical research subjects—an increasing number of practitioners, scholars, and journal editors in the fields of medicine and public health began asking pointed questions about the utility and stability of categories that often simply had been taken for granted. How many racial and ethnic categories are there? What about people who are multiracial or multiethnic? Are "races" and "ethnicities" the same thing, or are they different modes of classification? Is race primarily a social identity or a biological description? Who should determine the racial or ethnic identity of a patient or research subject—the clinician/researcher or the patient/participant? That such questions had not deeply troubled biomedicine previously is a testament to the aura of self-evident naturalness that continues to surround the phenomenon of race—within medical and health domains as well as in the broader culture. However, the emergence of public debate over these issues also reflected the entrance of critiques from the social sciences and humanities, where scholars had challenged the notion of race as a form of difference clearly fixed in biology and had demonstrated that systems of racial and ethnic classification varied significantly across societies and over time.

Even more specifically, in the early 1990s a range of scholars in social epidemiology, medical sociology, and related fields were objecting to the uncritical use of racial categories by physicians and medical researchers. For example, some presented evidence that the same individuals might be categorized as belonging to different races at various moments in their medical life history, as represented on birth certificates, hospital records, and death certificates.[3] Scholars such as David Williams also argued that the medical profession continued to hang on to discredited conceptions of the biology of race by retaining passages in medical textbooks that assumed underlying genetic homogeneity within races and distinctiveness between them.[4] At a workshop cosponsored by the CDC on the use of race and ethnicity for purposes of public health surveillance, Robert Hahn and Donna Stroup cited important strides in the collection and use of such data but also pointed to significant challenges that remained, including "questions of validity, lack of consensus on use, variability in terminology, misclassification, undercounting, diversity in popular understanding, and lack of reliability."[5]

Within mainstream medicine in the United States, controversy over the use of racial categories broke out into the open in 1992, with the publication in the *Journal of the American Medical Association* (*JAMA*) of a commentary by Newton Osborne and Marvin Feit entitled "The Use of Race in Medical Research." Part of the authors' argument focused on the problematic nature of categorization. "How white is white?" the authors asked. "Is a person who has only one grandparent of another race defined or categorized the same as one who has one great-grandparent or two great-grandparents? What happens if two grandparents are white, one is black, and another Asian?" But going beyond such critiques, the authors took aim at the deeper presumption that the discovery of a "racial difference" necessarily tells us something both about human biology and about the essential nature of races. The authors conclusions were blunt and provocative:

> When race is used as a variable in research, there is a tendency to assume that the results obtained are a manifestation of the biology of racial differences; race as a variable implies that a genetic reason may explain differences in incidence, severity, or outcome of medical conditions. Re-

searchers, without saying so, lead readers to assume that certain racial groups have a special predisposition, risk, or susceptibility to the illness studied. Since this presupposition is seldom warranted, this kind of comparison may be taken to represent a subtle form of racism.[6]

Letters in response to Osborne and Feit's salvo accused them of "an effort to impose an ideology of political correctness on medical research";[7] respondents also reminded their readers of the findings of racial differences in the effects of various medications. In reply, Osborne acknowledged the possibility of racial differences while insisting on the categorization dilemmas that rendered problematic any simple claims: "Yes, there may be racial differences in drug metabolism . . . among Asian Americans, blacks, and whites. However, Asia is a very big continent. Asian Americans, blacks, and whites come in many shades and from many backgrounds. . . . It is difficult to classify people as blacks, whites, or Asians in an actively changing population. Might not this biological mixture serve to contaminate the nice, neat framework the respondents describe?"[8]

By the latter part of the decade, more sustained critiques of the use of race in health contexts were being launched with some frequency. This was perhaps especially true in the field of public health, which is more attuned to understanding the social, economic, and political sources of health disparities. Indeed, a 1998 manifesto in the *American Journal of Public Health* by Mindy Fullilove recognized the salience of race to personal identity but called for the "abandonment" of race as a formal variable in public health research.[9] Within medicine, as well, a strong challenge was mounted by Harold Freeman, an oncologist at Harlem Hospital, who chaired a presidential panel on cancer for President Clinton. In a much-cited statement, Freeman noted the panel's conclusion that "the biologic concept of race is no longer tenable and . . . race should no longer be considered a valid biologic classification."[10]

By the latter part of the 1990s, medical journal editors also were paying increased notice to these contentious debates. In 1997 the major journals released the fifth edition of the "Uniform Requirements for Manuscripts Submitted to Biomedical Journals," a consensus document meant to guide authors in the preparation of manuscripts submitted to hundreds of medical journals. For the first time, authors were instructed that "the definition and relevance of race and ethnicity are ambiguous." When describing research subjects, "authors should be particularly careful about using these categories."[11] The instructions stopped there. According to George Lundberg, who was the editor of *JAMA* at the time, "There were strong differences of opinion in terms of making any more definitive statement than was made. Everybody agreed it was a problem. Everybody agreed it had to be dealt with somehow, and nobody knew how."[12]

One journal, the *Archives of Pediatrics and Adolescent Medicine*, announced a new policy in 2001 that authors simply "not use race and ethnicity when there is no biological, scientific, or sociological reason for doing so." According to two board members: "Ceasing to analyze data blindly by race or ethnicity is not an attempt to be politically correct, but rather doing so brings us closer to the underlying biological science on which medicine, and our care for patients, is firmly rooted."[13] In much the same spirit, a spokesperson for the National Library of Medicine responded in 2003 to criticism of its rather retrograde medical subject headings (such as "racial stocks") not only by announcing a revision of its terminology, but also by acknowledging the "larger and deeper question" about "the appropriateness of representing racial identities," given that "race is an unscientific concept."[14]

The Proliferation of Difference Findings

At the same time that scholars, journal editors, and practitioners increasingly worried about the usability of racial categories in medicine, reports proliferated about variation by race in the biology of disease and treatment. Some of these include findings of racial differences in susceptibility to illness. For example, in 1996 AIDS researchers discovered that a mutation in a gene called *CCR5* conferred greater resistance to infection with HIV or progression of disease by preventing the virus from latching onto its target cells in the immune system. The kicker was that the mutation was described as being unequally distributed across human groups.[15] The highest frequencies were among Europeans (particularly Ashkenazi Jews), with lower frequencies in Asia and the Middle East. "Outside of this region," said scientists, "the mutation is either absent or only present as isolated individual occurrences."[16] While scientific reports referred primarily to the geographic origins of blood samples, popular reports tended to describe the difference as a racial one.[17]

Another case of reported differential susceptibility by race concerns smoking. In 1998 researchers described differences in the levels of cotinine—a chemical derived from nicotine—found in the bodies of African American, Mexican American, and white American smokers, with African Americans having the highest concentrations. According to an editorial in *JAMA*, "the underlying cause of the higher cotinine concentrations in African Americans lies in a racially associated difference in cotinine metabolism."[18] Specifically, the conversion of nicotine into cotinine, as well as the clearance of cotinine from the body, depend in part on the activity of an enzyme called CYP2A6 (one of the enzymes in the cytochrome P450 family). However, the gene that controls production of the enzyme is polymorphic (that is, it may appear in variant forms), in certain cases causing individuals to be "poor metabolizers" who are slower to clear the substances from the body. Once again, the punch line was that the variant form of CYP2A6 was reported to be unequally distributed among racial groups, resulting, potentially, in racial differences both in addiction to tobacco and in the long-term health consequences of smoking.[19]

In addition to such studies of variation in vulnerability to disease, a growing number of investigators have been examining differences in responses to medical treatment. Some of the most oft-repeated claims concern drugs for various cardiovascular conditions, including hypertension, whose effects on African Americans have been the subject of much study.[20] As summed up by the NIH in the 2003 report of the Joint National Committee on Prevention, Detection, Evaluation, and Treatment of High Blood Pressure, not only is hypertension more prevalent and more severe among African Americans, but, in comparison to whites, their elevated blood pressure is less likely to be reduced by monotherapy with certain classes of drugs (beta-blockers, ACE inhibitors, and angiotensin-receptor blockers) and more likely to be reduced by other classes (diuretics and calcium-channel blockers). However, the comparative differences in response mostly vanish when African Americans are treated with drug combinations that include a diuretic as one of the medications.[21] Some have speculated that this variation reflects actual differences in the biology of hypertension across racial groups, with individuals of (west) African ancestry displaying distinctive patterns of salt sensitivity or renin levels.[22] However, others have questioned the biological link and have emphasized that, by and large, African Americans do respond to the same drugs as people of other races, though sometimes to lesser degrees.[23]

Reports of racial or ethnic differences in the effects of pharmaceutical drugs are not limited to hypertension. In a review published in *Nature Genetics* in 2004, Sarah Tate and David Goldstein compiled a list of twenty-nine medicines that "have been claimed, in peer-reviewed scientific or medical journals, to have differences in either safety or, more commonly, efficacy among racial or ethnic groups." About half of the list consisted of drugs for cardiovascular diseases, but the remainder included medications for hepatitis C, pain relief, mental illness, and other conditions. However, the authors characterized these claims about racial differences as "universally controversial" and observed that "there is no consensus on how important race or ethnicity is in determining drug response." Such uncertainties notwithstanding, the authors noted that of the 185 new drug products approved by the FDA from 1995 to 1998, 15 of them contained a statement in the drug labeling information about a racial or ethnic difference in the drug's effectiveness.[24] Putative or proposed mechanisms behind these racial or ethnic differences include genetic variations in the enzymes that metabolize these drugs, differences in immune response, and other differences in biological processes at the cellular or organ level. In their review, however, Tate and Goldstein classified ten of the twenty-nine cases as "possible false positives," either because the study had not been replicated, or because the findings from different studies had proven inconsistent, or because the reported racial or ethnic difference might actually be a consequence of differences in average body weight or other confounding factors, or because the racial or ethnic variation might be due to social factors, such as differences in the quality of health care or differences in prescribing practices. And of the remaining nineteen drugs, only in thirteen cases did the authors deem there to be evidence of either genetic causation or an underlying physiological basis.[25] As Jonathan Kahn has described, the nuances of Tate and Goldstein's discussion mostly have been lost on the media, who have repeated the simple claim of twenty-nine race-specific drugs as evidence of, and justification for, a broader move toward race-specific prescribing.[26]

The Clash over the New Genetics

Before turning explicitly to the issue of racial profiling, it is worth considering one last arena of controversy. A key step in understanding the varied claims about race-specific biological differences in disease expression and treatment is to appreciate how such claims have become closely intertwined with recent scientific debates over genetic diversity within the human species. These latter debates within the field of population genetics are often quite technical, and were it not for the presumption that they have biomedical relevance, they probably would receive considerably less attention than they have, at least outside the pages of journals such as *Nature Genetics*. Still, insofar as geneticists' arguments are deemed to tell us something about the "reality" of race, they have become the stuff of popular media reports in recent years.

An article from the Toronto *Globe and Mail* in 2005 suggests the stakes that many perceive in this research. "When the Human Genome Project was completed in 2000, its most touted result was that it showed no genetic basis for race," wrote Carolyn Abraham, a medical reporter for the newspaper. "In fact, some scientists went so far as to dub race a 'biological fiction.'" This was because the project found humans as a species to be 99.9 percent genetically identical: "A teeny 0.1 per cent, a mere genetic sliver, helps to account for all the profound diversity within the human race, with its freckles, dimples, afros and crimson tresses, its shy and bombastic types, its Donald Trumps and Dalai Lamas, Madonnas and Mr. Dressups, Bill Gates, Billie Holidays, George W. Bushes and Osama bin Ladens." According to Abraham, "It was a message of harmony: Hardly a hair of code separates us." But Abraham then went on to lay out the arresting paradox: "Five years later, one of scientists' main preoccupations has become to chart the genetic variations between and within racial groups—to parse that 0.1 per cent."[27] In fact, given the complexity of the human genome, that tenth of a percent represents several million potential points of genetic divergence between individuals, although the actual variations responsible for genetic differences in health or other observable traits are considerably fewer.[28]

Thus, on one hand, recent work in genetics has only strengthened the message about race that geneticists such as Richard Lewontin popularized in the 1970s—that humans are overwhelmingly similar at the basic level of the genome and that the degree of genetic diversity that does exist is actually greater within the conventionally recognized racial groups than it is between them. Unlike other species, including other primates, humans cannot be disaggregated into clearly defined genetic subspecies—meaning that the eighteenth- and nineteenth-century racist and imperialist conception of humanity as divided into biologically discrete groups simply has no basis in fact.[29] No less a figure than President Clinton celebrated the scientific affirmation of human commonality at the press conference announcing the completion of the mapping of the human genome: "I believe one of the great truths to emerge from this triumphant expedition inside the human genome is that in genetic terms, all human beings, regardless of race, are more than 99.9 percent the same. What that means is that modern science has confirmed what we first learned from ancient fates. The most important fact of life on this Earth is our common humanity."[30] Some have gone even further in drawing lessons from modern genetics: J. Craig Venter, who directed the privately funded initiative to map the human genome, has come out strongly in opposition to the use of racial categorization in genetic and medical research and has complained that "applying antiquated labels to the analysis and interpretation of scientific data could result in misleading and biologically meaningless conclusions."[31]

On the other hand, the drive to uncover the predictive significance of

the small fraction of the human genome that accounts for interindivid-
ual differences—by studying what are called single nucleotide polymorphisms, or SNPs ("snips")[32]—has given rise to renewed debate about the
degree to which those various tiny differences line up according to what
are conventionally called races. Careful analysts emphasize two crucial
points. First, the best way to understand genetic diversity is in terms
of geography. According to Rick Kittles and Kenneth Weiss: "Human
genetic variation is actually characterized by clines (spatial gradients)
of allele frequency[33] rather than categorical variation between populations, and the pattern varies among genes for the historic reasons of
drift, selection, and demographic history. . . . The pattern of variation
can generally be described as isolation by distance: Genetic differences
between populations are roughly proportional to the geographic distance
between them."[34] Second, and as a consequence of the preceding, population differences at the level of SNPs are invariably gradational rather
than absolute: there is no known example of a polymorphism that is
found exclusively in a single social group (as defined by race, ethnicity,
nation, continent, etc.) or found universally within it.[35] Hence, all of the
claims about group-relevant polymorphisms in the genes affecting drug
metabolism are actually statements about percentages.

For example, possession of the "null" allele of the gene *CYP2D6* affects
an individual's ability to metabolize many important drugs. (Those who
are homozygous for this polymorphism, having inherited it from both
parents, cannot convert codeine to morphine and therefore gain little
analgesic benefit from the drug.) But the median frequencies of the null
allele vary from 6 percent in "Asian populations," to 7 percent in "African
populations," to 26 percent of "European populations." Regardless of the
definition of these population descriptors (and leaving aside all the difficulties inherent in using them with accuracy), the point is that there is
no single racial or ethnic group within which everyone shares this—or
any other—genetic trait.[36] Similarly, there is no such thing as a racially
specific and exclusive disease. Even diseases such as sickle-cell anemia
that are caused by a mutation of a single gene have a prevalence that is
defined not by race but by geographic origin—in the case of sickle-cell,
African or Mediterranean ancestry, including many who would classify
themselves as white—and even this holds true only to the degree that human populations are "endogamous" (bear children with sexual partners of
the same ancestry).[37] Diseases caused not by a single gene but by multiple
genes in combination with complex environmental factors—that is to say,
most diseases—are even less plausibly characterized as "racial."[38]

But if these conclusions would seem to rule out of bounds a classical conception of races as discrete, mutually exclusive biological categories, they do still leave room for another possibility—one that has been highly significant for thinking about racial profiling in medicine. Given the salience of geography to an understanding of genetic variation, and given that our everyday conceptions of race do invoke geographic ideas of continental origin (from Africa, Asia, Europe, and the Americas), might not those "continental" categories of race work reasonably well in describing the clustering of certain SNPs among populations around the world? The point would not be that every individual within the racial group possesses the polymorphism, but rather that conventional racial categories function "well enough" in predicting which individuals will possess it. This has been the controversial claim of Stanford geneticist Neil Risch and his collaborators, and it is one with obvious relevance to the racial profiling debate. According to Risch, when humans are divided into clusters according to genetic similarities, these clusters roughly correspond to "continental" races (which he identified as Africans, Caucasians, Pacific Islanders, East Asians, and Native Americans). Therefore, "self-defined race, ethnicity or ancestry are actually more genetically informative than clusters based on analysis of random genetic markers."[39]

However, Risch's conclusions have been quite controversial among geneticists, and others have made contrary arguments. For example, David Goldstein, a population geneticist at University College, London, used a computer modeling program to assign individuals from eight populations to clusters based on genetic polymorphisms and then found that these clusters did not line up terribly well with conventional notions of race. Goldstein and coauthors noted that a majority of Ethiopians fell into a cluster that included Jews, Norwegians, and Armenians; 21 percent of Afro-Caribbeans clustered with Europeans; and individuals from China and New Guinea fell almost completely into separate clusters.[40] As a number of commentators in the field of science studies have observed, given the clear absence of consensus among geneticists, it is striking how much attention Risch's views have received in the popular press—what Lundy Braun has described as "the almost immediate credibility accorded to Risch's views and the subsequent marginalization of the views of other researchers, many of whom had been deeply engaged for decades in . . . theorizing and studying empirically the causes of racial and ethnic disparities in disease."[41] While Risch's professional reputation is clearly one factor in explaining his popular credibility, it is also worth considering the tendency for genetic (or otherwise biological) accounts of human difference to resonate widely in contemporary culture and to be embraced relatively uncritically.[42]

RACIAL PROFILING TAKES CENTER STAGE

Beginning around the year 2001, the controversies discussed above—about racial classification, difference findings, and the new genetics—began explicitly to feed into what suddenly became known as the "racial profiling" debate. A defining moment came in May of that year, when the *New England Journal of Medicine* published two articles investigating racial differences. What was noteworthy, however, was not these articles so much as the accompanying editorial, written by a deputy editor of the journal, Robert Schwartz, and bearing the none-too-innocent title "Racial Profiling in Medical Research." Commenting on the two research articles, Schwartz complained that they both "refer to 'race,' 'racial groups,' 'racial differences,' and 'ethnic background' but offer no plausible biologic justification for making such distinctions." Denouncing the "pseudoscience of race," Schwartz stated plainly: "I maintain that attributing differences in a biologic end point to race is not only imprecise but also of no proven value in treating an individual patient."[43]

Schwartz acknowledged that there may be medical benefit in understanding the uneven distribution of certain genetic polymorphisms among people from the same "geographic origin or culture." But such variation should not be labeled racial in the absence of "a plausible, clearly defined, and testable hypothesis" about why race might be related to disease. Race held considerable social significance, Schwartz argued, and hence "research to root out social injustice in medical practice needs continued support." But an uninformed or reflexive indulgence in subgroup analyses by race was a pernicious practice. Said Schwartz, "tax-supported trolling of data bases to find racial distinctions in human biology must end."[44]

An article in the *Chronicle of Higher Education* about the *New England Journal* controversy foreshadowed the debate that would play out over the next few years. On one hand, the reporter, Lila Guterman, cited several "critics of the studies [who] accuse the researchers of suggesting that biological differences underlie, and therefore reinforce, the social concept of race, implying genetic differences between races that may not exist." But Guterman also cited Jay Cohn, a coauthor of one of the *New England Journal* articles that Schwartz had criticized, who insisted: "Right now, we have only skin color to identify populations." Cohn added, "You'd have to blindfold yourself to say we're not going to pay attention to obvious differences."[45] Significantly, Cohn was just in the process of launching the study of BiDil in African Americans—the study that would result in the drug's marketing by the FDA in 2005. In an essay later that month by Sheryl Gay Stolberg, the *New York Times* picked up on the controversy as well as the BiDil story, asking, in its "Week in Review" section, "Shouldn't a Pill Be Colorblind?" Stolberg's essay noted that Cohn had the backing of the Association of Black Cardiologists and then quoted his astonishment at the critique launched by Schwartz: "Here we have the black community accepting the concept that African-Americans need to be studied as a group, and then we have the scientific community claiming that race is dead." Cohn added, "It seems to me absolutely ludicrous to suggest that this prominent characteristic that we all recognize when we look at people should not be looked at."[46]

Schwartz was not the first ever to use the term "racial profiling" in a medical context. According to the National Library of Medicine's PubMed database, the term appears in the abstracts of three medical journal articles published from 1993 to 1998 by Kenneth Jamerson, a hypertension expert at the University of Michigan Medical School who has been critical of some of the conventional wisdom concerning the differential effects of antihypertensive medications in African Americans.[47] But Schwartz dropped the phrase into the title of an editorial in the prestigious *New England Journal*, and he did so at a time when it was already on many people's lips because of debates in the domain of criminal justice. Although African Americans and Latinos had long been complaining of their vulnerability to being stopped by the police for the "offense" of "driving while black" or "driving while Hispanic," a New Jersey court attracted wide attention to the issue in 1996 when it found a policy of "selective enforcement" by troopers on the state turnpike, who targeted "blacks for investigation and arrest."[48] The next few years saw increasing attention to the problem, which even became a campaign issue in the 2000 presidential campaign when the Democratic candidate, Vice President Al Gore, vowed to address it: "If I'm elected President, ending racial profiling will be the first civil rights act of the new century," Gore promised during a speech in 1999 at the annual convention of the NAACP.[49] Four months after Schwartz's editorial appeared, with the terrorist attacks of September 11, 2001, the general issue of racial profiling became both more widely discussed and more controversial as the nation debated appropriate steps to prevent future attacks. The question of whether and how to profile for terrorists was taken to epitomize a deep tension between fairness to individuals and effective protection of the common welfare.[50]

By labeling race-specific medicine "racial profiling," critics sought not only to associate it with a widely suspect practice, but also to make a point about the similarities in the underlying logic—specifically, the use of group-based probabilities to make judgments about individual cases. Just as the racial imbalance in drug trafficking convictions tells us nothing specific about the likelihood that the next car on the New Jersey turnpike will contain cocaine, similarly racial correlations in medicine provide inevitably limited guidance to doctors when dealing with any individual patient. To imagine otherwise is to imagine an intrinsic relation between race and disease that is as illusory and as prejudicial as a presumed intrinsic relation between race and criminality.

To be sure, many have explicitly repudiated these concerns about racial profiling. Indeed, some have proudly taken up its banner. An interesting case is Sally Satel, a psychiatrist and fellow at the conservative American Enterprise Institute, who declared, in the headline of a *New York Times Sunday Magazine* commentary, "I Am a Racially Profiling Doctor." Wrote Satel, "In practicing medicine, I am not colorblind. I always take note of my patient's race. So do many of my colleagues. We do it because certain diseases and treatment responses cluster by ethnicity. Recognizing these patterns can help us diagnose disease more efficiently and prescribe medications more effectively. When it comes to practicing medicine, stereotyping often works."[51] What is striking here is that Satel was one of the harshest public critics of the NIH Revitalization Act. As I described in chapter 5, Satel had argued in the pages of the *New Republic* that the Congressional Caucus for Women's Issues "managed to turn the inclusion provision into a referendum on civil rights," irrespective of scientific fact.[52] Thus, Satel was firmly opposed to taking race into account to address what she deemed to be political concerns—which she characterized as the intrusion of political correctness into medicine[53]—but she was happy to make use of racial categories when they were understood as demarcators of biological difference.

Since Schwartz's editorial, there has been substantial discussion in medical and scientific journals and elsewhere—too much for me to recapitulate here—about the merits or drawbacks of racial profiling.[54] Importantly, the debate has become inextricable from the others I described previously: the meaningfulness of racial categories in medicine and the implications of population genetics for understanding the realities of race. The debate also has played out *within* organizations devoted to the health of racial and ethnic minorities in the United States, such as the National Medication Association (NMA). When an NMA Clinical Trials Consensus Panel reported in 2000 that "ethnic differences in the pharmacokinetics and pharmacodynamics of certain drugs have been shown in clinical trials" and that "racial and ethnic differences can also determine the biological course of certain diseases," the journal of the association published a blistering guest editorial in response by one physician, Okay

Odocha at the Howard University College of Medicine, who decried the use of unscientific, "racialistic constructs."[55]

Philosophers of science likewise have weighed in on the controversy. On one side, Ian Hacking has embraced profiling in cases where its medical utility can be demonstrated statistically. For Hacking, this includes the matching of bone marrow transplant donors and recipients by race, since doing so makes rejection of the transplant less likely, given the statistical association between race and human leukocyte antigen (HLA). It also includes racially differentiated drugs such as BiDil, even when the biological mechanism linking race to drug effect is uncertain: "Even if one is a complete skeptic about, for example, a genetic basis for the differential efficacy of the drug, the drug does appear to be statistically *useful* in treating the designated class of patients. That means that race may be a useful indicator to a physician of the potential effectiveness of this rather than another drug—under present social and historical conditions."[56] On the other side, Naomi Zack has maintained that "essentialist racialization" may hinder medical progress "by falsely implying that statistical associations of some debilities with social racial identities has explanatory force on a biological level." Moreover, since medical statements about racial populations do not apply to all members, when it comes to individual diagnosis and treatment, patients "have to be treated by medical practitioners as though they do not have a particular populations membership."[57] Similarly, Michael Root has argued against the use of "race as a proxy" for genetic difference, noting, among other things, that the genes associated with the observable physical characteristics that we routinely classify as "racial" are not related to the genes that are known to affect drug response.[58]

What are we to make of this controversy? Of course, there is nothing unusual, from a medical perspective, about the practice of forming medical judgments about patients according to their categories of belonging— "stereotyping," as Satel would have it. The centrality to biomedicine of profiling practices has been emphasized by Nikolas Rose, who has observed how much we now take for granted that doctors will allocate us to risk groups or assign us a risk profile on the basis of a slew of predictable characteristics: "age, weight, family history, smoking and so forth."[59] At times some perceive that group-based risk profiling treats individuals and groups unfairly—for example, there has been much controversy around the CDC's continued refusal to allow openly gay men in the United States to donate blood, a policy that may provide some statistical benefit in protecting the blood supply against contamination, but that stigmatizes gay men by suggesting an intrinsic connection between being gay and having HIV.[60] More often than not, however, we simply take for granted the application of a population-based logic to our individual condition.

The fundamental question in the case of racial profiling in medicine, however, is whether it makes sense to apply statistical generalities about the racial group to individual cases, when the rationale for the link between the biological process and whatever we take race to be is so tenuous and speculative. In my estimation, Troy Duster has made the crucial point: "It is possible to make arbitrary groupings of populations (geographic, linguistic, self-identified by faith, identified by others by physiognomy, etc.) and still find statistically significant allelic variations between those groupings. For example, we could examine all the people in Chicago, and all those in Los Angeles, and find statistically significant differences in allele frequency at *some* loci."[61] We could certainly prescribe different drugs to Chicagoans and Angelinos, but we might well be reluctant to do so, even if residents of the two cities on average had different polymorphisms affecting drug metabolism. After all, in the absence of a good hypothesis about *why* city of residence might matter, this would appear to be an arbitrary and medically meaningless basis for drawing a difference between groups. Why, then, does race "make sense" in a way that city of residence does not? My concern is that Jay Cohn has provided the answer, and it is a poor one: "You'd have to blindfold yourself to say we're not going to pay attention to obvious differences. . . . It seems to me absolutely ludicrous to suggest that this prominent characteristic that we all recognize when we look at people should not be looked at." The point here is that race stares us in the face: on one hand, we are socialized to treat race as a fundamental criterion of classification, one of the first things we notice about a person; on the other hand, there is a long history, both beneficial and disturbing, of attending to race in medical and health contexts. Thus, it becomes relatively easy for what I have termed "categorical alignment" to take place—for the categories that are so evident in everyday life to bleed over into medical and scientific settings.

Moreover, as James Jackson, a psychologist and the director of the Program for Research on Black Americans at the University of Michigan, described the problem, most people "have naive theories about race" that they are rarely obliged to articulate or defend, but which predispose them to expectations that racial differences have deep meaning. "So the literature is replete with descriptive findings of differences in race which bank on a shared sense of the essential differences . . . , which are never, ever brought up for any kind of discussion—and that's very problematic."[62] In short, in the society we live in, if we chop up the data in a way that causes a racial difference to emerge, then it becomes practically impossible *not* to see it as meaningful.

A pragmatically inclined reader might acknowledge my objections and still side with Ian Hacking. Such a reader might say, Who cares, ultimately, if race is an arbitrary way of dividing up the population? If it proves predictive in a statistical sense—if the knowledge that a person belongs to a racial group, however defined, helps us differentiate that person's diagnosis or treatment—then why not use that information, and bracket the question of *why* it works (let alone the question of what race "really is")? In my view, this position is not unreasonable, but the point is that those who hold to it do so on the pragmatic assumption that adopting it brings a clear benefit. My concern is that the overall dangers from racial profiling—to patients and to the society as a whole—may outweigh the benefits, in which case the appeal to pragmatism loses force. There are a series of such dangers, and I devote the remainder of this chapter to spelling them out.

The Problems with Profiling

Improper treatment. Racial profiling poses the serious risk of improper medical treatment of a patient who doesn't conform to the stereotype that pertains to his or her group. Even when we leave aside all the troublesome questions about how racial or ethnic group membership is defined in the first place—How do we handle those who are biracial or multiracial? Do "Hispanics" form a race? What about the differences between, say, Africans, African Americans, and Afro-Caribbeans?—can we really be certain that we will do the patient a favor by treating him or her as a representative member of the group? It is important to bear in mind that all claims of racial and ethnic differences in diagnosis or treatment are statements about differences on average, not hard-and-fast differences between groups. Indeed, many of the reported racial and ethnic differences appear to involve considerable overlap in response across racial or ethnic groups. Keh-Ming Lin, director of UCLA's Research Center on the Psychobiology of Ethnicity, has warned:

> Data suggestive of ethnic/racial differences could be easily misunderstood if and when interpreted in a simplistic manner. Statistical differences in the *means* are often misunderstood as indicating *absolute* differences. As a result, intra-group variability and overlaps across groups are neglected. Such misunderstanding could potentially lead to grave clinical conse-quences. For example, clinicians who learned that Asians tend to respond

to lower doses of neuroleptics may routinely prescribe only low doses of the medicine to *all* Asian patients, and by doing this fail to adequately treat a portion of their Asian patients whose drug response pattern may fall into the range that is similar to the majority of non-Asian patients.[63]

When individual cases are widely dispersed in relation to the mean, then the overlap between groups might actually be more meaningful than the differences between their averages. For example, one meta-analysis of data from fifteen clinical trials of antihypertensive drugs impressively found that even though whites on average responded better to beta-blockers and ACE inhibitors than blacks did, and blacks on average responded better to diuretics and calcium-channel blockers than whites did, overall 80 to 95 percent of blacks and whites had similar responses to these various drugs (see fig. 3). The author concluded that "race has little value in predicting antihypertensive drug response, because whites and blacks overlap greatly in their response to all categories of drugs."[64] In such cases, following rigid prescribing rules on the basis of a patient's racial identity could consign many patients to inferior treatment.[65]

Dubious associations between race and medical outcomes. Another way in which racial profiling in medical research and treatment could cause harm is by creating a tendency to routinely uncover questionable associations between race and medical outcomes. The risk here is related to Robert Schwartz's denunciation of "tax-supported trolling of data bases to find racial distinctions in human biology." By promoting subgroup comparisons by race and ethnicity, the NIH and FDA policies that make up the inclusion-and-difference paradigm have the inevitable effect of spurring the discovery of racial and ethnic difference findings. As biostatisticians critical of excessive subgroup analyses have emphasized, "the more questions asked of a set of data, the more likely it will yield some statistically significant difference even if the treatments are in fact equivalent."[66] (Following Duster, one could predict that if the NIH Revitalization Act had called for subgroup comparisons between Chicagoans and Angelinos, the medical literature would now be replete with findings of "city differences.") A classic example of this problem was offered by the British statistician Richard Peto and his collaborators in a large trial comparing therapies to treat heart attacks. The authors noted that subdividing the sample by the patients' astrological sign would yield the false conclusion that those born under Gemini or Libra are harmed by aspirin therapy, while those born under all other astrological signs benefited.[67] Particularly when a study results in a negative finding, the temptation can

FIG. 3 OVERLAP IN DRUG RESPONSE BETWEEN WHITE AND BLACK
PATIENTS WITH HYPERTENSION

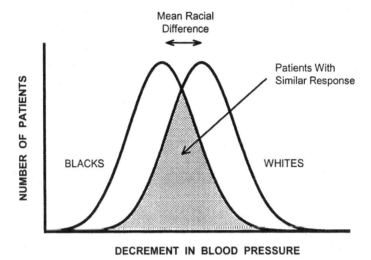

DECREMENT IN BLOOD PRESSURE

Source: Ashwini R. Sehgal, "Overlap between Whites and Blacks in Response to
Antihypertensive Drugs," *Hypertension* 43 (March 2004): 567.

be overwhelming to engage in post hoc subgroup analysis—that is, to
salvage some good news by finding a subgroup that experienced a benefit.
The problem, as described by one journal editor, is that such a subgroup
inevitably can be found, but its apparent difference is simply a result of
chance.[68]

Biostatisticians also warn that subgroup analyses of the data-trolling
sort are often disconfirmed by subsequent research. For example, a post
hoc analysis of the "non-white" subgroup of participants in a study comparing aspirin to the drug ticlopidine concluded that "ticlopidine is superior to aspirin for stroke prevention in non-whites."[69] Ten years later,
the African American Antiplatelet Stroke Prevention Study was stopped
prematurely when the data and safety monitoring board determined that
there was less than a one percent chance that ticlopidine would prove superior to aspirin in preventing recurrent stroke or major vascular events.
In the interval, if African Americans were given ticlopidine on the belief
that it was a superior treatment in their case, then they would have received the therapy with the greater potential to cause serious side effects.[70]
At an NIH conference in 2003, Lewis Kuller, the chair of epidemiology
at the University of Pittsburgh Graduate School of Public Health, pointed
to other examples of misleading findings from subgroup analyses, includ-

ing an incorrect claim that obesity is not linked to type 2 diabetes in blacks.[71]

Market incentives that may harm patients. Racial profiling may also create new opportunities for profit-making within the health sector, in ways that may work to the detriment of patients. There are a number of ways by which this can happen. First, several investigators whom I interviewed expressed worries that reports of racial differences in treatment effects could "collude with" other biases, as Keh-Ming Lin expressed it, in such a way as to provide people of color with less expensive but inferior products. "When you study the prescription pattern," said Lin, "there is always a tendency for African Americans—or patients from the public sector—to receive cheaper drugs, and so if you interpret some of the data stereotypi-cally, [the treatment data and the prescribing tendency] could go together and cause even more damage."[72] Similarly, Elijah Saunders, an expert on hypertension in African Americans, while claiming that racial differences in treatment response are real, nonetheless emphasized the importance of reminding "people that [African Americans] still should get [newer] drugs when they're indicated, and they should not be relegated to the . . . drugs that are cheaper, drugs that may get a good response but have loads of side effects which can lead to noncompliance."[73]

Alternatively, pharmaceutical companies may try to use reports of racial differences in the effects of medications to their financial advan-tage, in ways that may not be consistent with the public interest. For example, a 1993 report by the National Pharmaceutical Council, an in-dustry trade group, warned that cost containment strategies associated with managed care, such as the use of restrictive "formularies" (lists of drugs covered under a health insurance plan) or the mandatory use of generic drugs, might be particularly harmful to certain racial or ethnic groups. Such policies are based on the principle "that related medicines having the same general effect are almost identical in their actions and are therefore interchangeable." But "equivalent" drugs are not identical, and if, for example, they are cleared from the body by different enzymes, then individuals with genetic polymorphisms for those enzymes may in fact do better with one drug than another. And if those genetic polymor-phisms are unequally distributed in the population, then the insistence on standardized prescribing practices in the name of cost efficiency may unjustly sentence a racial or ethnic group to an inferior or ineffective therapy.[74] Nine years later, the author of this report, Richard Levy, was a coauthor of a similar report published in the *Journal of the National Medical Association* (the African American physicians' group), arguing against the restrictions on choice of pharmaceuticals built into many managed care plans, especially for an increasing number of patients on Medicare. The authors wrote, "There is good evidence to show that therapeutic substitution of drugs within the same class places minority patients at greater risk. This is because effectiveness and toxicity can vary among racial and ethnic groups."[75]

There may indeed be circumstances in which patients and doctors would be better off with greater freedom to choose among pharmaceutical drugs. However, it is difficult not to notice that such policy changes would also provide a boost to the profit margins of the pharmaceutical industry. Drug companies have been criticized for their emphasis on patenting and promoting "me-too drugs" that are substantially similar to products already on the market and for fighting to protect their expensive, name-brand medications against less expensive, generic substitutes.[76] Similarly, in 2003, when Congress sought to promote research on the cost-effectiveness of top-selling drugs, spokespersons for the Pharmaceutical Research and Manufacturers of America (PhRMA), the leading industry lobbying group, objected strenuously. Such studies, they argued, would indicate only which drugs were most cost-effective on average, while missing the benefit that some drugs might have for subgroups of the population, such as racial minorities.[77] Here, too, the strategic use of claims of racial difference rebounds to the benefit of the industry while increasing the overall costs of health care.

Another telling example of drug-company profit-making via racial profiling is provided by the case of BiDil, the first so-called ethnic drug to be approved in the United States. As Jonathan Kahn has described, "BiDil became an ethnic drug through the interventions of law and commerce as much as through medical understanding of biological differences that correlate with racial groups."[78] A compound of two previous pharmaceutical products, BiDil failed to demonstrate efficacy against heart failure in the overall population but was reinvented as an ethnic drug after a subgroup analysis of the clinical trial revealed that it provided benefit to the African Americans in the study sample. At that point, in what a science writer has called "a feat of creative repackaging," the company NitroMed launched a study exclusively in self-identified African Americans;[79] on the basis of a positive result, the drug was licensed in 2005.[80]

While the original patent would have expired in 2007—leaving the company only two years to earn a profit before competitors could enter the market—the reclassification of BiDil as a drug for African Americans permitted the company to obtain a new patent good through 2020. Upon acquiring the new patent, NitroMed went public, raising $66 million.[81]

And thus, as Gregg Bloche concluded in an editorial in the *New England Journal of Medicine*, "the emergence of the combination treatment as a race-specific drug was driven in large measure by regulatory and market incentives."[82] Moreover, although the FDA approved the product for use only in African Americans, U.S. physicians are permitted to prescribe any drug "off label" if they so choose—and the trial investigators have been quick to suggest that it is likely that BiDil has efficacy in people of any race.[83] Hence, the ability to patent a drug as race-specific will provide NitroMed with a much longer opportunity to profit from sales of its drug to the general population.[84] Indeed, the *New York Times* reported that "Wall Street is factoring use of the drug by people of other races into its forecasts for BiDil. Analysts' sales predictions range from $500 million to $1 billion by 2010."[85]

That other companies are savvy about the possibilities inherent in race-based marketing is suggested by the story of AIDSVAX, a once-promising AIDS vaccine developed by the biotech company VaxGen.[86] In 2003 VaxGen reported the disappointing news: 5.8 percent of the recipients of a placebo had become infected over the course of the trial, compared to 5.7 percent of the vaccine recipients—that is, the vaccine failed to have any impact.[87] But rather than admit defeat, the company played what an article about AIDSVAX in *Scientific American* referred to as "the race card."[88] VaxGen announced that the vaccine had been efficacious for the blacks, Asians, and other minorities enrolled in the trial: only 3.7 percent of them became infected, as compared to 9.9 percent of the minority controls. Immediately some experts leaped at the possibility that a magic bullet had been found for the skyrocketing HIV infection rate in the developing world. "We have to answer the questions," said José Esparza, a vaccine expert for the United Nations, "Why only in blacks? Would this vaccine work in Africa?" Meanwhile, AIDS treatment advocacy organizations criticized the claims of race-specific efficacy as "grossly premature."[89] Statisticians pored over the data, and some months later, an NIH official reported that the subgroup differences were "likely spurious."[90] According to an AIDS expert at Emory University's School of Medicine, "It was a desperate act by a company that was trying to save a failed product. . . . If they really cared about racial and ethnic differences, they would have structured a very different trial."[91]

In the examples of BiDil and AIDSVAX, the presumed beneficiaries of clinical attention to difference are racial and ethnic minorities, and the focus on race has been defended in those terms. Yet it is equally possible that the "BiDil strategy"—getting a drug approved by demonstrating its efficacy in a racial subgroup—may incline drug companies toward the outright *exclusion* of racial and ethnic minorities in clinical trials of some drugs. After all, if it is now deemed sufficient for drug approval to demonstrate efficacy in one group—and if there should be evidence suggesting that whites may be the most responsive to a given drug—then why not test it just in whites, the group that, after all, constitutes the largest market in the United States? In 2006 health activists realized this was no idle concern, when they learned that Schering-Plough was excluding African Americans from a Phase 2 trial of an experimental combination therapy to treat hepatitis C. African Americans are thought to respond poorly to many anti–hepatitis C treatments, including one of those used in the combination, and this consideration appeared to drive Schering-Plough's testing strategy. The irony, however, is that African Americans disproportionately suffer from hepatitis C. A coalition of advocacy groups sent a strong letter of protest to the FDA, expressing "outrage" at the exclusion and demanding that it "not set a precedent for future trials of other investigational agents."[92] Schering-Plough dismissed the criticism and promised that blacks would be included in the later, Phase 3 trials. But activists were not mollified. "We would understand if the exclusion was about safety," commented James Learned of the Hepatitis C Action and Advocacy Coalition, observing that instead the company's goal appeared to be that of generating "buzz."[93] The group issued a press release stating: "It is clear to us that Schering-Plough chose to exclude an entire racial group from the study to achieve the best efficacy results possible on the road to marketing the drug."[94]

Racial profiling as a permanent "temporary" solution. Criticism of racial profiling is often deflected by characterizing it as just a temporary measure—when that is not likely to be the case. The argument runs as follows: Phenotypic race serves as a proxy for underlying genetic differences in disease and treatment, and thus we need to take race into account "during our period of ignorance of the underlying causal factors."[95]

But in the not-too-distant future (it is claimed), profiling will be made obsolete by the new science of pharmacogenomics, which will permit truly individualized drug therapy according to each person's specific genetic polymorphisms. Doctors then will perform genetic tests before prescribing medications, in order to determine which particular drugs in which doses are most likely to be of maximum efficacy and minimum toxicity, given any individual patient's genetic profile.[96] "Knowing what's in your genes could . . . take some of the routine guesswork out of medicine," was how *Time* magazine expressed the promise of these techniques.[97] It could also go a good distance toward reducing so-called adverse drug reactions, many of which may be caused by drug company reliance on one-size-fits-all dosing.

In the terms of my analysis in this book, pharmacogenomics offers the hope of replacing the "standard human" not with a group-specific "niche standardization," but rather with a fully individualized or personalized medical practice—the opposite extreme from the logic of one size fits all. The distinction between niche standardization and individualized treatment is sometimes blurred by defenders of profiling, who gain rhetorical mileage by referring to the former as an "individualized" approach.[98] (Indeed, a news article in *Science* magazine on the approval of BiDil suggested that the FDA was thereby giving "another push to pharmacogenomics."[99]) But advocates are clear that a presumed virtue of pharmacogenomics is its ability to get us beyond the group. As a commentary in *Nature Genetics* expressed it, pharmacogenomics is "more than skin deep."[100] Or as an article on the pharmacogenomics of hypertension proposed: "Rather than empirically treating hypertension based on clinical experience and broad generalizations regarding such demographics as ethnicity or age, physicians eventually may perform genotyping of their patients, perhaps enabling identification of not only specific hereditary mechanisms of a patient's disease, but also more specific and rational therapies for that individual."[101] Opponents of racial profiling such as Craig Venter therefore argue that pharmacogenomics is the preferred strategy, for which profiling provides no reasonable substitute. As he and a coauthor wrote in *Science* in 2003, "Rather than reifying race by perpetuating its use as a variable, we encourage the practice of individualized medicine."[102] Meanwhile, proponents of profiling justify it as the logical next-best-thing until pharmacogenomic testing is widely available. For example, Sally Satel has written that "doctors look forward to the day when they can, in good conscience, be colorblind [and when] racial profiling by doctors won't be necessary. Until then, however, group identity at least offers a starting point."[103]

Pharmacogenomics is high on the agenda at the FDA, where experts speak of individualization as the "third great age of drug development," following upon previous successes in addressing first safety and then efficacy.[104] In 2005 the agency approved the first laboratory test to perform genotyping of patients for the purpose of selecting appropriate medications.[105] And at the NIH, the National Institute of General Medical Science has awarded grants to establish a Pharmacogenetic Research Network—a national consortium of research groups working to create a public database of genetic variation in response to therapies.[106] However, as Adam Hedgecoe has described, pharmacogenomics at present remains as much hype as hope, and we are far from the day when affordable genotyping will be regularly available in the average clinic, even in wealthy nations.[107] Indeed, a report by the United Kingdom's Royal Society in 2005 warned that "it will be at least 15 to 20 years before a patient's genetic make-up is a major factor in determining which drugs they are prescribed."[108]

The crucial questions, then, are what happens in the interim, and what predictions can be made about the future. Certainly, for quite some time, it is likely that the promise of pharmacogenomics will be a dream deferred, in which case the presumed rough correspondence between genetic polymorphisms and categories of racial belonging will be invoked to justify a continued reliance on racial profiling. But even in the long run, it is far from certain that pharmacogenomics will displace a concern with race. As Morris Foster and coauthors have observed, notions of racial and ethnic difference are already firmly embedded within the logic of pharmacogenomic research: "Because many pharmacogenetic studies use social classifications such as race and ethnicity as criteria for recruiting participants and as analytical variables in interpreting research results, these social classifications will likely continue to play a significant role in drug development and marketing."[109] Even more significantly, many commentators in the worlds of both research and industry have noted that, "from the industry perspective, the subdivision of a market into smaller markets is hardly ideal,"[110] and have questioned whether pharmaceutical companies will find it profitable to develop and market drugs at the level of genotypic difference. According to Robert Temple, a high official at the FDA's Center for Drug Evaluation and Research, "It's not absolutely clear to me that drug companies *want* to narrow the population that can get their drug. So it remains to be seen how vigorously that will be pursued."[111]

As Troy Duster sees it, the implications of those financial pressures are clear: "The mantra of pharmacogenomics is that drugs will be fine-tuned for the individual . . . , but individuals are not a market. Groups are a market."[112] Hence, it is entirely possible that the reliance on race-based prescribing will only be solidified in coming years. If so, then the claim that racial profiling is being used only as a short-term stopgap— and therefore we need not worry overmuch about its limitations—is false reassurance. Again quoting Duster: "Race is such a dominant category in the cognitive field that the 'interim solution' can leave its own indelible mark once given even the temporary imprimatur of scientific legitimacy by molecular genetics."[113]

Inaccurate and problematic understandings of race. Yet another problem with racial profiling is that it disguises the racial categorization problem, thereby encouraging misleading views of the nature of race. The history of racial ideologies is a history of attempts to argue that precise racial identities can be attributed to persons—that a color line can be drawn. Despite widespread awareness that racial "pure types" do not exist in the real world, racial profiling both presumes and reinforces a notion that each individual belongs to a category and can be diagnosed and treated accordingly. The convoluted logic that may follow from this proposition is well demonstrated by an example reported in the *Washington Post* concerning Elyse Frazier, a 56-year-old woman with heart failure who was enrolled in NitroMed's study of BiDil: "When research coordinator Jackie Rayford asked her if she might be interested in the study for African Americans, she was puzzled. She considered herself black in matters of politics, but it was not a question she had ever been asked before in a health context. Frazier's mother is half black, half Cherokee Indian. Her father is half black, half Blackfoot Indian." To resolve the dilemma, Rayford asked Frazier: "Do you consider yourself African American?" When she replied in the affirmative, Frazier was enrolled in the BiDil trial.[114] Needless to say, the findings from the trial were not taken to represent the effects of the medication in people who might be a bit of this and a bit of that, still less in people who consider themselves black in matters of politics. The trial presented conclusions about African Americans, presumed to be a distinct group. More problematically still, the marketing of an ethnic drug only reinforces the idea that blacks have inherent, presumably biological, characteristics that serve to distinguish them from all others. The complex sociopolitical processes by which someone might come to call herself African American are then thoroughly disguised from view.

Dangerously inaccurate understandings of the causes of health disparities. One final consequence of racial profiling merits attention: By clouding the relationship between the biological and the social, racial profiling interferes with our attempts to understand and eliminate health disparities. Defenses of racial profiling in medicine nearly always are set forth in biological terms, and a reliance on profiling inevitably "encourages the belief that race is a genetic category."[115] But when racial differences are attributed to biology and to genetics, what questions are left unasked? A wealth of evidence suggests that health differences between socially defined groups, such as races or ethnicities, are structured in powerful ways by social and cultural factors. Awareness of these factors is crucial for any serious attempt to address the problem of health disparities. The danger of the racial-differences discourse, as Sandra Soo-Jin Lee and coauthors have noted, is that it will "disguise other explanations of disparities." Meanwhile, "more and more diseases will be 'racialized,' and at the same time, the idea that racial differences exist and are inherent is reinforced."[116]

The point here is not that racial differences in health are *really* social and cultural *rather than* biological, or *really* environmental *rather than* genetic. Any either/or formulation would be equally problematic and would ignore the complexities of what it means to be an embodied person. Scholars have developed a range of theoretical approaches to thinking about this issue in a sophisticated way. For example, Nancy Krieger's "ecosocial" theory calls for "taking literally the notion of 'embodiment,' [to understand] how we literally incorporate biologically—from conception to death—our social experiences and express this embodiment in population patterns of health, disease, and well-being."[117] Similarly, in their call to move "beyond the binary trap," Pilar Ossorio and Troy Duster assert that "race is a set of social processes with biological feedbacks that require empirical investigation."[118] Approaching the problem from a somewhat different angle, Anne Fausto-Sterling has invoked "dynamics systems and developmental systems approaches" to develop an interactive model of how genes and environments come together in the production of human capabilities—a formulation that, as she puts it, permits us "to work with the idea that we are always 100 percent nature and 100 percent nurture."[119] This is the kind of complexity that is obscured by the practice of racial profiling and the proliferation of claims about biological and genetic racial differences. The problem of biological and genetic reductionism is particularly apparent in mass media discussions of race and genetics, which tend to reinforce popular understandings of genes as wholly determinative of developmental outcomes.[120]

In fact, numerous examples demonstrate that racial differences in health that typically are presumed to be genetic or otherwise biological may have more complex causes. One arena in which this is evident is in reports of the prevalence of diseases by racial group. For example, black people are often considered to have the highest rates of prostate cancer. However, according to two specialists, Oscar Streeter and Mack Roach, "it is noteworthy that Gambians from West Africa have the lowest rates, and blacks in Connecticut have lower rates than those who live in the state of Utah, which has very few blacks." Moreover, among Asians, it has been found that the incidence of prostate cancer increases upon migration to the United States.[121] Presumptions about inherent racial differences have inclined observers to attribute the poorer survival rates of African Americans with prostate and other forms of cancer to genetic differences, when in fact the issue may be one of suboptimal care and the co-occurrence of other diseases.[122] Another example is provided by hypertension, which frequently is asserted to be especially prevalent among black people because of physiological differences. But as Richard Cooper has observed, "a very sharp gradient of hypertension risk exists from 12 percent to 15 percent in rural Africa to about 35 percent in Chicago."[123] A growing body of work suggests the relation between life stresses and hypertension—including the stress associated with experiencing racism.[124] In addition to data on disease prevalence, mortality data also reveal considerable variation among people with the same African ancestry, suggesting the limitations of purely biological explanations. For example, a study of New York City death records found substantial differences in numbers of deaths from cancer between blacks born in the U.S. South and those born in the Caribbean. Indeed, Caribbean-born blacks had lower overall death rates from cancer than did whites in New York City. As the authors noted, genetic explanations for such differences pale in comparison to stark differences in diet, housing, and smoking rates.[125]

What about treatment differences? Can differences in the effects of taking medications be affected by anything other than biology? A study in 2003 found evidence that black patients with hypertension are less likely than whites to take their medications as prescribed—a finding that not only points to the presence of complex social factors in constructing racial disparities, but which also sounds an important caution about the interpretation of findings from clinical trials. When a subgroup difference is reported, is it because the same medication has different effects, or because medications are being consumed in different ways by different groups?[126] In another example, Tate and Goldstein have described how "one study found significant differences in response to treatment of childhood acute lymphoblastic leukemia among racial or ethnic groups, with greatest response in Asians, followed by Europeans, Hispanics and African Americans. Other investigators, however, found no difference in outcome when African Americans and Europeans Americans were given equal access to the most advanced therapies."[127]

As Gregg Bloche aptly noted in his editorial on BiDil in the New England Journal, the problem is not simply that "we have hardly begun to elucidate" the mechanisms by which "a miasma of psychosocial, economic, cultural, environmental, and other determinants affects human physiology in ways that are poorly understood"; more problematically still, the "focus on race as a genetic placeholder risks discouraging us from trying."[128] Biologically reductionist explanations, as Lundy Braun has noted, "naturalize racial and ethnic difference and create a conceptual barrier to developing a research program that explores the complex ways in which social inequality and experiences of racial discrimination interact with human biology to influence patterns of disease."[129] A crucial corollary to these arguments is that it makes no sense to throw out race as a variable in medical research, insofar as the social experience of race may have powerful bodily effects. The question is not whether to study race, but how to study it.[130]

Historical Parallels and Differences across Differences

By describing six potential unintended consequences of racial profiling in medicine, I have argued that the very "obviousness" of its utility is exactly what should cause us to slow down and ask questions.[131] One way to make sense of the problem is from the vantage point of history. In some respects, the repudiation of one-size-fits-all medicine, the substitution of what I have called niche standardization, and the adoption of profiling might seem like déjà vu—a return to the medical thinking of previous centuries. After all, as I described in chapter 2, the perception that members of different races are biologically incommensurate has been with us for quite a long time. However, what is crucial to observe is that these earlier assertions of medical difference were manifestly elitist and hierarchical and functioned to legitimize prejudice and reinforce social exclusions: it was in comparison to the European white male ideal that other bodily types typically were found wanting.

Thus, it needs to be said that history does not simply repeat itself, even if the present brings echoes of the past. After all, most modern-day defenders of attending to medical difference offer their arguments in ostensibly nonjudgmental fashion and would repudiate any link to racist or colonialist mentalities. If, for example, certain medications are deemed less likely to be efficacious in certain racial groups, few pharmacologists would invoke this fact as evidence for the innate biological superiority of some races over others. Indeed, as I have noted, representatives from within communities of color, such as the Association of Black Cardiologists, have embraced racial difference findings. And, as Fatimah Jackson has described, other African American scientists have pursued research on African Americans in domains such as genetics precisely to counter practices of exclusion in which whites have been taken to be the standard.[132]

Yet the debate over racial profiling demonstrates that concerns over the potentially harmful downstream effects of the medical reliance upon certain categories have by no means vanished in the present era. By tracing various potential consequences of racial profiling, I have argued that the philosophy of difference that lies behind the inclusion-and-difference paradigm can have deeply problematic consequences when applied in an uncritical fashion to an understanding of disease, health, and treatment. Those consequences may be experienced on the level of the individual patient, whose health may suffer; but they also may be felt at the level of the society, where the strengthening of a perception that race is biologically meaningful tends to legitimize social inequalities by naturalizing them, thus making it harder, rather than easier, to solve the problem of health disparities. These social consequences are primarily what distinguish this case from the more generic—and ultimately unavoidable—issue that medicine very often relies on probabilistic knowledge about groups that may not accurately characterize all of those groups' individual members.

I therefore find myself in deep sympathy with comments expressed in 1992 by Patricia King, who (with reference to blacks and whites) wrote about the "dangers of difference" in compelling terms: "An appropriate strategy should have as its starting point the defeasible presumption that blacks and whites are biologically the same with respect to disease and treatment. Presumptions can be overturned, of course, and the strategy should recognize the possibility that biological differences in some contexts are possible. But the presumption of equality acknowledges that historically the greatest harm has come from the willingness to impute biological differences rather than the willingness to overlook them."[133]

So far I have addressed these issues only with reference to race, because that is the category on which the medical profiling debate has focused. In the next chapter, I take up a parallel set of questions concerning the new biomedical research on sex and gender differences. In what ways are these two cases analogous in terms of the issues that they raise? In what ways is each one distinct?

CHAPTER ELEVEN

Sex Differences and the New Politics of Women's Health

The prescription drug terfenadine (sold as Seldane) was a modest break-through of recent pharmaceutical science: the first antihistamine not to cause drowsiness. In 1989, as pharmacology expert Raymond Woosley re-called, Seldane was selling briskly by prescription and was soon to be made available over the counter, when a woman in Bethesda, Maryland, who was taking the drug blacked out and ended up at Bethesda Naval Hospital. Physicians there detected a cardiac arrhythmia and wondered if it might be caused by an interaction between Seldane and another of her medi-cations. The physicians reported the potential "drug-drug interaction" to FDA officials, who then uncovered other such cases involving Seldane. FDA officials contacted Woosley, who had been studying a life-threatening drug toxicity called *torsades de pointes*, a form of arrhythmia associated with prolongation of the "QT interval" (the time period needed for the heart to recharge between beats). Thus, the stage was set for Seldane's eventual demise—it was formally taken off the market in 1998—but also for a spate of research by Woosley and others on the various medications associated with *torsades de pointes*.

In 1993 Woosley noticed something that had escaped his attention previously: about two-thirds of the cases of arrhythmia from Seldane and several other drugs were in female patients. "It was a bit embarrassing" not to have recognized the gender disparity earlier, said Woosley, "but we then started studying it." Soon the NIH's Office of Research on Women's Health and the FDA's Office on Women's Health had taken an interest and were supporting Woosley's efforts. It turned out that, after puberty, the QT interval becomes fractionally longer in women than in men—by about 20 milliseconds—perhaps because of effects of sex hormones on heart functioning. As a result, women are more vulnerable to medications that prolong the QT interval than are men, and therefore are more likely to experience, and sometimes die from, *torsades de pointes*.[1]

The sex difference in this case is not absolute: men are also vulnerable to drug-related arrhythmia. However, the link between women's elevated statistical risk and an observable physiological difference between the sexes (the length of the QT interval), along with the presence of a reasonable hypothesis about a sex-linked cause of that physiological difference (hormones), confers a powerful plausibility on the claim of a medically relevant sex difference. Nor are QT-prolonging drugs the only such example. In June 2005 *Science* magazine ran a special issue on women's health, featuring a series of articles, news reports, and commentaries on research into the health differences between females and males. A news report in the issue, entitled "Gender in the Pharmacy: Does It Matter?" suggested that the answer to that question more than occasionally was yes. For a variety of reasons, or for reasons unknown, the same medication might affect women and men differently—moreover, women might be more inclined to suffer the consequences in the form of increased risk of adverse drug reactions.[2]

Medically relevant biological difference findings by sex, like the corresponding difference findings by race, are both cause and consequence of the inclusion-and-difference paradigm. On one hand, advocates of change used early reports of such differences as one rationale for their proposed inclusionary reforms; and on the other hand, the establishment of new inclusionary policies and procedures for subgroup comparisons has resulted in the proliferation of difference findings. Thus, when Viviana Simon, Director of Scientific Programs at the Society for Women's Health Research, wrote an editorial for the special issue of *Science* about the "increasing awareness of significant biological and physiological differences between the sexes, beyond the reproductive ones," she attributed that awareness to the new "federal mandates" and the abandonment of "the old paradigm of the '70-kg white male'" as the normative patient.[3]

However, while new policies and regulations have resulted in findings about both sex differences and race differences, there is a noteworthy distinction to be drawn between the two cases: reports of biological difference by race have sparked a heated medical and public controversy about "racial profiling," but no corresponding debate seems to have arisen as yet with regard to biological differences by sex. A few commentators have suggested that "gender in the pharmacy" is not the problem it is made out to be, because most drugs have a relatively wide "therapeutic index"—that is, a substantial margin of safety between the effective dose and the toxic dose in each individual.[4] And Sally Satel, the inveterate critic of "political correctness" in medicine, has responded with a "not so fast" to what she calls the medical slogan of "Vive la Différence."[5] But for the most part, there has been little public discussion of the merits or risks of "sex profiling" in medicine—indeed, the phrase does not even exist.[6]

To what extent, if any, is the case of biological differences by sex or gender analogous to that of biological differences by race and ethnicity? What does it mean that racial profiling in medicine has become an intellectual battleground while sex profiling has not? These questions have received little direct discussion.[7] To the limited extent that analysts (in academia and elsewhere) have addressed the comparison, it has been to contrast the "tricky" case of race with the "easy" case of sex: obviously men and women are biologically different, while racial difference at the biological level—and even the determination of which racial categories to work with or whether "race" exists at all—is contested terrain. Thus (the argument goes), while choosing a medication on the basis of the patient's sex may be sensible and commendable, making such determinations according to race is deeply problematic. Even those who differ on the merits of racial profiling, such as the philosophers of science Ian Hacking and Michael Root, are in agreement when it comes to this point. Hacking has observed that "many medical differences between males and females are uniform, but medical differences between races are almost always only statistical."[8] Root has warned that some seek to endow racial profiling with legitimacy via the suggestion that racial differences in medicine have the same status as sex differences. In opposition to this appeal for legitimation, Root makes a careful argument about "the differences between the categories of race and sex":

> A gene X that regulates drug metabolism can vary with a gene Y on a sex chromosome, but there is no race chromosome or race gene Y for X to vary with. As a result, doctors have a reason to study sex differences but not racial differences in drug response and a reason to use sex but not race as a proxy for response when deciding how best to treat an individual patient. Sex has more explanatory and predictive power in the clinic because there are genes for sex and good reasons to believe that the genes for sex and some genes for drug metabolism are concordant.[9]

As the views of Root and others suggest, many critics of racial profiling in medicine have engaged in "boundary work," erecting a wall between sex and race in order to designate the study of sex differences as good science and the study of race differences as bad science.[10] Is this boundary work a problem, or is it commendable?

Certainly, the biological significance of sex and race are quite different cases. It is true that females as a class are biologically different from males as a class in easily identifiable respects. It also appears true that men and women *on average* are biologically different in a number of well-known as well as less obvious respects. To the degree that Hacking, Root, and others are correct about the differences across types of difference, then the tendency of the policies of the inclusion-and-difference paradigm to treat all forms of difference in a standardized way—to "flatten" or commensurate differences, as I described in chapter 7—deserves critical scrutiny.

However, it immediately bears saying that biological sex is *not* an either/or—not at the anatomic, the hormonal, or the chromosomal levels. There are no truly dichotomous variables in nature, and, as many scholars have shown, there is no precise or fully satisfactory biological means of demarcating all males from all females.[11] And if so, then the problems associated with profiling—such as the risk of treating individuals improperly on the basis of their group affiliations—may apply to medical research on sex differences, too, and not just to research on differences by race.

THE NEW MEANINGS OF SEX DIFFERENCES

In this chapter, my expository strategy is to follow the general logic of the previous chapter on race. After considering the plethora of reports of biological sex differences in medicine in recent years, I will describe the emergence and development of a movement calling for "sex-based biology" (or "gender-specific medicine"), and I will locate it in relation to other recent research on the biology and genetics of sex difference. While sex-based biology has not provoked a debate analogous to that over racial profiling, it is implicated within the tensions that have emerged between sectors of the broader women's health movement, and I will analyze what is at stake in those strategic disagreements. Then, I will proceed one-by-one through the various critiques that I launched at racial profiling in the previous chapter. In each case, I will ask whether and to what degree the critique might also apply to the case of sex profiling.

The Explosion of Difference Findings

Emphasis on sex differences in medicine is part of a larger trend toward claiming or assuming the overriding significance of biology and genetics in understanding the behavior of males and females, in domains ranging from brain functioning to mating behavior.[12] As with race, arguments about sex differences drawn from genetics can cut both ways, and occasionally reports of fundamental genetic similarities make their way into public view. For example, in 2001 *The Scientist* magazine reported: "Genetic studies are revealing that men and women are more similar than distinct. So far, of the approximately 31,000 genes in the human genome, men and women differ only in the two sex chromosomes, X and Y, and only a few dozen genes seem to be involved." However, the notion that our usual distinction between "pink and blue" might be replaced with "a blurred rainbow of confusion"—as the article's author put it—runs up against the vast wave of commentary that assumes or reports on stark differences between the sexes.[13]

Nowhere is the attention to biological sex differences more pronounced at present than in biomedicine, and the concern with the effects of pharmaceutical drugs is an especially important example. An interesting aspect of the case of Seldane is that it concerns a group-specific difference related not to the more typical issue of the *pharmacokinetics* of a medication (how it is metabolized, absorbed, and ultimately cleared from the body) but rather to *pharmacodynamics* (the actual effects of a medication on bodily organs and processes). Over the course of the 1990s, a range of reports in the medical literature described differences in drug effects of both sorts, building on earlier research dating back to the early 1970s. A review in 2001 by pharmacologist Mary Berg noted a wide variety of sex- or gender-related differences, significantly including the effect of oral contraceptives in increasing or decreasing the speed of clearance of drugs such as aspirin, caffeine, and morphine. Berg also described research in "chronopharmacology"—the effect of bodily rhythms, such as the menstrual cycle, on how drugs are processed.[14] Another review essay—by Monica Gandhi and coauthors, published in 2004—attributed pharmacokinetic differences by sex not only to variation in the cytochrome P450 enzymes but also to a number of other factors, including body weight and gastric emptying time.[15] Gandhi and coauthors also discussed the burgeoning literature on sex differences in response to pain medications (believed to reflect differences in how men and women actually experience pain), as well as the evidence on differences in the effects and side effects of antipsychotic and antidepressant medications.[16] Antiviral drugs targeting HIV have provided yet another important example: women appear to have more frequent and more severe side effects with several classes of anti-HIV medications, though some research also indicates that such drugs may also be more efficacious for women in terms of keeping the virus in check.[17]

"We now know that gender is one of the most important factors that influences and predicts response to all kinds of treatments," FDA Commissioner Mark McClellan said in 2003 in a speech at a Society for Women's Health Research event. "The FDA is working to better define the genetic differences between men and women that influence how they are going to respond to a particular medication."[18] Indeed, research on these various differences in the effects of medications has been a priority at the various women's health offices, which have organized conferences and developed research agendas.[19] A particular concern has been the issue of adverse drug reactions, estimated by the FDA to affect women at least one and a half times as often as men.[20] In April 2004 the Agency for Healthcare Research and Quality (a DHHS agency) held a two-day meeting of experts to consider the problem of adverse drug reactions and to focus on the goal of "Improving the Use and Safety of Medications in Women through Sex/Gender and Race/Ethnicity Analysis."[21]

The growing literature on biological sex differences in medicine extends beyond the important issue of pharmacology to include attention to many other kinds of differences in biological processes with health implications. According to the "statement of editorial purpose" of an electronic journal devoted to women's health research, "It is increasingly evident that sex-based differences exist in a range of conditions, including heart disease, cancer, stroke, depression, HIV/AIDS, autoimmune disorders, neurologic diseases, bone and joint disorders, as well as in reactions to drugs."[22] Heart function and cardiovascular disease provide an excellent example, as the case of Seldane already has suggested. According to an editorial published in *Cardiovascular Research* in 2004 (entitled "A Radical Idea: Men and Women Are Different"), "gender has a pronounced influence on the type and severity of cardiovascular disease that will likely ensue during one's lifetime. Sex differences have been noted in most major cardiovascular diseases including coronary heart disease, stroke, and hypertension."[23] Women also tend to develop heart disease at a later age than do men, and women and men are reported to have different symptoms prior to heart attacks—indeed, the canonical symptom of chest pain "was notably absent or was described differently by the women," according to research reported in 2004.[24] Women are more likely than men to have a hidden form of coronary disease;[25] and women with coronary artery disease and implantable cardioverter-defibrillators also have been reported to develop a form of arrhythmia more often than do men with the device.[26] As described in a recent article in *Science* on the "Molecular and Cellular Basis of Cardiovascular Gender Differences," many of these differences may be linked to hormones, and some may be traced to developmental pathways laid down *in utero*.[27]

Given the story told in this book, perhaps the most interesting of the recent cardiovascular difference findings concerns the protective effects of aspirin. In chapters 4 and 5, I described how the Physicians' Health Study, a randomized trial of low-dose aspirin to prevent heart attacks, tested in male doctors over 40, became a *cause célèbre* in the congressional debate over women's health research and a prime example in the General Accounting Office's damning report in 1990 on the underrepresentation of women in clinical trials. While the Physicians' Health Study demonstrated the efficacy of aspirin for men, it left open the question of whether the finding could be extrapolated to women. However, the investigators were by no means unaware of this issue, and they launched a separate study with 40,000 female participants, called the Women's Health Study. In March 2005 the verdict finally was in: although aspirin protected women from a major form of stroke—something that had not been demonstrated in the trials in men—it failed to prevent the occurrence of first heart attacks in women younger than 65.[28] As an editorialist commented in the issue of the *New England Journal of Medicine* that reported the study's findings, this "difference between the sexes in the cardiovascular response to aspirin . . . is at once a puzzle and a coda to the recent crescendo of demands that clinical research must always be organized to account for the biologic differences between women and men."[29] Newspapers around the country ran the story on the front page. The Associated Press called it a "stunning example" of "polar opposite" medical findings by sex, while the *Washington Post* concluded that the study added "powerful new evidence to the growing body of data showing that men and women differ in fundamental ways on various aspects of health, and that research on men does not necessarily translate directly to women."[30]

The Philosophy of Sex-Based Biology

On April 25, 2001, the Institute of Medicine (IOM) of the National Academy of Sciences announced the forthcoming publication of a book-length report entitled *Exploring the Biological Contributions to Human Health: Does Sex Matter?* This 288-page volume was the product of a lengthy review by a sixteen-member panel of experts, and it was sponsored by a range of government agencies, advocacy groups, and pharmaceutical companies. The report answered the rhetorical question—"Does sex matter?"—emphatically in the affirmative: "Sex does matter. It matters in ways that we did not expect. Undoubtedly, it also matters in ways that we have not begun to imagine."[31] Calling for medical researchers to study sex differences "from womb to tomb," the panel reviewed the literature on sex differences in the efficacy of pharmaceutical drugs, sex differences in the etiology and pathogenesis of autoimmune conditions, sex differences in the experiencing of pain, sex differences in coronary heart disease, and so on. The panel also offered a raft of recommendations, including the quite radical one that researchers should "determine and disclose the sex of origin of biological research materials" and that "journals editors should encourage researchers . . . to specify the extent to which analyses of the data by sex were included in the study."[32]

By coincidence, the announcement of the IOM report preceded by only about a week the publication in the *New England Journal* of Robert Schwartz's editorial on racial profiling.[33] But where reports of medically relevant biological differences by race provoked controversy, the IOM report seemed almost universally to be praised. For example, in a 15-minute segment on the *NewsHour with Jim Lehrer*, the story was presented straightforwardly as an episode in the forward march of medical knowledge.[34] Particularly keen to promote the IOM's conclusions was the Society for Women's Health Research (SWHR), one of the groups that had sponsored the report. In the early 1990s, the SWHR had coalesced around the goal of inclusion of women in research and had campaigned for the NIH Revitalization Act. By the late 1990s, the Society's raison d'être was the furtherance of research on differences between men and women that bore medical significance. "This report substantiates everything we've been saying for six years," Phyllis Greenberger, the president of SWHR, told the press. "Many scientists see the emphasis on sex and gender differences as a passing fad, reflecting some kind of political agenda. But the Institute of Medicine has validated this as an important field of research."[35] Sometime later, at a conference sponsored by the NIH's Office of Research on Women's Health, Sherry Marts, the SWHR's scientific director, repeated the rhetorical question in the report's subtitle and suggested that the most pithy executive summary to the report might be the single word *yes*.[36]

The SWHR has been a key proponent of a social movement within biomedicine on which the IOM report conferred crucial legitimacy.[37] Along with academic medical researchers, NIH scientists, and scientists at pharmaceutical companies invested in women's health, the SWHR has sought to establish a new field of study known as "gender-based biology" or (more recently, in an attempt to clarify their interest in what they understand to be biological and not social processes) "sex-based biology." Others, such as the cardiologist Marianne Legato at Columbia University, have used the term "gender-specific medicine." As distinct from more generic proposals for the development of a women's health specialty in medicine, advocates of sex-based biology emphasize fundamental, thoroughgoing, biological differences between men's and women's bodies, from the heart to the brain to the immune system. Those who subscribe to this movement believe that women—and men—deserve separate medical scrutiny because they are biologically different at the level of the cell, the organ, the system, and the organism.[38] Indeed, one of the chief rhetorical strategies of its proponents is to insist on physiological sites of difference that seem far removed from parts of the body traditionally coded as "female" or "male." As Florence Haseltine, the NIH scientist who was central to the founding of SWHR and who claims credit for the invention of the term "gender-based biology," told me, "I always say the liver is the sexiest organ." She meant by this that men's and women's livers metabolize medications at different rates because of differences that affect the presence and function of metabolizing enzymes.[39] Marianne Legato's organ of choice is the heart, though she also has written on gender dimorphism in the brain and a variety of other sites of bodily difference.[40]

On its Web site, the SWHR defines *sex-based biology* as "the study of biological and physiological differences between men and women." The organization notes: "Sex differences have been found everywhere from the composition of bone matter and the experience of pain to the metabolism of certain drugs and the rate of neurotransmitter synthesis in the brain. Sex-based biology has revolutionized the way that the scientific community views the sexes."[41] Sex-based biology first became the topic of a national meeting in 1995, when this society made it the theme of its Scientific Advisory Meeting.[42] The journal published by the Society, the *Journal of Women's Health*, also has served as an important forum for the dissemination of this agenda.[43] Since the mid-1990s, the term *sex-based biology* and its variants have surfaced in a wide range of settings, and diverse collection of actors have gathered beneath its banner. This includes not only researchers who convene at conferences organized by SWHR, but also researchers and other representatives from many of the leading pharmaceutical companies. According to Sherry Marts, an irony of the term's growing ubiquity is the erasure of its origins: "This phrase keeps coming up and Phyllis [Greenberger] gets a little frustrated; she says, 'They aren't giving us any credit. Don't they know we invented that?' And I say, 'Phyllis, this is what we want. We want it to be a household word.' . . . In effect, you want people to forget who invented it, because by then you know it's out there."[44] To be sure, the SWHR's goals extend well beyond the simple diffusion of the concept. "In another 10 years," Marts told a reporter for *The Scientist*, sex-based biology "is going to be like neuroscience, [which] started out as a few physiologists and a few biochemists, and pretty soon you've got a core group that's really moving the field forward. Then folks start to realize that this is actually something you can build a career on."[45]

In 1997 Marianne Legato opened up what a reporter described as a "second front in the movement,"[46] founding the Partnership for Women's Health at Columbia University (renamed the Partnership for Gender-Specific Medicine in 2002). The Partnership also puts out an academic journal, the *Journal of Gender-Specific Medicine* (renamed *Gender Medicine* in 2004), and has published a medical textbook on the principles of gender-specific medicine.[47] Legato also has founded an Association for Gender-Specific Medicine,[48] which helped organize the First World Congress on Gender-Specific Medicine in Berlin in 2006.[49] Meanwhile, across the country at Stanford, the university's medical school has revamped its women's health program to include attention to research on sex-based biology. The Web site of "Women's Health @ Stanford" asserts: "When it comes to the way our bodies fight off and process disease, sex truly does matter."[50]

The ORWH also has provided important institutional backing to the emphasis on sex-based biology. In 2000 the agency cosponsored a program, called Building Interdisciplinary Research Careers in Women's Health, that funds universities to recruit junior researchers to the study of medically relevant sex differences.[51] The following year, the ORWH advertised a new funding initiative, cosponsored by the NIH and the FDA for $11 million dollars per year for five years, the creation of "Specialized Centers of Research on Sex and Gender Factors Affecting Women's Health," designed to "develop a research agenda bridging basic and clinical research on sex/gender factors underlying a priority health issue."[52] Advocacy groups have kept up the pressure to institutionalize sex-based biology within the DHHS. For example, the SWHR has combed the database of NIH-funded grants to prepare a report on the funding of research into sex differences by the different NIH institutes, and it has used the findings to push for increased efforts by those institutes perceived as lagging.[53] In a noteworthy victory for the Society, the Senate Appropriations Committee, at the urging of the SWHR, placed "report language" in its version of the fiscal 2005 funding bill that urged the NIH to "include sex-based biology as an integral part" of research conducted as part of a transinstitute initiative on brain research.[54]

As Peter Keating and Alberto Cambrosio have observed, "biomedicine does not have a stable division of labor corresponding to an unproblematic partition of the object of work, namely the human body." While many specialties are formed with reference to an organ or system, others are defined by bodily functions, life stages, occupation, or other criteria.[55] This variety of ways in which specialties may emerge and be defined leaves the door open for all sorts of medical innovations to become institutionalized over time. By midway through the first decade of the twenty-first century, there were many signs that sex-based biology was on its way to becoming, if not a full-fledged specialty, then at least an established and entrenched intellectual movement within the biomedical sciences and within the U.S. health research infrastructure. One indicator was the endorsement by the American Medical Association in 2000 not simply of increased research on women's health but also of the "sex-based analysis of data."[56]

Feminism, Difference, and the New Politics of Women's Health

One of the most striking aspects of the movement for sex-based biology is its unabashed embrace of a thoroughgoing conception of difference between women and men. A publicity video put out by the SWHR in 1998 opens with the voice of a teenage girl:

> When I was young, I didn't like boys very much. But now that I'm grown up, I know that men and women are just different. Boy, are they different! My mother says [Mother's voice], "Men are from Mars, and women are from Venus." My dad says [Father's voice], "Vive la différence!" But he doesn't even know how different we really are. Men and women may have been created equal, but we were not created alike. Our brains, our hearts, our immune systems, even our livers work differently. From conception to death, we live separate biological lives.[57]

This short segment does several bits of ideological work. It grounds the difference between the sexes in biology, even while establishing a domain of bodily difference far more extensive than the reproductive organs. It hastens to remind the viewer that "different" does not mean "unequal." It associates the new scientific findings with conventional wisdom from popular culture—"Men are from Mars, and women are from Venus," and "Vive la différence!" And it renders the fact of difference as something timeless, universal, and unchallengeable by its expression in the voices of parental authority and tradition.

Making the logic of sex-based biology comprehensible to a broader public by resting it on cultural stereotypes about gender difference is a common strategy in public representations of this scientific movement. According to the Web site of "Women's Health @ Stanford," "The differences between men and women are well-known: we think and act differently at almost every level. However, medical researchers are now realizing that those same sex differences extend to every cell in the human body."[58] One author, writing in the magazine *American Health for Women*, observed: "Everyone knows men and women have different shapes, hormones, and psyches. It seems obvious then that illnesses and medications would affect us differently too."[59] Here, phrases that gesture at an irrefutable common sense—"everyone knows" and "it seems obvious"—seek to root sex-based biology within an everyday discourse of gender essentialism, while at the same time laying the groundwork for a reformulation of that common sense in the language of modern biomedicine.

These strategic moves in the construction and public representation of sex-based biology raise important questions about the politics of women's health and about the broader feminist currents within which the women's health movement has swum. With the rise of second-wave feminism in the late 1960s, and throughout the 1970s, many women devoted considerable energy to preaching the philosophy of sameness, challenging gender stereotypes and demanding equal treatment in all walks of life. "Men and women are, of course different. But they are not as different as day and night, earth and sky, yin and yang, life and death," wrote the feminist theorist Gayle Rubin in a classic statement from the period that sought to rethink the conventional wisdom suggested by the ordinary, but very problematic, phrase "the opposite sex."[60] Many considered it important to argue that to the extent that women and men exhibited different behavioral characteristics or personalities in modern society, those differences were the product of nurture, not nature, and would largely disappear in an egalitarian society.[61] However, there also were strong expressions of "difference feminism" within the broader women's movement of the 1970s, including among those who valorized women's characteristics or even argued for women's innate superiority.[62] And by the 1980s, as the theorist Lise Vogel has analyzed, struggles in the domains of law and public policy around issues of particular concern to women, such as pregnancy and childbirth, had raised questions about whether a philosophy of sameness really made sense in the struggle for social justice: "Faced with the specificities of women's lives, equality suddenly appeared inadequate as a goal of social policy."[63]

Thus, at different moments and to varying degrees, feminists (like many other challenging groups) have pursued either "symmetric" or "asymmetric" approaches to the pursuit of social change: they either have insisted upon their fundamental sameness with the dominant group (and hence their right to be treated as equal), or they have emphasized their fundamental difference (and hence their special claim for attention or special grounding for social critique).[64] In recent years, the pendulum swing toward embracing difference has been pronounced. Some social commentators have tried to dislodge the dominant frame of Mars versus Venus. According to Katha Pollitt, for example, "It would be truer to say that men are from Illinois and women are from Indiana—different, sure, but not in ways that have much ethical consequence."[65] Yet it seems that whenever bodies and biology are brought into the discussion, the notion of the two sexes as "opposites" tends to win out.

Medically oriented proponents of the new wave of women's health research, like Bernadine Healy, the former director of the NIH, locate it broadly within the legacy of feminism—in Healy's historical reckoning, it constitutes the third stage of modern feminism, after the suffrage movement and women's liberation. In the two previous stages, explained Healy, women were obliged to present themselves as really just like men. But this time women "could acknowledge that they are different from men without giving up any of the rights gained."[66] As opposed to Healy's stage theory, perhaps a better way of classifying the current oscillation toward difference in women's health research advocacy would be to associate it with so-called postfeminism. That is, such views appear to reflect a perception that the fruits of previous feminist struggles are now being reaped, that those victories are safely entrenched, that women need no longer be concerned about establishing their claims to social equality, and, indeed, that "strident" discourse about "the patriarchy" and suchlike is counterproductive and passé. "It's safe to talk about sex differences again," was how Hara Estroff Marano expressed it in her essay on sex-based biology in *Psychology Today*. "Of course, it's the oldest story in the world. And the newest. But for a while it was also the most treacherous. Now it may be the most urgent. . . . Do we need to explain that difference doesn't imply superiority or inferiority?" Citing feminist icon Simone de Beauvoir's dictum, "One is not born a woman but rather becomes one," Marano effectively drew a separation from an earlier generation of feminism by asserting, "Science suggests otherwise, and it's driving a whole new view of who and what we are."[67]

Leaders of the sex-based biology movement have addressed the sameness/difference debate in somewhat more reflective terms than this, but also in ways that mark their distance from a previous feminist moment. Marianne Legato has written, "It is important to address the concerns of women who resist our concentrating on the differences between the genders, fearful that such an emphasis will once again define women as less fit and able than their male counterparts. In fact, it is important to tell women that our research does not prove them less competent than men. Quite simply, we are finding only that they are different."[68] Similarly, Sherry Marts, the scientific director of SWHR and a sociologist by training, noted the concern among feminists that claims about biological differences "seem to hearken back to that whole 'biology is destiny' thing." But, she added, "the thinking is that hopefully we've come far enough along now that it won't turn into another way to ghettoize women or to cast gender differences in concrete."[69]

In 2005 the question of the extent of innate differences between women and men burst into public consciousness again after Lawrence Summers, the president of Harvard University, was quoted speculating about the reasons why relatively few women were represented in the highest ranks of the sciences and mathematics. Perhaps it had something to do with innate differences, Summers suggested, to the consternation of many, not least among his own faculty.[70] While many commentators were outraged by the suggestion that this social outcome of gender inequality had biological causes, Legato embraced the controversy as an opportunity to advance the agenda of gender-specific medicine. Wrote Legato, "Despite the personal cost to Harvard's president, nothing could have been healthier for the new science of gender-specific medicine than the flurry of discussion his remarks provoked." Legato noted the divergence in public reaction between claims about biomedical differences and claims about differences in intellectual abilities, but her general message was that we should all put emotions aside and embrace the new science of sex:

> Saying that the ingredients and flow rates of our saliva differ as a function of sex is politically neutral; no one is going to be outraged by the fact that the salivary flow rates of males are higher and the sugar content lower than that of their female counterparts. But to point out the many sex-specific differences in brain anatomy and chemistry and in the systems involved in cognition is a different story. And to hypothesize that we are not equally gifted or that we at least excel at different things—and to say so—is the equivalent of loping across a minefield and expecting to reach the other side without incident. Despite the dangers of traveling this path, many institutions are investing huge sums of money and effort into expanding the whole realm of neurobiology—my own university, for one.[71]

Citing the furor that greeted past scientific heroes such as Darwin and Freud when they first proposed their new theories, Legato cast the new science of sex differences as a dragon-slayer that ultimately would succeed in displacing "old and entrenched systems."[72]

At a time when the broader women's health movement has become increasingly heterogeneous, the willingness—indeed, eagerness—to embrace findings or assertions of biological differences by sex is a characteristic way in which the new women's health research advocacy groups distinguish themselves from the politics of those organizations that emerged directly out of the feminist women's health movement of the 1970s and 1980s.[73] However, it is not the only such point of divergence. As Sheryl Burt Ruzek and Julie Becker have described, where groups like the Boston Women's Health Book Collective (the publishers of *Our Bodies, Ourselves*), the National Black Women's Health Project, and the National Women's Health Network have remained tied to other progressive movements for social change, the new advocacy groups have a narrower focus; where the earlier groups often sought to "demedicalize" women's experiences, the new advocacy, often led by women inside medicine and science, seeks to extend scientific scrutiny of their bodies; where the earlier activism sought to empower women as consumers and as patients, the newer advocacy embraces professionalism; and where the earlier activism steered clear of corporate ties (and mostly continues to do so), the new groups depend heavily on funding from the pharmaceutical industry.[74] (Confirming this last point, the SWHR's Corporate Advisory Council reads like a Who's Who of the drug industry, and the financial dues paid by these corporations to the SWHR provide that organization with a substantial part of its operating budget. In addition, Legato's research center at Columbia University was supported by a $2.5 million donation from Proctor & Gamble.[75])

Spokespersons such as Vivian Pinn, the director of the ORWH, are quick to credit the pivotal accomplishments of the feminist women's health movement of the 1970s and 1980s and to point out that "a focus on women's health didn't just start in 1990."[76] However, others have warned that this history is indeed in danger of being lost and its present-day descendants marginalized. According to feminist scholars of medicine Paula Treichler, Lisa Cartwright, and Constance Penley, "this new women's health agenda is founded upon a well-documented history of feminist politics and women's health activism; yet it achieved its present prominence only by obscuring or obliterating its problematic political roots in struggles over abortion, reproductive choice, patient autonomy, and egalitarian ideals of health access for women across class, race, and employment status."[77] A trenchant critique by Anne Eckman has linked the transmutation of women's health politics and the foreshortening of its history precisely to the new emphasis on the pervasiveness of sex differences and a corresponding de-emphasis on reproductive rights. According to Eckman, the shift in attention away from women's reproductive organs and toward bodily differences that are less obviously sex-linked—in the heart, the liver, and so on—"has ironically positioned women's reproduction . . . as peripheral to current efforts to secure equal health and health care for women."[78] At the same time, the presumption of pervasive biological difference between women and men has presupposed a forgetting of feminist critiques of much previous research into sex differences: "Biological sex, extended throughout the whole of a woman's body, has been repositioned as the foundational truth from which women's health research should start. . . . As a result, important questions about the construction of sexual difference as a category of analysis within research—questions at the heart of a well-elaborated feminist and radical critique of science . . . —have not been linked to the production of new biomedical knowledge."[79]

THE NONDEBATE OVER SEX PROFILING

The ideological divides within the broader women's health movement and the concerns about the politics of sex-based biology suggest that there are political stakes in the questions that I posed at the outset of this chapter. Even if there is little public debate over the science of sex differences analogous to that over the science of racial differences, the topic of sex profiling in medicine does merit critical scrutiny. In what ways are the cases of racial profiling and sex profiling similar and in what ways are they different? In the last chapter, I developed six points of critique of racial profiling. In the remainder of this chapter, I consider the applicability of the same potential critiques to determine what we can learn about sex profiling.

The Problems with Profiling

Improper treatment. Much as with racial profiling, sex profiling poses the risk of improper medical treatment of a patient who doesn't conform to the stereotype that pertains to his or her group. It is noteworthy that so many claims in the sex-based biology literature are framed, at least rhetorically, as universal observations about all women and all men. Florence Haseltine has written that "the female body has more fat and less water"; Marianne Legato's book is called *The Female Heart*.[80] Representations of medically relevant sex differences in the popular press likewise use the language of blanket differences. According to *USA Today*'s magazine, "women are less active and consume less oxygen than men. Rib cages are smaller in women, resulting in lower lung capacity." Also, "Women say 'ouch!' to pain before men do, but tolerate the pain better."[81] At least at the level of rhetoric, such claims appear to divide the universe of human experience into two utterly separate camps, while thoroughly homogenizing all that which lies within each one. Because of the binary and either/or nature of the discourse on sex differences, such claims seem even more all-encompassing and less nuanced than those about racial and ethnic differences in medicine.

Certain sex differences, such as sex-linked traits linked to genes on the X chromosome, may indeed function to demarcate half of humanity from the other half—leaving aside, just for the moment, those individuals whose chromosomal sex is nonstandard. But most of the claims about sex differences are, once again, statements about differences between averages. Clearly it is not the case that all women have smaller rib cages than all men, or that all women say "ouch!" first. Just as the science of statistics has constructed diseases as racial, so statistical processes also result in the sexing of diseases. Stefan Hirschauer and Annemarie Mol have described how this process works using the example of anemia:

> There is nothing inherently sexed about this disease. . . . [A] normal hemoglobin level differs from one person to the next and has no sex. . . . Statistical practice turns anemia into a sexed disease. Statistical practice builds on the anatomical differentiation between the sexes and clusters hemoglobin levels of hundreds of people identified anatomically as either males or females. Two curves emerge. The median and cut-off point of the first are a little higher than those of the second. Thus "men" have a higher normal hemoglobin level than do "women."

As Hirschauer and Mol observed, "the sex generated in this way is not one of bodies but is one of populations."[82]

Particularly in the case of the pharmacokinetics and pharmacodynamics of medications, usually the best that can be claimed is a statement about probabilities. Raymond Woosley, the pharmacology expert who has researched the harmful effects of drugs that prolong the QT interval, noted that certain of those drugs affect men and women in strikingly different ways, while, with other drugs, "the most sensitive male [is] equal to the average female, so there is considerable overlap; . . . it's a mean difference."[83] Thus, sex profiling in the clinic—drawing a decision about treatment based on knowledge of the patient's sex—may function quite reliably in certain circumstances, while in other circumstances it might raise the familiar problem of taking statistical generalities about a group and applying them to individual cases. In other words, Hacking's claim, cited at the beginning of this chapter, that "many medical differences between males and females are uniform, but medical differences between races are almost always only statistical," fails to ask the crucial question of just how many medical differences between males and females are statistical as well.

As Judith Lorber has argued, the overriding mistake of so many "epistemologically spurious" studies of sex differences in both the biological and the social sciences is that they begin simply by assuming that "men" and "women" are the relevant groups to compare, look for differences between them, and then attribute whatever they find to the underlying sex difference. Lorber observed: "These designs rarely question the categorization of their subjects into two and only two groups, even though they often find more significant within-group differences than between-group differences."[84]

People and groups differ in an unlimited variety of ways. The problem here—as with race—is when we assume that the ways of differing that are most socially salient and "obvious" are necessarily the ones that carry the most explanatory weight.[85] In the context of clinical care, this becomes dangerous. The unavoidable risk is that some individuals might receive the wrong diagnosis or treatment if they are approached as a representative member of their social group. The hard-and-fast language of binary sex difference makes it particularly difficult to catch sight of this limitation, while the reliance on the group stereotype then serves to reinforce that "hardness" and "fastness."

The ideology of sexual binarism may have additional problematic consequences in the world of medical research. On one hand, it might function to obscure commonalities. In an example suggested by Barbara Hanson, it is not inconceivable that breast cancer and prostate cancer could have a causal factor in common, but the emphasis on studying women's and men's diseases separately makes it less likely that researchers would uncover it.[86] On the other hand, binary logic might work to obscure differences within each sex—by race, class, sexuality, age, or health status. As Sheryl Burt Ruzek, Adele Clarke, and Virginia Olesen have observed, "differences between groups of women may well be as salient as gender status itself in both the production and experience of health and healing."[87] While certain institutional actors within the inclusion-and-difference paradigm, such as the ORWH, are closely attuned to the diversity of women's experiences, many advocates of sex-based biology seem to privilege the universal category of female, while treating aspects of difference largely as an afterthought. For example, a book by the cardiologist Nieca Goldberg entitled *Women Are Not Small Men* makes many essentialist claims about women as a class—that their hearts are different, that they have different symptoms from men, and so on—but then devotes only two pages to "special considerations for women of color."[88]

Dubious associations between sex/gender and medical outcomes. Another way in which sex profiling could cause harm is by creating a tendency to routinely uncover questionable associations between sex/gender and medical outcomes. The arguments made in the previous chapter about race and ethnicity would seem to apply equally well here. As biostatisticians who are suspicious of an automatic turn toward subgroup analyses have argued, "the more questions asked of a set of data, the more likely it will yield some statistically significant difference even if the treatments are in fact equivalent."[89] With sex differences as with race differences, NIH and FDA policies calling for subgroup comparisons may inadvertently promote the generation of spurious findings that may bring about inappropriate or inferior medical care. In the process, the claim that women and men are utterly different becomes a self-fulfilling prophecy. Susan Leigh Star made this point in 1979, in relation to her study of sex differences in the brain: "The very fact of dividing subjects into male and female categories for research purposes may serve to reify and perpetuate a socially created dichotomy. The search for differences can help to create the differences; if you are looking for something you are likely to find it."[90]

Market incentives that may harm patients. Sex-based medicine also may create new opportunities for profit-making within the health sector, in ways that may work to the detriment of patients. In 2002 Zelnorm, a drug made by Novartis to treat irritable bowel syndrome, became the first of two drugs so far approved by the FDA for use only in women, for a condition that affects both sexes. The drug's advantages over a placebo in a mixed-sex population could not be demonstrated with statistical significance.[91] Is Zelnorm the "BiDil" of sex-based prescribing? Again, it is interesting that the advent of the first "ethnic drug" created a stir, while the marketing of the first "gender drug" went unnoticed—no doubt because so many other drugs, such as hormones and most contraceptives, have long been marketed only to women. For advocates of sex-based biology like Sherry Marts, the sex-based marketing of drugs like Zelnorm is a victory that validates their whole approach: if subgroup analyses had not been performed, a drug that brings demonstrable benefit to women would simply have been lost.[92] But of course, in the clinical trials that led to marketing, Zelnorm did not bring benefit to all women, while it did bring benefit to some men. One wonders, then, how often the ability to market to a subgroup will function primarily to provide a pharmaceutical company with a strategy for salvaging products that do not perform adequately in humans overall but, statistically, do so in subpopulations to some degree. If the drug truly brought benefit to women as a class, say, because of a difference related to sex chromosomes, then there would be no argument with sex-specific drug approvals. But if sex is merely a proxy—a crude way of distinguishing some of the drug responders from some of the nonresponders—then our enthusiasm to embrace such marketing might be diminished substantially.

Sex profiling as a permanent "temporary" solution. Just as with racial profiling, advocates of sex profiling describe it as a step on the way toward truly individualized medicine. "Researchers foresee a world in which they will be able to read a patient's DNA to gauge the likely course of the person's disease or response to drugs," wrote Viviana Simon, the Director of Scientific Programs at SWHR, in the special issue on women's health in *Science*: "Until that degree of individualization is possible, patients and doctors must continue to rely on the results of studies carefully designed and analyzed by patient type—including by sex—to obtain the clinical results that are useful and meaningful to the health of both women and men."[93] However, if indeed there are limitations with sex-based prescribing, then the future promise of pharmacogenomics is not guaranteed to mitigate the harm. Pharmaceutical companies are likely to be much more interested in marketing to a "niche" that constitutes half the population than to tiny, genetically distinct segments of the market. And to the extent that sex-specific drug development becomes institutionalized, it is highly questionable whether companies will want to abandon it in favor of more finely individualized treatment. In the meantime, while genetic screening remains unavailable and unaffordable to most people, the characterization of sex-based prescribing as the "next best thing" may endow the latter with a legitimacy that it does not deserve.

Inaccurate and problematic understandings of sex and gender. Yet another problem with sex profiling is that—like racial profiling—it disguises the problems of categorization. The result is to promote misleading views of the nature of sex. In the case of race, the problem of maintaining a stable scientific categorization system is obvious to many, and most will acknowledge it if pressed, even if in practice researchers and policymakers typically charge forward anyway, as if the meanings of categories were clear and settled. In the case of sex, the categorization problem is of a different order. Sex categories do have an obvious biological grounding in the body. But the precise ways in which sexed bodies correspond to our social categories—or fail to do so—are obscured by an overwhelmingly strong ideology of sexual dimorphism: the belief that males and females are utterly distinct, if not opposite, and that no middle ground exists. Thus, sex poses another sort of categorization problem, one that is less easily discernible than that resulting from our classifications by race and one that perhaps is even more deeply inscribed, both historically and cross-culturally.

In biomedicine as in our culture generally, sex is almost always treated as if it were a simple dichotomous variable. The presumptions are that one is either male or female and that the correct designation is not hard to determine—it can, in effect, be "read off" the body. But nature knows no absolute distinctions. There is no unambiguous dividing line between the two sexes, and every criterion of differentiation that might be invoked, from genitalia to hormones to chromosomes, fails to perform a strict demarcating function. According to Anne Fausto-Sterling:

> Are there *no* sex differences? I usually start by saying that there are repro-
> ductive differences, although even there the extreme borders get blurred.
> There are men who produce no sperm and women without ovaries. There
> are hermaphrodites who have some organs of each sex. . . . XY females and
> XX males may not abound, but they exist with a frequency high enough to
> worry the International Olympic Committee. They require chromosome
> tests of their female athletes, even though many believe these tests to be
> useless for telling male from female.[94]

Conventional notions of "male" and "female" fail to do justice to hu-man variation—indeed, according to Fausto-Sterling, "no classification scheme could more than suggest the variety of sexual anatomy encoun-tered in clinical practice."[95] Nor are intersexuals and hermaphrodites "really" just somewhere "in between" the natural poles of male and fe-male.[96] Rather, as Alice Dreger has argued, modern scientific attempts to understand hermaphroditism were part of the process of defining biolog-ical sex in the first place.[97] Similarly, as Joanne Meyerowitz and Stefan Hirschauer both have shown, the medical creation and management of the transsexual has involved the practical transformation of the meaning of sex.[98]

Drawing on feminist analyses from the 1970s, social scientists some-times think of "sex" as the biological bedrock and "gender" as a social and cultural edifice constructed on top of it—or, to use another metaphor, we imagine that sex provides the "raw materials" for the cultural work of defining and performing gender. However, as a range of feminist and science studies scholars have argued in the 1990s and since, cultural ideas about gender attributes have filtered into and shaped scientific conceptions of biological sex itself—in the process endowing sex with the strictly dichotomous character that we take for granted.[99] Nelly Oudshoorn's analysis of early research on sex hormones makes this point elegantly by showing how ideas about masculinity and femininity were attributed to sex hormones by scientists, and how those early-twentieth-century scientists were forced to grapple with the disconcerting realization that women also possessed "male" sex hormones and vice versa.[100] Thus, the classification of individuals into dichotomous sex categories inevitably involves cultural work made possible by a history of definitional acts.

Various authorities, from doctors who perform surgeries on intersexed newborns to the athletic committees referenced by Fausto-Sterling that debate whether athletes compete as male or female, perform the social control function of fitting individuals into categories. Yet the active labor that goes into making sex appear dichotomous is generally invisible to the broader society, or at least, rarely remarked upon. Despite the recent political agitation on the part of intersexuals insisting on their right not to be either male or female, and despite the emergence of surgical options to transform the sex of adults, this notion of clear and reliable sex differences endures.[101] Sex profiling, like racial profiling, both presumes and reinforces a problematic notion that each individual belongs to a category and can be diagnosed and treated accordingly.

Dangerously inaccurate understandings of the causes of health disparities. By clouding the relationship between the biological and the social, sex profiling may interfere with our attempts to understand and eliminate health disparities. Nearly every point that I made about racial profiling applies equally well here—in particular, that the focus on biological differences encourages the inaccurate belief that health disparities by sex are mostly a function of biology and also disguises the role of cultural and social factors. Again, to avoid being misunderstood, it is important to clarify that the point is not that sex differences in health are really social and cultural rather than biological, or really environmental rather than genetic—any "either/or" formulation would be equally problematic and would misconstrue the tight interactive links and developmental loops connecting "nature" and "nurture."[102]

It also bears saying that, within the inclusion-and-difference paradigm generally, the increasing use of the "slash" concept of "sex/gender" (in place of the confused use of "gender" in the early years of the paradigm) functions to create space for research into both biological and social causes of men's and women's illnesses. For example, a 2003 call for funding proposals on "Women's Mental Health and Sex/Gender Differences Research" issued by the National Institute of Mental Health observed that the "pattern of disparities in the epidemiology of mental disorders in males and females provides indirect evidence of hormonal, biological, social, cultural and developmental factors in etiology and course."[103] Often, however, the research program of sex-based biology is as skewed toward the biological as the name would suggest. Yet there is good reason to insist on the serious limitations of biological explanations for health disparities between women and men—beginning with the fact that the most striking disparity of all, women's greater longevity in developed societies, is likely due significantly to social factors.[104] The fact that male "excess mortality" from cardiovascular disease appears to have emerged, in the United States and Britain, only in the 1920s should sound a further cautionary note about the growing tendency to attribute differences between "the male heart" and "the female heart" primarily to consequences of estrogen.[105]

To take another example from the cardiovascular arena, if women's heart attack symptoms are reported to be different from men's, why might this be so? Little discussion has focused on the possibility, supported by research conducted in Scotland, that "women were concerned that reporting their chest pain wasted the doctors' time."[106] Not only do accounts that privilege the biological often deflect our attention from the social organization of gender relations, but sometimes such accounts also serve to naturalize the conditions of gender inequality that in and of themselves may be bad for women's health and well-being.

Race, Sex, and the Politics of Difference

Sex differences and race differences are *different differences*, and invocations of biological explanations in the two cases clearly do not pose precisely the same dilemmas. Nevertheless, my argument has suggested that many of the critiques of racial profiling apply to sex profiling as well, at least in some respects and to some degree. Indeed, although sex profiling is often more defensible then racial profiling, the extremity of many claims about sex differences—the glib imagery of Mars versus Venus, the presumption of fundamental difference at the level of every cell—is a particular point of concern. In my view, therefore, the tendency to engage in sharp boundary work between race and sex, and to accept sex profiling as "obviously" sensible in contrast to the problematic character of racial profiling, is both intellectually misguided and seriously mistaken in terms of health care interventions.

Why is it that, at the present moment in the United States, sex differences are thoroughly reified and naturalized in biomedical research, while the use of race as a proxy has been contested, within the research community and outside of it? Certainly some of the answer lies in the contrast between sex and race as kinds of difference, but perhaps some of the answer has to do with the broader political environments within which claims about sex and race circulate. My reflections on this latter point are necessarily speculative, so I will keep them brief. As I described, while an insistence on equality as sameness was a typical strategy of feminist movements in past decades, in more recent years notions of essential difference appear to provide a strategic wedge especially to certain sectors of the women's health movement. But which sectors? This particular wave of mobilization on women's health research reflects the professionalization of the women's health movement and the concomitant rise of some women (often white and middle-class) to positions of authority and influence within Congress, the Department of Health of Human Services, and biomedical research institutions. This was the constellation of forces that was positioned to press for measures such as the NIH Revitalization Act. For these women, whose relative social equality has been affirmed, conceptions of essential or biological difference appear to pose no substantial political risk. Instead, such essentialism serves as a foundation for their professional agendas.

By contrast, in an era of general retrenchment against affirmative action by race, advocates of biomedical research to benefit people of color stand in a less secure position. Especially given the historical suspicion of clinical research on the part of communities of color, it is not surprising that efforts to promote attention to minority health concerns through an emphasis on biological difference would war against profound concerns that difference will be construed in pejorative terms—indeed, as new justifications for racism. Finally, as social movements organize on behalf of multiracialism and as the discourses of multiracialism become more prevalent in popular culture,[107] racial categories gradually are coming to lose some of their obviousness and appear more arbitrary. Thus, it makes sense that the transposition of social categories of race into biological categories of difference would come under increasing scrutiny. By contrast, despite the efforts of intersexuals and transgender people to "queer" the meanings of "male" and "female," categories of sex and gender are rarely presented in the mass media and popular culture as anything but fixed and natural.

These reflections point to the importance of locating the policies, practices, and philosophies of the inclusion-and-difference paradigm within the broadest possible social and political context, in order to understand what is at stake in the changes that they represent. In the next chapter, I adopt a broad view in order to examine the likely future of the inclusion-and-difference paradigm.

CHAPTER TWELVE

Whither the Paradigm?

Where might the inclusion-and-difference paradigm be heading? Having explored the history of its emergence and consolidation, and having investigated its consequences and implications, we can now ask: What is its likely future? In this chapter, I take up three issues that are central to assessing that trajectory. First, I examine the degree to which these reforms establish a model that can be extended to other groups: aside from women, people of color, children, and the elderly, who else will "qualify" as full biopolitical citizens under its framework? And to the extent that such extensions may be resisted, what accounts for the opposition? As part of this discussion, I pay special attention to attempts by lesbian, gay, bisexual, and transgender (LGBT) health advocates to jump on the inclusion-and-difference bandwagon—so far with limited success.

Second, I consider the durability of the paradigm in hostile political climates, as well as the internal tensions that hostile scrutiny may bring to light. Is the inclusion-and-difference paradigm necessarily dependent on politically liberal defenders? Finally, I consider the paradigm's likely capacity to "travel" across international borders. Are other countries adopting, or are they likely to adopt, these particular ways of thinking about biomedical identity and difference? Together, these analyses suggest the staying power of this means of administering and ministering to bodies and groups, but they also point out some of the practical limits on its extension.

DOMAIN EXPANSION

Who gets to become a "special population"? Once particular ways of conceiving of biomedical difference are institutionalized, to which kinds of groups can the model be extended? I argued in chapter 7 that the initial emergence of the policies, practices, and offices that make up the inclusion-and-difference paradigm begged some crucial questions: Why were certain means of social differentiation deemed to be medically relevant? Why sex and gender, race and ethnicity, and age, and why not social class, or religion, or other markers of identity and difference? It took work—what I called categorical alignment work—to make the former set of social markers play a dual role as categories of both political mobilization and biomedical analysis. Furthermore, I postulated that—abstractly speaking—the inclusion-and-difference paradigm is well disposed to recognize categorical identities in certain circumstances: when the identity is already socially salient, when the representative group is highly mobilized, when the group lays claim to a form of difference that is already authorized by state classifications, and when proponents are able to convincingly deploy frames that link justice arguments to biological difference claims.

But suppose that a group more-or-less "qualifies" according to these considerations. What kind of work is necessary to turn that potential into the reality of new forms of biopolitical citizenship? And how does the prior existence of the paradigm affect the possibilities of its own extension? These questions can be approached by means of the sociological literature on "domain expansion," which looks at how and when policies come to be applied to more and more social groups and categories over time. For example, Valerie Jenness and Ryken Grattet have described the gradual expansion of the "domain of the 'condition-category'" in federal hate crime legislation, which over time came to protect individuals from attack based on their religion, race, ethnicity, gender, and sexual orientation.[1] Similarly, in his study of the "minority rights revolution," John Skrentny has analyzed both successful and unsuccessful attempts to extend federal affirmative action policies and protections to groups beyond the originally designated racial minorities; while Mary Katzenstein and Judith Reppy have described the historical parallels in attempts to open up the U.S. military first to blacks, then to women, and most recently to gays and lesbians.[2] Domain expansion is often propelled by the power of the successful example: social movements may be inclined to adopt strategies and approaches that have already proven successful for other groups, while organizations not only are shaped by past choices but also are likely to adopt ways of confronting external pressures that have proven efficacious in the past.[3]

More specifically, it appears that several processes may facilitate domain expansion.[4] First, the splintering often attributed to identity politics—a tendency for each identity-based group to subdivide, as smaller identities within the group assert their difference—can propel subgroups to press their claims for attention. (I provide an example below, in my discussion of how lesbians positioned themselves as a subgroup of women whose differences were medically relevant.)[5] Second, successful attention to specific differences can reveal new gaps—for example, some scholars have pointed to the medical invisibility of adolescents, who may fall between the cracks by failing to meet the age cutoffs either for pediatric research or for trials conducted on adults.[6] Third, as Jenness noted in the case of hate crime legislation, new paradigms, once institutionalized, tend to create their own momentum. Thus, while initial passage of a law protecting a group may require significant political mobilization, "later in the process, social movement involvement . . . is no longer critical" in all cases.[7] Fourth, as Skrentny has described, once government offices are established to promote a policy, those offices become "beachheads" of a sort.[8] For example, the staff of existing offices serving "special populations" may often be sympathetic to the claims of other groups and may be willing to work on their behalf.

Finally, a number of scholars, particularly Skrentny, have emphasized the role of analogies in the expansion of policy domains.[9] In his analysis of the creation of the "official minorities" in the "minority rights revolution," Skrentny described how government officials "quickly classified some groups as 'minorities'—a never-defined term that apparently meant 'analogous to blacks.'" Judgment calls about the degree of analogical similarity to African Americans fueled perceptions of where the boundaries of affirmative action policies appropriately lay.[10] And as Jenness noted, groups have employed strategies to construct comparability across categories— for example, emphasizing the "innateness" of the condition—in order to extend a statutory mandate.[11] Precisely because the inclusion-and-difference paradigm tends often to "flatten" differences (as I argued in chapter 7)—to conceptualize sex/gender, race/ethnicity, and age as ways of differing that are all analogous to, or commensurate with, one another from a policy standpoint—it may lend itself to extension via analogy-making of this sort.

At the same time, there are several likely sources of resistance to domain expansion in cases such as the one I am considering. Groups may sometimes encounter ideological resistance to the claim that their position is analogous to others who were incorporated earlier. For example, in his account of the extension of civil rights to various groups in the 1960s and 1970s, Skrentny notes that "rights for the disabled were included easily and without debate, [while] gay rights were a political non-starter." In that time period, being gay simply was not seen by enough lawmakers as sufficiently analogous to being black.[12] Thus, the likelihood of domain expansion may depend significantly on what Anne Schneider and Helen Ingram have called the "social construction of target populations"—the public characterizations and images of groups affected by public policy.[13] In addition, once policies are in place, there may be resistance to revising or extending them in ways that appear to complicate standard operating procedures. More than one DHHS insider suggested that it would be harder for each successive group to call for improved numerical representation in clinical studies because of a disinclination to lay additional reporting burdens upon biomedical scientists.[14]

One explicit attempt to invoke the DHHS inclusionary policies by analogy demonstrates the political stakes that may sometimes be implicated in analogical arguments. In 2002 a DHHS official sought to include unborn human fetuses in the definition of "human subjects" deserving protection from research risk. While the move appeared consistent with other attempts by the George W. Bush administration and its allies to tear down ideological supports for women's rights to abortion, a DHHS spokesperson explicitly invoked the history of inclusionary policies to justify the proposal. "Not long ago," explained the spokesperson, "clinical trials included only white men. Recognizing this, the scientific community moved to expand the number of those who can be included in such research." Expanding the categories of protected human subjects to include the unborn, the official maintained, was a natural implication of this shift in perspectives and procedures.[15] However, the social category of "fetus" possessed only some of the features I described earlier as being generally necessary for incorporation within the paradigm: the category was only partially cemented into state classifications, and political mobilization on behalf of fetal rights, while certainly strong, was counterbalanced by strong mobilization against. But while there has been no general move to extend the inclusion-and-difference paradigm to encompass fetuses, the incident is telling: it demonstrates that diverse political actors, and not simply those situated toward the leftward end of the political spectrum, can appropriate the logic of inclusion and difference for their purposes.

The Plight of Pregnant Women

This incident of fetal politics aside, in recent years there have been two primary cases of attempted domain expansion within the inclusion-and-difference paradigm. The first of these involves pregnant women. As I described previously, before the 1993 removal of the FDA's restriction on the participation of women in clinical trials, women had been kept out of many trials out of the fear that, if they became pregnant, the drug being tested might harm the fetus. The restriction was lifted out of the eventual recognition that it was not fair to treat women as a class as if they existed in a state of perpetual potential pregnancy.[16] However, the new rules that were then implemented had the effect of placing women who *were* pregnant in medical limbo. According to a study by the FDA, women under the age of 35 take three prescription medications on average during their pregnancies, while pregnant women over 35 take five on average.[17] Yet because of the exclusion of pregnant women from drug testing, there is a near total absence of knowledge about the effects of these medications, either on the course of the pregnancy or on the offspring. Nor are there clear guidelines on how dosages ought to be adjusted in light of the physiological changes associated with pregnancy. Instead, most drug labeling in the United States simply states: "There are, however, no adequate and well-controlled studies in pregnant women. Because animal reproductive studies are not always predictive of human response, this drug should be used during pregnancy only if clearly needed." As a result, in the words of the authors of a chapter on pregnant and nursing women in a medical textbook on pharmacology, "the pregnant woman is perhaps the last true therapeutic orphan."[18]

A number of scientists, NIH officials, and members of Congress have sought to address this problem. The existence of offices promoting the interests of women's health has helped ensure that the concerns of pregnant women find expression; for example, the NIH's Office of Research on Women's Health (ORWH) sponsored a conference in 1999 on sex differences in pharmacology that took up the issue of pregnancy and, in a report recommendation, urged the inclusion of pregnant women in clinical trials.[19] The NIH's National Institute of Child Health and Human Development has also taken an interest in the issue.[20] Several pharmaceutical companies, such as GlaxoSmithKline, have established "pregnancy registries" tracking the effects of their products when taken by pregnant women; and the FDA has issued draft guidelines governing such registries.[21] And in 2002 Senator Tom Harkin of Iowa and Rep. John Dingell of Michigan introduced the "Smart Mom Act," which, if enacted, would have (among other things) sought "to expand knowledge about the safety and dosing of drugs to treat pregnant women with chronic conditions and women who become sick during pregnancy."[22]

At the same time, the goal of including pregnant women in clinical trials has not gained significant traction, perhaps because the case does not appear sufficiently analogous to that of other groups that have been recognized under the paradigm. Pregnant women are not generally thought of as a group subject to injustice or discrimination; and since the goal of safeguarding them from harm often appears to outweigh other social considerations, a more protectionist ethic may prevail in their case. Here, too, the contested politics of abortion and "fetal rights" casts a shadow. Legal and medical controversies on issues ranging from fetal surgery to drug or alcohol consumption by pregnant women have revealed sharp political cleavages over whether and when the "rights" and "interests" of the fetus trump those of the mother.[23] In some jurisdictions in the United States, prosecutors have sought to jail or fine women who take actions that bring theoretical risk to their unborn children. Thus, in the present political environment, it seems unlikely that inclusionary policies will be extended to cover pregnant women if any risk to their fetuses is perceived to follow as a consequence.

Sexual Orientation as a Research Variable

The other case of attempted (and partially successful) extension, which I have described at greater length elsewhere,[24] concerns health research focused on lesbians, gays, bisexuals, and transgenders (LGBTs). In the 1990s, activists, researchers, and physicians made concerted efforts to institutionalize LGBT (or, more often, just lesbian and gay) health as a formal concern of public health and health research bureaucracies. At the crux of this advocacy lay the claim that lesbians, gay men, bisexuals, and transgendered persons have distinctive health concerns and that they would benefit from research that takes categories of sexual and gender identity as the foundation of a health promotion and biomedical research strategy. These efforts met with some success in the late 1990s. However, the replacement of Bill Clinton's administration by that of George W. Bush in 2000 mostly put a halt to the forward march. The story is interesting, therefore, both in suggesting what sorts of analogies are "sellable" and in pointing to the political tensions within the inclusion-and-difference paradigm.

Just as other groups have approached biomedicine with mistrust or ambivalence, LGBTs often have found themselves caught, in public health scholar Ronald Bayer's terms, "between the specter and the promise of medicine."[25] A foundational success in the history of the nascent gay liberation movement in the United States in the early 1970s was the campaign to pressure the psychiatric establishment to cease classifying homosexuality as a disease.[26] The legacy of such conflicts also informed gay activists' responses to the medical profession upon the emergence of the AIDS epidemic in the 1980s.[27] In reaction against the biomedical tendency to construe sexual difference as pathology, patients and activists have found a variety of ways to "talk back," as Jennifer Terry has described in her historical analyses.[28] Yet surely one of the most significant responses has been a pervasive distrust of medical expertise and wariness about homophobia in health care settings. Often, lesbians and gay men either have avoided seeing physicians as much as possible or have practiced "a necessary secrecy and segregation of any sexual or personal issue when dealing with the mainstream health care system"—undoubtedly with negative consequences for their health.[29]

Although gay and lesbian AIDS activists had been crucially involved in promoting the inclusion of women, people of color, and children in trials of antiviral drugs, throughout the 1980s and much of the 1990s, LGBT communities were not typically considered "special populations" covered under the rubric of the inclusion-and-difference paradigm. Substantial amounts of NIH funding went to grants that listed homosexuality as a primary or secondary focus. But as one analysis of funding patterns has revealed, most of these funds (totaling about $20 million a year on average from 1982 to 1992) were directed at the HIV epidemic, with only about $532,000 per year devoted to all other health issues affecting gay men and lesbians.[30] In the 1990s, activists sought to change this. Having learned from AIDS and breast cancer activism that they could successfully transform biomedical research practices through direct engagement with the state, advocates proceeded to make the argument to DHHS officials that sexual orientation was a distinct form of difference to which researchers and physicians needed to attend, just like sex and gender, race and ethnicity, and age.[31] Advocates insisted that gay men and lesbians experienced a range of health disparities, and they cited examples linked to social oppression, such as higher rates of alcoholism and teen suicide, but also examples related presumably to behaviors, such as anal cancer among gay men and breast cancer among lesbians. At the same time, proponents of transgender health also pointed to the need for serious research on biological processes related to the life circumstances of transgenders. At what age, for example, would it be appropriate to begin mammography screening for someone who has been on high-dose estrogen and progesterone therapy since their mid-20s?[32] In light of the consumption of hormones by transgenders, with what regularity should health care providers order blood work to check blood sugar and cholesterol levels or liver functions?[33]

Crucially, proponents of lesbian health research were able to benefit from positioning themselves as a specific subgroup of women to which the new DHHS infrastructure devoted to women's health ought reasonably to attend—that is, women's health provided a strategic wedge for lesbian health advocates. The capacity of lesbians to make use of this wedge was not foreordained; in fact, the 1985 task force report on women's health that had helped to kick off the inclusion-and-difference paradigm had made no explicit mention of lesbians.[34] However, many DHHS employees within the newly established offices promoting women's health were sympathetic to domain expansion. In one telling victory, lesbian health advocates eventually were successful in adding a question on sexual orientation to the demographic data collected on participants in the Women's Health Initiative—though only following upon what Deborah Bowen, a health psychologist, described as a "bloody battle." According to Bowen, "reactions ran the gamut from 'Why bother studying lesbians, they are just like heterosexual women?' to 'I wouldn't ask my wife these questions, so I'm not going to ask my participants these kinds of questions.'"[35] Similarly, a question about sexual orientation was added to the Nurses' Health Study, the large, NIH-funded observational study of cardiovascular disease in women, after a lobbying campaign in which nurses were encouraged to write to the study investigators and demand such a question.[36]

That lesbian health activists appreciated the opening provided to them by the emphasis on women's health at the DHHS was made clear in a 1993 report on lesbian health by the National Gay and Lesbian Task Force (NGLTF), a prominent lobbying group. Noting that federal health policy documents had called for consideration by DHHS agencies of the unique health conditions affecting women or "some subgroups of women," the authors, Peri Jude Radecic and Marj Plumb, argued that lesbians constituted one such distinct subgroup of women. They proposed, therefore, that lesbians be included "as subjects, reviewers, and principal researchers in all women's health and mental health research initiatives," that future and ongoing longitudinal health studies funded by the NIH be stratified according to sexual orientation, and that the DHHS create a "fully funded office on Lesbian Health Care."[37] The NGLTF also organized a meeting between advocates for lesbian, gay, and bisexual health and DHHS Secretary Donna Shalala, who appointed one of her assistants, Patsy Fleming (who became President Clinton's "AIDS czar" the following year) as a lesbian and gay health liaison.[38] At this and subsequent meetings with DHHS officials, ORWH Director Vivian Pinn by all accounts played a supportive role, encouraging the notion that lesbian health should be included in the agenda of her office.[39]

Building gradually over the course of the 1990s, momentum on behalf of lesbian health research grew sharply with the decision by the Institute of Medicine (IOM) of the National Academy of Sciences to prepare a report on the state of lesbian health. The report piggybacked on DHHS interest in women's health in several senses. First, an earlier IOM report on the inclusion of women in biomedical research had been pivotal in directing attention to women's health issues,[40] and therefore it seemed logical to advocates of lesbian health to try to replicate that success. Second, funding for the report was provided by the ORWH, as well as by the CDC's Office of Women's Health.[41] Published in 1999 by the National Academy Press, the book-length report *Lesbian Health: Current Assessment and Directions for the Future* notably went to some pains to clarify what might be meant by a "lesbian health issue." On the basis of the data available, the report concluded, lesbians experienced greater health risks. But there were no grounds to maintain that lesbians were at higher risk for any health problem than heterosexual women "simply because they have a lesbian sexual orientation." It was not that being a lesbian was somehow intrinsically unhealthy; rather, certain specific health risks, such as nulliparity (not giving birth), stress effects of homophobia, and avoidance of health care, apparently were overrepresented among lesbian women.[42] Precisely whether these greater risks were resulting in worse health for lesbians was a question that required additional research, and the call for such research was one of the chief thrusts of the report.

Attempts to follow up on the IOM report reflected not only the further involvement of DHHS agencies but also the explicit attempt by advocates to piggyback on the inclusionary emphases of legislation like the NIH Revitalization Act. The DHHS Office on Women's Health, together with NIH's ORWH, the Gay and Lesbian Medical Association (GLMA), and the Lesbian Health Fund, organized a "Scientific Workshop on Lesbian Health 2000" to develop specific recommendations based on the report. Participants at the workshop drafted a document that in many ways reflected the goal of following in the footsteps of other groups incorporated within the inclusion-and-difference paradigm. For example, the Cancer Working Group urged that "sexual minority status . . . be incorporated in the list of 'special populations' or 'medically underserved' persons as defined by the Office of Special Populations Research" at the National Cancer Institute and further proposed that the NIH Guidelines for Inclusion of Women and Minorities as Subjects in Clinical Research be "amended to include sexual minority status."[43]

Another key instance of this attempt at domain expansion was the struggle for inclusion of sexual orientation in *Healthy People 2010*. Running more than eight hundred pages, this planning document prepared by the DHHS was meant to establish the nation's health priorities for the first decade of the new century.[44] Initially, LGBT groups were not included in the consortium of advocacy groups convened by the DHHS to participate in the *Healthy People 2010* planning process. Nevertheless, early drafts of the document did name sexual orientation up front as one dimension of health disparity: along with "disability," sexual orientation was added to the list of forms of disparity that had been used in *Healthy People 2000* ten years before, namely, gender, race and ethnicity, income and education, and geography. As one DHHS employee commented, this set a nearly irreversible precedent: it is hard to imagine that sexual orientation would get deleted from *Healthy People 2020* or *Healthy People 2030*.[45]

An early draft of the document also included sexual orientation as a demographic item to be tracked in twenty of the tables corresponding to specific health objectives in the document. However, when the near-final "conference edition" of *Healthy People 2010* was released in January 2000, these specific mentions of sexual orientation mysteriously had been deleted, and only a paragraph in the introduction to the draft of *Healthy People 2010* about sexual orientation remained: there was then no mention of sexual orientation in relation to any of the report's 467 health objectives.[46] In response to vociferous protests from GLMA and other groups and negative publicity in the lesbian and gay press, DHHS Secretary Shalala designated her appointment secretary, Martin Rouse, on openly gay man, to serve as liaison to the LGBT community in relation to *Healthy People*; and Rouse traveled around the country giving presentations to LGBT groups about the *Healthy People* process. In the end, the final version of the document incorporated sexual orientation into the "data templates" for 29 of the 467 health objectives. In addition, words like "gay," "lesbian," "bisexual," "men who have sex with men," and particularly "sexual orientation" appear in the text of the report at a number of places along the way (as revealed by a text search conducted by GLMA).

Meanwhile, advocates of LGBT health sought additional, formal mechanisms for institutionalizing their concerns within the DHHS bureaucracy. Most significantly, in 2000 they attempted to convince DHHS officials to establish an Office of Lesbian and Gay Health that would parallel the Office on Women's Health and the Office on Minority Health. Painfully aware that if the Republican candidate won the presidential election in November, the prospects for such an office would dim considerably—and hopeful that, in an election year, the Democratic administration would be anxious to curry favor with gay and lesbian voters—advocates pressed hard for the DHHS to take action quickly.[47] Responding cautiously, Assistant Secretary for Health David Satcher appointed a "Steering Committee on Health Disparities Related to Sexual Orientation." Consisting of representatives from each major DHHS agency, the Steering Committee took an inventory of how lesbian and gay issues were treated within DHSS and drafted a strategic plan.[48]

However, with the change in administration in 2000, these efforts effectively were placed on the shelf. In the fall of 2002, in response to pressure from the National Coalition for LGBT Health, nineteen members of Congress wrote a letter to DHHS Secretary Tommy Thompson, asking the DHHS to "identify the actions that have been taken or will be taken across the department to ensure that health disparities due to sexual orientation and gender identity are being addressed and reduced."[49] But in fact, the progress of LGBT health advocacy within the Bush administration has been minimal. By October 2002, after the DHHS withdrew $75,000 in funding previously earmarked for a lesbian health conference, researcher Judy Bradford was complaining that LGBT health concerns were moving "off the radar screen" at DHHS.[50]

In modest ways, however, the incorporation of LGBT concerns within the inclusion-and-difference paradigm has continued within the DHHS.[51] In May 2001 the NIH issued a program announcement entitled "Behavioral, Social, Mental Health, and Substance Abuse Research with Diverse Populations."[52] Sponsored by a series of DHHS agencies, the program announcement invited principal investigators to apply for up to five years of grant support, for amounts of up to $250,000 per year in direct costs, for research on "lesbian, gay, bisexual, transgendered, and related populations." However, the program announcement developed out of a workshop that took place prior to the change in administration, and the fact that words like *gay* and *lesbian* do not actually appear in the title are indicative of caution in a changed political environment. While skillful career civil service employees enjoy a certain room to maneuver in promoting policies that they favor, LGBT health advocates have achieved few explicit victories during the George W. Bush administration. And to the degree that the success of this advocacy has depended on the accidental presence of LGBT persons employed within "the belly of the beast" who have been willing to take stands on LGBT health issues, then it matters that fewer such employees have felt emboldened to speak up.

There can be little doubt that incorporation of LGBT health and health research concerns within the inclusion-and-difference paradigm has been decidedly partial, as compared with other groups that have more fully been encompassed within its framework. As a group, LGBTs possess some of the characteristics I listed as prerequisites, such as possession of a socially salient identity and a history of strong political mobilization. Moreover, the ability of lesbians to position themselves as a subgroup of women has permitted them to build on the advances of women's health research within the DHHS. But in other respects LGBT health advocates have had trouble establishing the analogy between themselves and other groups recognized by the paradigm. In biomedicine as elsewhere in U.S. society, LGBTs have proven unable to establish full citizenship.

Obviously, the antipathy toward gay rights on the part of many within the George W. Bush administration—and the unwillingness of a Republican-controlled Congress to force DHHS to move forward in this case, as Congress did on behalf of other groups previously—is central to the story. Key presidential appointments—such as that of Claude Allen, a staunch social conservative and former aide to homophobic Senator Jesse Helms, to the post of Deputy Secretary of Health and Human Services in 2001, also helped to set the tone.[53] But it is worth considering additional reasons why LGBT health advocates have been unable to make a stronger case.[54] Some critics simply have not been convinced that LGBTs confront health issues that are specific to their sexual or gender identities. In addition, the absence of a prior history of the institutionalization of sexual orientation categories within the federal bureaucracy means that LGBT demands for inclusion are a bit trickier than those of other groups. By contrast, when racial and ethnic minorities pressed for inclusion as subjects in biomedical research in the 1990s, the fact that race and ethnicity categories were already in long use on the U.S. census and on health surveys meant that it was easier to operationalize inclusion of these groups. Government officials are far less used to thinking about categories of sexual orientation—and categories such as "transgender" are considered simply too "out there" by federal officials, who are hardly prepared at present to replace the standard "Male/Female" demographic item with one that includes a third option.[55]

By comparison with transgender, sexual orientation categories such as "homosexual" (and "heterosexual") might seem to lend themselves to straightforward operationalization. (And perhaps "bisexual" does as well, though some view this as a suspect category because of its apparent in-between status.) But these categories also pose difficulties for a different reason: the lack of clear correspondence between identity and behavior. Surveys that ask respondents to name their sexual orientation will produce one set of mappings of individuals onto categories. Surveys that ask respondents who they have sex with will produce a different set of mappings, and questions about the object of desire will produce a third. As we know from empirical research, these mappings will overlap but will not coincide.[56] This disjuncture between identity, practice, and desire necessarily complicates the operationalization of sexual orientation.

Advocates of LGBT health have tended to emphasize identity rather than behavior or desire, probably for strategic reasons. The focus on identity reinforces a perception that LGBT individuals are distinct classes of people with unique health concerns and research needs. In a climate in which claims about the biological bases of sexual and gender orientations are increasingly common—in which "gay genes" and "gay brains" are the stuff of common discourse—advocates are thus able vaguely to suggest biological or quasi-biological differences between LGBTs and straight people. This move aids in the construction of an analogy between sexual identity and other categorical identities recognized within the inclusion-and-difference paradigm, such as gender and race. Similarly, it allows advocates to invoke the biological-differences frame, at least by implication. The tacit appeal to biology may enhance the claim for legitimate domain expansion—though it may have problematic consequences in other respects.[57]

However, the biological-differences frame does not fit perfectly in the case of sexual orientation, and this may be another reason why lesbians and gay men have not fully been incorporated into the paradigm. Many "lesbian and gay health risks" simply reflect a statistical propensity of gay men and lesbians to engage at higher or lower rates in specific sexual or social behaviors. If it does turn out that lesbians, as a group, are at greater risk of breast cancer, then this may have little to do with their identity as lesbians—except insofar as lesbians bypass mammography screening to avoid homophobic treatment by medical professionals—but instead may perhaps be due to the fact that lesbians are more likely not to have children. If gay men, overall, are at greater risk of anal cancer, then this may be a consequence of engaging in anal sex—an activity that is neither universal among gay men nor restricted to them. Some have argued that it might instead be more helpful to insist that the only health issues that are specific to LGBT people *as lesbians, gay men, bisexuals, or transgenders* are those that stem from the oppression directed at them as such. As Jennifer Terry has speculated in the case of lesbian health: "Perhaps a specifically *lesbian* agenda for health would disappear if equity and respect were extended to all women, regardless of their class, color, or sexual practices."[58] This observation might provide a powerful alternative basis for biomedical politics, but one that would employ a rather different logic from that of the inclusion-and-difference paradigm.

The disjuncture between identity, behavior, and desire points to yet another reason why LGBT health has not fully been accepted within the fold of the inclusionary reforms. While an emphasis on behaviors might often be a more precise way of talking about health risk in the case of lesbian, gay, and bisexual health, speaking of identity tends to keep the focus on personhood, while emphasizing behavior inevitably would mean talking explicitly about sexuality. It can be argued, in fact, that the political viability within the DHHS of LGBT health politics to date has depended substantially on avoiding explicit discussion of sexuality. In the corridors of Washington, it is far less threatening to speak of "sexual orientation as a demographic variable" than it is to speak of actual sexual practices.[59]

In recent decades, Republicans in Congress have torpedoed the funding even for survey research related to sexuality, and federal agencies have shown a distinct lack of interest in health research that seems "too gay," such as research on anal condoms or rectal microbicides.[60] Under the George W. Bush administration and simultaneous Republican control of the U.S. Congress, hostile scrutiny of sexuality research has intensified (as I have described in more detail elsewhere[61]). In July 2003 the U.S. House of Representatives came within two votes of revoking the funding previously granted by the NIH to four research projects on topics related to sexuality and health.[62] Soon thereafter, a "hit list" of 157 sexuality researchers—compiled by the Traditional Values Coalition, a self-described "grassroots church lobby" based in Southern California and renowned for its attacks on "the gay agenda"—was winding its way through Congress and the NIH.[63] Other recent episodes in the annals of federal policing of sexual health promotion include a crackdown by the Centers for Disease Control and Prevention (CDC) on the use of federal funds by community-based AIDS prevention organizations perceived to be "promoting" sexuality,[64] an unwillingness on the part of the CDC to endorse the efficacy of condoms in preventing the spread of HIV,[65] and a decision by the Food and Drug Administration (FDA) to overrule its expert advisory panel and refuse to license over-the-counter sales of a morning-after contraceptive pill.[66] Thus, the extraordinary discomfort in the United States with sexuality in general and nonnormative sexualities in particular, combined with a concerted right-wing attack against sexual freedoms and sexuality research in recent years, likely has much to do with the stalling out of the incorporation of sexual orientation within the inclusion-and-difference paradigm.[67] The example clearly demonstrates how contingent, group-specific factors may affect the capacities for domain expansion, especially at unpropitious political moments.[68]

NATIONAL AND TRANSNATIONAL DIRECTIONS

Entrenchment and Partisan Politics

In thinking about the consolidation of the inclusion-and-difference paradigm and its likely future, one important question, very well suggested by the debates over sexuality and LGBT health research, concerns the impact of alternations in the political party controlling the executive branch and the Congress. Was the inclusion-and-difference paradigm just a temporal "blip" corresponding to a liberal political moment? Will it disappear if the United States government continues to veer in a conservative direction? Here, the evidence appears equivocal but does tend to suggest a fair measure of stability overall.

On one hand, there can be no doubt that the Clinton administration was sympathetic to the inclusion-and-difference paradigm. Not only were the inclusionary policies popular among its support base, but they also meshed closely with the strongly voiced commitment of Assistant Secretary for Health David Satcher (who also served as Surgeon General) to the reduction of health disparities, particularly disparities by race. On the other hand, the paradigm actually originated during the Republican administrations that preceded Clinton: such actions as the establishment of the task forces on women's health and minority health, the creation of the DHHS's Office of Minority Health and Office on Women's Health, the drafting of the first NIH policies on inclusion, the publication of several FDA guidelines on analyses of subpopulation differences, the appointment of Bernadine Healy as director of the NIH, and the approval of the Women's Health Initiative all took place between 1983 and 1992, during the Reagan and George H. W. Bush administrations. (To be sure, some of these developments benefited from the strength of Democrats within Congress and the legislative organizations that they supported, such as the Congressional Caucus for Women's Issues. The caucus, which played such a pivotal role in promoting women's health research, was essentially eliminated once Republicans took control of the House of Representatives in 1995.[69])

Moreover, the paradigm has survived into the presidency of George W. Bush. Rumors voiced in 2001 about the impending elimination of the DHHS Office of Minority Health and Office on Women's Health did not translate into reality,[70] and when the administration announced in 2002 that it would suspend the FDA's rule, imposed in 1998, requiring drug companies to test new drugs in children, the suspension was reversed a month later in response to a public outcry.[71] Other cornerstones of the paradigm, including the mandate and funding of the NIH-level offices and the current NIH policy on inclusion of women and minorities, are authorized by statute and necessarily will remain in place until Congress says otherwise.[72] Thus, the halting of domain expansion in controversial cases such as LGBT health does not necessarily mean that the paradigm as a whole is at risk.

Barring a substantial reframing of the DHHS mission, it may be the case that the new classificatory standards and standard operating procedures of the inclusion-and-difference paradigm are sufficiently institutionalized at this point that the political costs of dismantling the framework override any perceived ideological gains from doing so. As scholars have observed, there is an "inertial" quality to standards that often helps to cement policies into place.[73] Political sociologists, using terms such as "policy legacies" and "policy feedback," have described the "path-dependent" character of policymaking and how "decisions at one point in time can restrict future possibilities by sending policy off onto particular tracks."[74] The inertial qualities of biopolitical paradigms may also be given a boost by the discretionary powers of civil servants. For example, employees within the offices serving "special populations" may find creative ways to quietly advance their agendas and safeguard past victories, even in the face of opposition from political appointees located higher in the DHHS hierarchy.

Of course, there are always competing tendencies within a biopolitical paradigm, and changes in administration may lend support to one side in that competition. For example, it could be argued that the Clinton administration attempted to move the inclusion-and-difference paradigm beyond an emphasis on "differences" between groups and toward a concern with health "disparities." Whereas "differences" can be construed as a neutral term, "disparities" is a more manifestly political designation that points to an analysis of social inequalities. As noted above, Clinton and his appointees explicitly embraced the goal of reducing health disparities. DHHS agencies responded with concerted efforts to target disparities, in some cases creating new offices, such as the National Cancer Institute's Center to Reduce Cancer Health Disparities, which in 2000 absorbed that agency's former Office of Special Populations Research.[75] Since the beginning of the George W. Bush administration, however, DHHS concern with disparities—though promoted by the NIH's National Center on Minority Health and Health Disparities, created by Congress in 2000— has subsided somewhat overall, even while attention to "differences" continues.[76]

Transnational Extension?

A final question about the trajectory of the inclusion-and-difference paradigm concerns the extent to which other nations adopt similar policies and approaches. I have suggested that there is something "characteristically American" about the inclusion-and-difference paradigm, which seems to reflect the salience of the politics of identity in the United

States, as well as the politicization of biomedicine here. But in the world of biomedicine, the United States often has been the source of standards that are taken up and adopted elsewhere. Especially given the increasing degree of international collaboration in biomedical research, it makes sense to wonder whether other nations are finding their way to arrangements similar to the inclusion-and-difference paradigm, whether by intentional importation and adaptation of U.S. policies, or by a looser sort of diffusion, or by some process of relatively independent invention.

The field of science studies has traced how particular knowledge claims travel from place to place: Can we also speak of the spread of larger frameworks of knowledge production?[77] I have not investigated this question through a systematic inquiry into research practices in other countries, so I cannot answer it in an exhaustive way. The evidence available to me suggests a limited, but perhaps increasing, spread of inclusionary goals—particularly with regard to women—from the United States to a number of Anglophone and European countries. However, this expression of an inclusionary intent mostly has not translated into a new regulatory framework, and formal policies with mechanisms of enforcement are mostly absent outside the United States.

The country that has come closest to the United States in its concern with inclusion and difference in the biomedical research arena is Canada. In 1996 Health Canada, the Canadian government's health ministry, announced that its Drugs Directorate would "require the enrollment of a representative number of women into clinical trials for those drugs that are intended to be used specifically by women or in populations that are expected to include women."[78] The following year, Health Canada issued a broader policy statement on the "inclusion of women in clinical trials," affirming the importance of studying female subjects in all stages of drug development, and also calling for subgroup analyses to detect differences in how drugs may affect women and men.[79] In 1999 the agency adopted a policy of conducting "gender-based analysis" as "an organizing principle . . . to bring forth and clarify the differences between women and men."[80] Health Canada also contains a Bureau of Women's Health and Gender Analysis, first established in 1993 and emphasizing policy in its mission.[81]

The similarities between these policies and offices and their analogues in the United States are not altogether surprising, given the close ties between the two neighbors (and despite the stark contrasts in their health-care financing systems). To a large degree, they are due to direct communication between the two countries. Ruth Merkatz, the former head of the FDA's Office of Women's Health, recalled discussions between the government officials and the advocacy groups in the two countries,[82] and Health Canada's inclusion statement noted that their policy was "consistent with that taken by other regulatory agencies that have taken steps to encourage the study of all subpopulations in their countries."[83] At the same time, the differences are interesting: Canadian inclusion-and-difference policies are less extensive and less coercive than their U.S. counterparts. Despite making the general argument that "drugs should be studied prior to approval in subjects representing the full range of patients likely to receive the drug once it is marketed," Health Canada's inclusion policy focuses on women; it has little to say explicitly about other dimensions of identity and difference, such as age, race, or ethnicity.[84] It may be relevant here that the Canadian government collects less information about its citizens by race: the census only began asking a sample of respondents to indicate their "visible minority" status in 1996, although a question about the ethnic origin of one's ancestors dates back to 1961.[85] In addition, critics have complained that officials at Health Canada do little to enforce the guideline. According to two researchers writing in 2001, "they have failed even to collect data by sex or to monitor the inclusion of women in drug trials."[86]

Other English-speaking countries, such as the United Kingdom and Australia, also have promoted the inclusion of women in general terms, though without adopting any regulations actually mandating such inclusion. The United Kingdom's Medical Research Council does not have formal guidelines on gender inclusion or gender analysis but does recommend that clinical trials be conducted in a way that permits generalizability to all populations.[87] In addition, according to two researchers writing in the *BMJ* (*British Medical Journal*), "concerns of low participation by minorities in randomised trials have led to calls for the adoption of a similar standard" to that instituted by the NIH.[88] Similarly, Australia's National Health and Medical Research Council has declared it "the responsibility of researchers to systematically collect gender-specific data as part of every clinical trial in order to identify any clinically important differences between men and women that may, or may not, exist."[89]

Elsewhere in Europe, there appears to be less attention to these issues—and perhaps even some skepticism.[90] One U.S. expert on clinical trials returned from a period of living in Brussels in 1998 and reported that biomedical researchers there "just 'pooh, pooh' [the NIH guidelines] and think [that Americans] are obsessed with political correctness and so on."[91] French researchers have suggested to me that the U.S. concern with difference is inconsistent with the French emphasis on citizenship as a universal status; they note that the French state simply does not collect data on anyone's racial identity.[92] In addition, pediatricians have claimed that European countries have been less aggressive in promoting studies of the effects of medications on children.[93]

At the same time, the development of supranational governance is having important effects in Europe. Not only is it bringing about more standardization of research procedures and drug regulation across the continent, but also, it may be moving Europe more in the direction of the United States in these matters. For example, a European Union "guidance for the request for authorisation of a clinical trial on a medicinal product" requires researchers to indicate the numbers of subjects they intend to recruit, broken down by age and by gender.[94] However, perhaps the strongest indication that the European Union may be taking some cues from the United States came in 2005, when the European Parliament approved a law explicitly modeled on U.S. practice that compels pharmaceutical companies to test new drugs in children. Before any new drug can be approved, the sponsoring company must submit a pediatric investigation plan to a thirty-five-member advisory committee whose membership will be independent of industry.[95]

The work of the International Conference on Harmonisation of Technical Requirements for Registration of Pharmaceuticals for Human Use (ICH), a transnational body created in 1990 whose goal is to "harmonize," or standardize, the registration of pharmaceutical products in the European Union, Japan, and the United States, is also likely to encourage the concern with identity and difference. In chapter 7 I described the ICH's attempt—not altogether successful—to grapple with the impact of "ethnic factors" in the acceptability of foreign data. In addition, the ICH has issued guidelines on the study of geriatric populations that call for an end to improper exclusions of the elderly from clinical trials.[96] Another ICH document, on the evaluation of new antihypertensive drugs, recommends: "Patients from relevant demographic subsets should be studied, including both men and women, racial/ethnic groups pertinent to the region, and both young and older patients. The very old or 'fragile elderly,' i.e., patients >75 years old, should be included."[97]

To the extent that the ICH succeeds in its goal of standardizing clinical research practices internationally, inclusionary policies may eventually spread throughout Europe as well as in Japan. However, the precise categories that are invoked in such policies are likely to vary, and, again, the policies may well prove to lack the enforcement "teeth" of those adopted in the United States. In this limited way, it is certainly possible that versions of, or parallels to, the inclusion-and-difference paradigm will eventually become visible in diverse locations around the world.

Identity, Difference, Disparities, and Biopolitical Citizenship

UNDERSTANDING BIOPOLITICAL REFORM

Recap

Beginning in the 1980s, a diverse set of reformers developed a critique of an exclusionary and homogenizing, one-size-fits-all approach to biomedical knowledge-making as well as the medically problematic and socially unjust logic that underpinned it. The alternative orientation toward biomedical research that they have promoted—an inclusive but group-specific one—has attracted broad support at both elite and popular levels in the United States. It mattered little that the charge that medical researchers had studied only middle-aged white men, and had taken this group to be the "standard human" and the basis for generalization to all others, was an oversimplification. Though this claim truncated complex histories of scientific medicine, biomedical ethics, and the study of racial and gender differences, it did still manage to capture something important about the biases and blind spots of biomedical researchers. By criticizing those biases and blind spots, reformers drew needed attention to the health needs of their constituencies.

This heterogeneous collection of political actors—including members of health advocacy groups and grassroots social movements, medical professionals and scientists, government officials, and elected politicians—mounted an "antistandardization resistance movement." Representatives of different social groups, such as women, racial and ethnic minorities, and children, mostly acted separately, but they took advantage of similar political opportunities, and their argumentation overlapped significantly. Reformers proved able to bring pressure to bear simultaneously from several directions: from sympathetic "insiders" within government health agencies, from aggressive external advocacy groups, from experts and professionals, from the media, and from the U.S. Congress. Their strength derived in part from their location on both sides of the boundaries between science and policy, state and society, and "insider" and "outsider" politics. In addition, these various advocates successfully framed their concerns in a variety of ways that bridged questions of citizenship and biology. And they fused different meanings of *representation* (statistical, social, political, and symbolic) to construct a multirepresentational politics.

In the end, reformers succeeded in promoting a new set of meanings about medical research in the United States—indeed, in creating a new common sense. This cultural work—the invention of a sort of bio-multiculturalism—went hand in hand with institutional change, reflected in the creation of laws, policies, practices, and state bureaucratic offices. I have described this new set of beliefs and practices as an example of a biopolitical paradigm, and I have called it the "inclusion-and-difference paradigm" to emphasize its two key principles: the inclusion of members of diverse groups as research subjects and the measurement of outcome differences across medical subgroups.

Advocates of such policies helped bring that reality into being by encouraging the alignment or superimposition of categories used in biomedicine, identity politics, and bureaucratic administration—what I have called "categorical alignment." The unspoken agreement to assume that the categories of political mobilization and state administration also functioned as the categories of biomedical differentiation was given crucial support by federal health officials. DHHS officials took ways of thinking about group inequality and systems of group classification used elsewhere in government (such as the census) and transposed them onto the biomedical research domain, inscribing the categories into policies, forms, and surveillance systems that prescribe biomedical work practices. In the process, other ways of classifying health risks, such as by behavioral practices, and other ways of classifying populations, such as by social class, received far less attention—and the question of why the categories of political mobilization and administration should also be viewed as the categories of greatest biomedical relevance was effectively bypassed.

By endorsing specific social categories as the official targets of governance and scientific inquiry, reformers thereby promoted what I have termed "niche standardization"—an alternative to either complete generality (a one-size-fits-all embrace of the "standard human") or full particularity (a focus on the individual) that instead treats designated social categories or groups as the standardized formal units of analysis. Though proponents of group-specific policies gained rhetorical mileage by aligning their approach with concepts such as "personalized medicine," their actual policies displaced standardization to an intermediate level—that of the census category, the social identity, and the market niche—located in some sense between individuality and universality.

Reformers confronted significant opposition from many researchers, politicians, and biostatisticians, who framed the issues quite differently. Opponents challenged reformers' empirical claims, worried about damage to the biomedical enterprise, and sometimes warned of "quotas" or "affirmative action." But the new approach proved capable of speaking to the interests of at least some representatives of several constituencies: health advocates concerned with promoting more research on specific sociodemographic groups, thereby to improve their health and reduce health disparities; defenders of equality of opportunity and affirmative action who came to see biomedical research as a new domain in which citizenship rights could be pursued; pharmaceutical companies interested in niche marketing to women, children, or racial and ethnic minorities; clinical researchers studying specific groups; and federal health officials staffing new offices in areas such as women's health, for whom the paradigm provides a mandate. Others who started out with less enthusiasm, including many biomedical researchers, state actors, and pharmaceutical companies, also found they could live with requirements that were less onerous and that impinged less on their autonomy than they initially had feared.

Closure of controversy in this case had much to do with the flexible and often creative approaches taken by DHHS officials in charge of implementing political mandates. These officials translated the insistent but sometimes vague mandates of Congress into workable policies. Jockeying between competing pressures, these officials helped solidify the paradigm through boundary work—drawing new lines between "science" and "politics"—in ways that substantially appeased both reformers and their critics while preserving the autonomy and discretion of DHHS agencies.

As a consequence, over time, the inclusion-and-difference paradigm has assumed an important place within U.S. health research policy and practice. In particular, its logic has diffused through the DHHS. While most closely associated with the NIH Revitalization Act of 1993, the paradigm in fact is manifested in a whole series of laws and policies established from the mid-1980s to the present, as well as in special offices created within the DHHS. New standard operating procedures for the conduct of federally funded research and pharmaceutical drug development have become institutionalized, and federal officials have developed systems intended to track compliance. The pressure to carry out more inclusive and representative research also has sparked the development of the auxiliary science that I have termed "recruitmentology"—new, scientific approaches to the recruitment of human subjects, particularly from previously underrepresented groups—and a concomitant reconsideration of issues of risk, trust, and community participation in medical research. Spillover effects of the paradigm are evident elsewhere in the world of biomedicine, such as in the policies of medical journals, the curricula of medical schools, and the marketing practices of pharmaceutical companies. There also has been some movement toward "domain expansion"—extending ideas of inclusion and difference to encompass other social groups conceived of as comparable or analogous—with limited success for lesbian, gay, bisexual, and transgender health advocates, among others. Finally, the inclusion-and-difference paradigm may even be spreading across national borders, at least in some countries and to a limited extent, and despite considerable uncertainty about the definitions of ethnic and racial categories at a global level.

Inclusionary policies bring needed attention to groups that historically have been at a disadvantage in the medical domain (whether through statistical underrepresentation in medical research or by other means), and they merit praise on those grounds. Moreover, the new concern with studying outcome differences between groups has sometimes brought obvious benefit. Few would dispute the virtues of obtaining better knowledge, for example, about the doses of medications that ought properly to be administered to children—though, to be sure, pursuing such data inevitably increases the risk of harm to those children who participate as research subjects. Yet the institutionalization of the inclusion-and-difference paradigm highlights—and sometimes masks—many important and difficult questions, both practical and normative, about its real-world consequences, both intended and otherwise. While critics maintain that the policies have gone too far and have enshrined a simplistic, bean-counting approach to questions of medical difference, many supporters of the new policies charge that reform has stalled out. Noting that inclusion remains an elusive goal for certain diseases and that subgroup analyses are not always performed when they should be, these supporters of inclusion argue that further pressures and sanctions are needed to realize the original intent.

By one reading—not an implausible one—a formally rational and technical approach to monitoring the compliance with inclusionary policies and a preference for symbolic rituals of compliance often have taken precedence over a substantive concern with the issues that originally motivated the reform wave. Yet at the same time, symbolic politics may have real effects—not least in forcing researchers at least to think about a set of important issues that otherwise they might simply avoid. Moreover, criticism of the formalistic aspects of DHHS monitoring of inclusion can miss the extent to which informal work-arounds often lead to reasonable outcomes at the end of the day.

Meanwhile, to the extent that the policies indeed have succeeded— in the sense of actually redirecting research practices—my analysis has suggested additional dangers. By displacing attention away from other ways of grouping people and by focusing on categorical identities rather than on social practices and social structures, the inclusionary policies adopted by the U.S. government may distract us from addressing key pathways that lead to ill health in general and to unequal health outcomes in particular. And by promoting subgroup analyses, they may inspire a proliferation of findings of racial and sex differences whose causes and significance are unclear.

Furthermore, insofar as the policies reinforce a problematic under-standing of differences in health as matters of biology, then they may actually get in the way of addressing health disparities. And by encouraging racial profiling, the reliance on racial identification as a proxy in medical decision-making, they may lead to inappropriate care in individual cases. Related, though not identical, questions can be raised about the consequences of reinforcing ideas about the biological bases of health disparities by sex and gender. In fact, I have argued that the tendency to engage in sharp boundary work between race and sex, and to accept sex profiling as "obviously" sensible in contrast to the problematic character of racial profiling, merits reappraisal. Thus, the new policy framework may be coming together with new biomedical approaches to the study of race and sex to create a self-reinforcing system of meaning and practice, within which questions about inequalities in the domain of health are addressed reflexively with reference to the biological. In the process, other ways of thinking about health, illness, and risk are occluded.

Clearly, this is a complicated story, centering on a policy shift with complex causes and on double-edged and sometimes unintended consequences that make it hard to reach a simple conclusion about "success" or "failure."[1] What can we learn from it that goes beyond the specifics that I have recounted? In the remaining pages of this book, I approach this question from two angles. First, I briefly consider the lessons of this historical episode for how we think about the relationship between biomedicine and politics, and I argue for the virtues of studying what I have called biopolitical paradigms. Second, at somewhat greater length, I address the issue of paths not taken: How might things be otherwise?

What alternative ways of conceiving of the problem and its solutions might we consider?

Studying Biopolitical Paradigms

Although the everyday domains of scientific work and political action are constantly crisscrossing, it is often hard to anticipate the specific ways in which they can become woven together through words and deeds. Who would have expected that technical questions about the methodologies used by medical researchers and political struggles about group rights would come to be seen as inextricably linked? A contingent set of historical circumstances in the United States prompted an eclectic set of reformers to bring these issues into joint focus—and to assume not only that political pressure should be brought to bear to make science function better, but also that clinical research was an appropriate arena in which to pursue equality, justice, and full rights of citizenship. Yet the bridging of concerns made cultural sense, and in that respect this story says something more general about the relations among biomedical institutions, state administration, and social movement activism in countries like the United States at the present historical moment.

I have called the inclusion-and-difference approach a "biopolitical" paradigm to reflect this intriguing fusion. The point here is not that the domain of science was "invaded" by the political machinations of lay health advocates and state administrators and transformed from without. Neither is the point that biomedical science was yoked into administrative service by those outsiders. Rather, the inclusion-and-difference paradigm is biopolitical because it promotes ways of defining, knowing, and governing populations that are derived from, and serve to shape, both governmental and scientific practices simultaneously. Biomedical science is linked to governance in this case not simply because the health of the people has become conceived of as a matter of crucial public concern, but because academic medical researchers, pharmaceutical company scientists, federal health bureaucrats, and lay health advocates have collaborated in deciding upon the basic population subunits for biomedical purposes.

Processes of classification and standardization, therefore, lie at the heart of this story.[2] Indeed, three broad historical tendencies converge in placing categories and standards at the center. First, the agencies of modern democratic states have become increasingly involved in naming and singling out subgroups of people for policy purposes, assigning social rewards (or punishments) according to administrative categories, and thereby placing phenomena such as race and gender at the heart of the state's maintenance of social order.[3] Second, social movements have become ever more likely both to assert demands on the basis of claimed social identities and to elaborate new collective identities through their very activism.[4] Third, scientific experts progressively have developed new technologies and understandings that result in the segmenting or classifying of the human species, sometimes creating new lines of cleavage or bases of solidarity.[5] Not infrequently, these three developments collide, resulting in competition over symbolic power, as state actors, political activists, and scientific experts vie for the authority to say who counts as what and struggle to determine whose categories will rule. By contrast, the case of the inclusion-and-difference paradigm is largely one of categorical convergence or alignment, rather than categorical competition. (Only those who fought the passage of new inclusionary polices challenged the idea that the self-descriptors of identity politics, the bureaucratic categories of state administration, and the subgroup designations of clinical research might all come together into a single standardized set of classificatory labels.)

Because my empirical case is situated on the terrains of "the state," "medical science," and "social movements" and yet confounds attempts to distinguish clear borders between these theoretical entities, it demands a hybrid set of theoretical approaches and conceptual tools. I have borrowed freely from science studies, political sociology, racial and ethnic studies, and gender and sexuality studies, among other bodies of literature, in order to analyze the nexus of science/state/society relations.

In a sense, I have built my analytical toolkit "outward" from a basic starting point, the question of extrapolation of medical findings that is at the heart of this case: How can the knowledge obtained by studying a designated group of people participating in clinical research be applied to others outside the experimental situation? Within science studies, much analysis has focused on the capacity of scientists credibly to generalize findings beyond the restricted domain of the laboratory so as to make those findings broadly relevant.[6] Such work on the part of scientific spokespersons demands not only the attribution of likeness across diverse cases, but also, as Bruno Latour has described, the dissolving of boundaries between what is "inside" and "outside" the laboratory.[7]

In the case analyzed here, however, what is at stake is not only the construction of similarities but also, quite centrally, the definition of human differences. Therefore, it becomes crucial to consider the intertwining of biomedical fact-making with processes of racial formation and gender formation—that is, how the unstable and contested meanings of race and gender temporarily congeal into particular forms through the representational work of individuals and organizations.[8] In this case, ideas about the very meaning of race, gender, and other forms of difference were co-constructed with ideas about the proper inferences that might be drawn from biomedical experiments. At the same time, as the representatives of groups that were organized around categorical identities put forward their own claims about the meanings of *sameness* and *difference*, the issue of generalizability also became interwoven with debates over identity politics and multiculturalism. And as these actors made claims about their rights vis-à-vis the institutions of biomedical research and health policy, they put forward new conceptions of biopolitical citizenship.[9] Thus, a debate over scientific generalizability ended up being about much more.

Further complicating the analytical task, this broadened story of generalizability and difference-making has unfolded within a complex political field marked by a hybrid reform coalition of state and nonstate actors. To understand an interpenetrated movement that is both inside and outside the state and to track its attempts to institutionalize changes within the formal organizations that make up biomedicine and health policy, I have relied on sociological literatures that span the gap between the study of social movements and organizations. This structural analysis of the relation between scientific and other institutions—combined with a cultural emphasis on frames of meaning, institutional schemas, and work practices—is consistent with the move to elaborate a "new political sociology of science," as described recently by Scott Frickel and Kelly Moore.[10] The goal here is to understand the material production of knowledge—not just the construction of facts, but what Karin Knorr Cetina has called the "construction of the machineries of knowing"[11]—while embedding that scrutiny within a close analysis of the mechanisms of power, hierarchy, and social organization.[12] The concepts that I have put forward in the service of that analysis—categorical alignment, niche standardization, multirepresentational politics, and biopolitical paradigms—lend themselves to potential application in a wide range of cases involving the modern politics of bodies, groups, and populations.

Analyses of interpenetrated movements that take up questions related to science and technology point us in the direction of a larger theoretical and empirical project. On one side, scholars have suggested models for understanding the mutual constitution of state and society that abandon reified and holistic notions of "the state" as well as any simple notion of a divide between it and "society."[13] On the other side, a central project of science and technology studies has been to theorize the mutual constitution of the state and science and to describe the tight historical intertwining of technoscientific development and modern state formation.[14] Case studies of interpenetrated technoscientific movements demand that we find ways of bringing these literatures together to understand the ever-evolving relations among—and the redefinitions of the boundaries between—science, society, and the state.

This is a large project, but the concept of the biopolitical paradigm presents a useful point of entry. Additional studies can reveal the manifold ways in which science and government come together, conceptually and practically, in the definition and management of bodies, groups, and populations in different societies at different historical movements.

ALTERNATIVE PATHWAYS

While pointing toward new theoretical syntheses, the story of the inclusion-and-difference paradigm also raises practical, political, and theoretical dilemmas for all those who care about the promotion of health and the eradication of social inequalities. I have suggested throughout this book that the changes encompassed within this reform wave help achieve those two goals to a limited degree, but also generate new obstacles. How might things be otherwise? What alternative paths might be pursued? The point here is not to engage in utopian fantasizing that is divorced from on-the-ground practicalities, but rather to examine the alternative models that inhere within existing social developments: What other languages exist for speaking about inclusion, participation, identity and difference, and health inequalities? I address these four concerns in turn.

Beyond "Inclusion": What Conceptions of Research?

The debate over inclusionary research policies begs a number of questions about the conditions under which clinical research most effectively can shed light on the relations between difference, inequality, and health. Drawing on the critiques developed by various analysts, I propose a number of concrete suggestions. As a starting point, it is important not to exaggerate the capacity of clinical trials to provide fully trustworthy knowledge about *any* population. For example, an interesting, and worrisome, finding from recent reviews of clinical trials is that drug trials funded by industry are statistically more likely to yield positive results than trials funded by nonprofit sources.[15] It is conceivable, in other words, that effects having to do with who sponsors a trial may swamp any differences potentially detectable between population subgroups.

Additional problems built into the structure of drug testing and approval also have implications for how critiques of one-size-fits-all medical research are considered. For example, Jay Cohen has described how drug companies are inclined to use unnecessarily high doses of experimental drugs in clinical trials in order to generate sufficiently convincing evidence of the efficacy of their products—but these doses then cause problems for many patients that may become widely apparent only after a drug has been marketed. Thus, the adverse effects of medications that often are cited as a rationale for separate study of groups who disproportionately suffer them, such as women and the elderly, may in part be attributed to contingent aspects of how drug companies marshal evidence for presentation to the FDA.[16]

Other difficulties with clinical trials are even more fundamental to the experimental technique. As the biostatistician critics of the NIH Revitalization Act correctly emphasized, the problem of how to generalize from human subjects (who, being volunteers, rarely approximate a representative sample) to actual groupings of people outside of the experimental setting is intrinsic to the clinical trial and never fully resolvable. No methodology (short of studying everyone) ultimately guarantees the "external validity" of trial findings for the mass of humanity, let alone for any specific subgroup or individual.[17] And no policy of inclusion or subgroup comparison can make the uncertainties go away. In short, when considering how to improve clinical research for any particular group, it is worth bearing in mind the ultimate limits of the technology to provide us with the knowledge that we crave.

Second, it might be valuable to focus expert and public attention less on the issue of the "efficacy" of therapies (as measured in the experimental situation) and more on their "effectiveness" in the broader context of everyday use.[18] For example, if the ultimate effectiveness of a therapy depends on the ability of a patient to obtain and consume it on a regular basis according to schedule, then concern might appropriately be directed to issues of pharmaceutical pricing and health care financing. Outside the experimental setting, such matters may have more impact on whether a drug "works" for a particular group than, say, genetic differences affecting the metabolizing of the drug. The biological-differences frame employed by reformers can potentially obscure this important consideration, one that goes to the heart of what we mean by social equality in the domain of health care.

Third, it is important to think beyond the conceptual limits of the models of health and illness that have tended to accompany the inclusionary policies. A number of critics have suggested rightly that such policies are, at best, a starting point. According to Chloe Bird and Patricia Rieker, in a critique of the biomedical study of gender differences in health, simply including women and performing subgroup analyses is not enough: "these

287 Biopolitical Citizenship

efforts alone will not clarify whether differences in men's and women's health (e.g., morbidity, mortality and their relative responsiveness to particular medical treatments) are due to social or biological factors." Their point is not that we need to choose between the two, but rather that we always should be studying their complex interaction.[19]

Similarly, Londa Schiebinger, in her book *Has Feminism Changed Science?* has judged medicine to be one of the clearest cases where the answer is yes—but she has insisted that just adding women to studies is insufficient, unless the dominant explanatory models are supplemented by community, social, and ecosocial models.[20] Janet Shim also has provided an important critique by noting how the "operationalizing" of identity categories—the transformation of such phenomena as race, class, and gender into health research variables—not only strips the phenomena out of their social context but also changes what we imagine them to be: "Race, class, and gender are thus seen not as relational constructs but as individualistic attributes, as located solely *in* the biological bodies of individuals rather than also in the social spaces *between* them."[21] The disembedding of race, class, and gender from their social context also makes it harder, as Shim has argued, to examine the complex ways in which these social relations *intersect* in everyday life and help to constitute one another.[22] (These intersections are taken seriously by some DHHS agencies, such as the ORWH, though certainly not by biomedical institutions generally.) Together, these analysts have suggested the need to think outside the box of "difference" as it has tended to be construed in discussions of health research. Simply including various groups as research subjects within mainstream research is insufficient unless some of the presumptions of mainstream research are questioned simultaneously.

Fourth, it is crucial for researchers to proceed beyond the simple identification of outcome differences. As Shim also has observed, research on sex/gender and race differences has a tendency to halt prematurely, with the simple identification of a difference. But this "terminal analysis," as Shim has called it, stops short of investigating "exactly *how* such inequalities are produced"—the key question to be addressed.[23] Because the injunction to perform subgroup analysis inevitably will result in more and more difference findings, it is important—as advocacy groups such as the Society for Women's Health Research indeed have emphasized—that such findings serve as the starting point for investigation, not the final word.

Fifth, as I have suggested throughout this book, there is great virtue in constantly questioning the premise that categories with high visibility and political salience in the United States, such as sex/gender, race/ethnicity, and age, necessarily and automatically are the most relevant in under-standing health disparities in every case. Examples cited in previous chapters—about hair color and height, among others—suggest the range of bodily factors that can have medical significance in particular cases. And in many instances, categories of identity may simply be less rele-vant than the particular practices in which individuals engage. Jacqueline Stevens has made the provocative proposal that the NIH expand its defi-nition of "minorities" beyond racial and ethnic groups when interpreting the mandate of the NIH Revitalization Act. According to Stevens, a re-vised regulation "should specify that federally funded medical research study many populations, including those that vary by childhood resi-dence, current residence, occupation, diet, exercise, age, wealth, income, and regularity of medical care." While studying all such subgroups would not be feasible or desirable, Stevens is right to challenge "the intuition that hereditary identities confer the most important differences among us."[24]

Finally, given the tendency of the policies within the inclusion-and-difference paradigm to presume and construct equivalences across the various forms of difference recognized within it, it is advisable to keep sight of the differences that exist across differences. Chapter 11 empha-sized the importance of considering sex/gender and race/ethnicity com-paratively when thinking about the practical utility of making prescribing decisions based on social membership. Other ways of differing, such as age and sexual identity, likewise pose unique questions and complica-tions.[25] We should be wary of the presumption that a common set of research practices or policy guidelines can do justice to the particular-ities of alternative systems of social differentiation, collective identity, or social hierarchy. In fact, we also should be cautious about presuming that a single set of practices or guidelines can do justice even to a single social group, given the inevitable differentiation within it. As Lise Vogel has argued more generally, "diversity should be recognized as relentlessly heterogeneous."[26]

Beyond "Participation": What Kinds of Political Interventions?

A different set of strategic dilemmas concerns the sort of political orga-nizing done and the kinds of democratizing or participatory claims made by those who seek to reform biomedical research practices. Several issues are worth considering. First, how should disruptions of the scientific pro-cess be viewed? How problematic is it for new criteria—simultaneously scientific and political—to be introduced into the peer review and drug approval processes? An interesting analogy—though perhaps an unlikely one on first glance—might be made to the debates that have ensued in recent decades about disruptions to the military as a result of pressures for racial integration, inclusion of women, and acceptance of open gays and lesbians. As Mary Katzenstein and Judith Reppy have argued, these debates typically have been "framed as a trade-off between the goals of egalitarianism and the requirements of military excellence." Against this way of conceiving the problem, they proposed that military efficacy and social equality be viewed "as values that inform each other." Rather than object that the military is no place for "social experiments," Katzenstein and Reppy's point is that militaries constantly are in the business of adapting simultaneously to changes in strategic needs and changes in society.[27] Similarly, there is no reason to presume that changes in biomedical research policies must be viewed as a trade-off between social equality and scientific excellence and no reason to view the imposition of such policies as an unnatural intervention into an otherwise pristine and unchanging realm of scientific practice.

Still, one might well worry that attempts to introduce new criteria for the judgment of biomedical research priorities and methods can have the practical effect of opening the floodgates for all sorts of interventions into the scientific domain—and it can be hard work to determine criteria for when such pressures are appropriate.[28] This concern was amply demonstrated in 2003, when (as I described in the preceding chapter) the Republican-dominated U.S. House of Representatives came within two votes of revoking the funding previously granted by the NIH to four research projects deemed a waste of federal tax dollars, all on topics related to sexuality and health. This intervention turned out to be spearheaded by the Traditional Values Coalition, a self-proclaimed "grassroots church lobby" well known for its attacks on gay rights.[29] To its credit, the Society for Women's Health Research was one of many health advocacy organizations that objected to this effort to impose the criteria of the Christian Right in the evaluation of research proposals. However, their response, which mirrored that of most others who rose to the defense of sexuality research, hit on the theme of protecting the autonomy of science and insulating the NIH peer review process from public pressure—a note that rang a bit hollow when sounded by a group that had had so much to say about how biomedical research should be done and how the NIH should go about its business.

To be sure, the SWHR was not being hypocritical when arguing that "it is inappropriate for Congress to dictate to NIH which individual grants are deserving of support by the agency": the SWHR has not focused on criticizing individual research projects (except perhaps completed ones, such as the Physicians' Health Study), and it certainly has never sought to defund any grants already approved by NIH study sections. Still, it seemed at least a bit disingenuous for an advocacy group that was founded to promote the inclusionary mandate of the NIH Revitalization Act and that consistently has sought additional legislative and administrative means to strengthen its effects to declare: "Political interference in scientific research sets a dangerous precedent. . . . Every effort must be made to ensure that the scientists at NIH and other federal agencies are allowed to pursue important research without the burden of undue government interference."[30]

In a political environment in which groups across the political spectrum, on issues ranging from climate change to evolution to health and medicine, seek to evaluate and influence scientific research, it seems unlikely that calls to shore up the autonomy of science will be heeded. Moreover, if some sort of public participation in relation to science and technology is considered a virtue in a democratic society, and if the real question is how such participation best can be organized so as to promote, rather than impede, effective research, then the simple notion of a dividing line between science and politics is unlikely to be helpful.[31] I have suggested elsewhere, drawing on the example of AIDS treatment activism, that certain styles of lay participation—based on the acquisition of a hybrid expertise that combines useful local knowledge with a decent understanding of the relevant scientific knowledge base—are most likely to increase the practical benefits of medical research.[32] A related approach has focused on the need to develop what Alison Wylie has called "a framework for understanding how, far from compromising epistemic integrity, certain kinds of diversity (cultural, racial, gender) may significantly enrich scientific inquiry, a matter of urgent practical and political as well as philosophical concern."[33] However, in the absence of perfect solutions to these conundrums concerning the politics of knowledge, it seems important that there be open discussion and careful consideration of the virtues as well as the pitfalls of different sorts of political interventions in the biomedical research process.

If the above questions concern the impact of political pressures on scientific research, another set of concerns has more to do with the transformation of health advocacy. Building on the work of other scholars, I suggested in chapter 11 that the professionalization of women's health advocacy in recent decades and its focus on issues of inclusion and difference comes at a potential political cost and may reflect a turning away from some of the goals and philosophies of the feminist women's health movement. Additionally, Carol Weisman has suggested that "the heightened visibility of women's health issues" in the 1990s made it possible for a range of politicians and medical organizations to adopt and co-opt the theme of women's health, "fram[ing] an issue as 'women's health' to garner support, even if their initiatives or issues were not endorsed by women's groups."[34]

The case of LGBT health activism also demonstrates some of the dilemmas posed by a state-targeted health advocacy of this sort. To the limited degree that LGBT health has been incorporated within the framework of the inclusion-and-difference paradigm, then the turn toward the state on the part of health advocates has posed complications for some grassroots activists. For example, activists who have promoted a "sex-positive" approach to gay health issues have been made uncomfortable by the implicit requirement of incorporation within the inclusion-and-difference framework—namely, that sexual orientation should be treated as a dimension of identity that distinguishes different subgroups of people, but that sexuality itself should be mentioned as little as possible.[35] It may prove inadvisable for social movements to ignore what the political theorist Wendy Brown has described as the "dangers in surrendering control . . . to the state, as well as in looking to the state as provider, equalizer, protector, or liberator."[36] It is also worth considering the long-term impact of building up new state bureaucratic structures, as well as the irony, described by the political scientist James Morone, that, in the United States, reforms with a democratizing intent so often have the effect of "expand[ing] the scope and authority of the state, especially its administrative capacity."[37]

Beyond "Identity versus Difference"

The empirical case analyzed in this book also sheds light on the much-discussed and oft-maligned notion of identity politics. I have argued that a style of politics based on promoting the rights and interests of categorical groups, such as "women" or "people of color," was central to the call for inclusionary reforms in biomedical research. Indeed, as I have suggested, the greater attractiveness of these reforms in the United States as opposed to other countries likely has something to do with the higher salience of, and greater cultural familiarity with, identity politics in the United States. While identity politics has been both defended and attacked from many quarters,[38] this case calls attention to the particular resonances of identity politics in a biomedical context: What happens when familiar debates about universalism and particularism or sameness and difference take shape in relation to bodies and diseases? How does a tendency to construe identities and differences in biological terms affect the dynamics of identity politics?

As I have described, an important body of work, premised on a critique of liberal notions of both individualism and universalism and supportive of group-based rights, is broadly consistent with the logic of the inclusion-and-difference paradigm. For example, the political theorist Iris Marion Young has argued that "sometimes recognizing particular rights for groups is the only way to promote their full participation."[39] Against the notion that citizenship properly implies a homogenizing sameness in the formal treatment of everyone, Young has maintained that "the inclusion and participation of everyone in public discussion and decision making requires mechanisms for group representation."[40] As Young has noted—drawing on what feminist theorists have called the "dilemma of difference" or the "equality versus difference debate"—sometimes genuine social equality requires treating different groups differently, rather than (as traditional liberalism would have it) treating everyone just the same.[41] The idea that individual rights may need to be supplemented with group rights in order to ensure fair treatment also has been advanced by Will Kymlicka and others seeking to promote new models of "multicultural citizenship" that can be made compatible with democratic institutions.[42] Analysts of the fight to include more women in clinical research have noted the relevance of these discussions. For example, Lisa Eckenwiler has invoked Young's work in declaring: "The goal of social equality, therefore, calls for the public affirmation of particularity. Research policies that attend to the situatedness of groups and their members, that recognize persons as physiologically unique and socially situated (relational, informed in their knowledge and moral commitments by group membership, and modified by complex and often oppressive social relations and processes), can offset or counteract historical disadvantages and promote social equality and justice."[43]

In health policy as in other domains, agencies of the state increasingly are confronting the question of whether to endorse differential treatment according to the logic of "group rights."[44] In a recent comparative analysis, Frank De Zwart outlined a range of potential responses by modern states to such demands for group rights. One option is "accommodation," where state actors "designate beneficiaries of redistributive policies according to membership in groups that state and society take for granted," and where policymakers, having formalized the list of official groups, effectively "treat the social categories as real groups." While De Zwart's example of accommodation is affirmative action policy in the United States, the approach toward medical research policy described in this book also illustrates this framework. Quite a different response is "denial," the insistence that, "despite inequality between social or cultural groups, redistribution policies do not benefit any particular group."[45] Here, as De Zwart has noted, a "textbook example" is the "philosophy of republican citizenship" in France, a country that does not collect data on race or ethnicity and whose government has proclaimed (remarkably) that "France is a country in which there are no minorities."[46]

As the analyses by Young, Kymlicka, and De Zwart all make clear, notions of group rights often are linked to claims about access to resources and rewards. Similarly, in their attempt to redirect medical research resources toward previously under-studied groups, the inclusionary reforms represent more than simply a "politics of recognition," as identity politics are often characterized as being.[47] When *The New Republic* gave the name "Group Therapy" to a 1993 article that was highly critical of the NIH Revitalization Act's subgroup analysis requirement, the magazine effectively associated the group-specific approach toward clinical research with a kind of self-absorbed, psychotherapeutic turn often seen as a risk in identity politics—a turn "away from engagement with institutionalized structures of power, toward a kind of apolitical introspection," in L. A. Kauffman's terms, or what Wendy Brown calls the danger of "the steady slide of political into therapeutic discourse."[48] But the program for biomedical inclusion was characterized not by an inward-looking obsession with wounds and victimization, but rather by what Mary Bernstein has called the strategic "deployment" of identity.[49] Although "cultural" demands for recognition of difference sometimes have been juxtaposed with the "political" pursuit of redistributive goals through institutional change, with the suggestion that these approaches are mutually exclusive,[50] the actions of the reformers I have studied would support the position of those who claim that the opposition has been exaggerated and that these approaches may often coincide.[51]

Identity politics also has been accused of promoting a "balkanization" of protest, through the fragmentation of a potential oppositional bloc into ever more finely characterized subdivisions based on narrow, though heartfelt, identities that are treated by their bearers as personal "essences."[52] At the same time, identity politics has been criticized for just the opposite problem of projecting an essentialist, monotone sameness that ignores crucial intragroup differences.[53] In both cases, critics have argued that these defects have implications for the capacity of the group to construct alliances, articulate a broader vision of social change, or otherwise rise above its particularistic interests. There is much to be said for the invention and promotion of alternative models of solidarity—rooted, perhaps, as Donna Haraway has suggested, "in friendship, work, partially shared purposes, intractable collective pain, inescapable mortality, [or] persistent hope."[54] However, as the work of scholars such as Mary Bernstein and Paul Lichterman has shown, the broad-brush charges against identity politics are also problematic: they reflect unwarranted generalizations that typically fail to consider the contingent effect of political circumstance on the diverse ways in which groups make use of identities.[55] Therefore, I would like to consider the specific forms in which identities are asserted and deployed in biomedical contexts. While there may be nothing inherently essentialist about identity politics, there may indeed be particular risks of a rigid essentialism when difference is biomedicalized.

As Craig Calhoun has noted, "a particularly troubling version of [the] impulse to find universally acceptable grounds for distinctive identities is the recurrent—and currently resurgent—urge to naturalize in the sense of finding a fixed biological basis for human identities."[56] Although it is common to view biological reductionism as an approach favored by those well to the right on the political spectrum—those who might, for example, assert the belief that scores on I.Q. tests reflect biological differences in abilities between racial groups—sometimes liberal social movements may biomedicalize themselves: they may invoke a belief in biological difference, or even assert a medical self-diagnosis, to provide strategic leverage in advancing their claims. They may argue, for example, that because homosexuality is innate (and rooted in a "gay gene" or in distinctive brain structures), gay people should not be expected to change their sexuality and, indeed, are entitled to legal protection of their rights;[57] or that women with postpartum depression are entitled to special consideration by legal and economic institutions precisely because the condition has been defined by experts as a legitimate and objective medical category. "The medical field is uniquely positioned to recognize the vocabulary of female difference spoken among American mothers who historically have gotten remarkably little support from the state," Verta Taylor noted in her analysis of the latter example.[58] Embracing a biomedical conception of identity is "a way of getting there," according to Carol Tavris—an effective, if problematic, route to legitimacy in certain social contexts.[59] Indeed, in an era of backlash in which it is increasingly difficult to articulate a compelling rationale for promoting social equality that is not tagged as "reverse discrimination,"[60] it is understandable that political actors would turn to medicalized notions of bodily difference to ground their demand for group rights and recognition in the authoritative language of modern science.

Yet there is tremendous irony in the turn to the biological and the medical, given the historical role of medical theorizing and practice in helping to construct the otherness of socially disenfranchised groups. In light of the long history within medicine of conceptualizing difference as pathology,[61] it may be highly problematic for groups that in the past have borne the brunt of such pathologizing—women, racial and ethnic minorities, sexual minorities, and the disabled, among others—to invoke biomedical notions of difference to legitimate their claims vis-à-vis biomedical institutions. As Matthew Waites has argued in a critique of essentialist "fixity claims" by identity-based social movements such as the lesbian and gay movement, "far from 'biomedical knowledge' and '[social] movement knowledge' . . . being distinct and opposing, . . . they have been overlapping, deeply intertwined and mutually sustaining to a considerable degree."[62] Hence, the very meanings (both formal and ordinary) of concepts such as race, sex, gender, and sexuality are hybrid historical outcomes of repeated cycles of interactive loops between expert labeling and the self-assertions of those being labeled.[63] In a sense, medical spokespersons and institutions helped to consolidate the social categories through which actors have come to challenge the biomedical establishment—to speak what Michel Foucault called a "reverse discourse."[64] That history does not preclude the possibility that those actors might change the cultural meanings of biological differences and wrest them out from under the shadow of pathology. But it does suggest that "positive" assertions of biological difference may readily backfire or lend tools to those who seek to reinforce old hierarchies. They also may provide a beachhead to those whose interest is to convert social identities into "market niches" for profit-making purposes.

Furthermore, the recourse to biological essentialism and reductionism manifested in the argumentation of many advocates of the inclusionary reforms not only encourages the spread of the idea that group differences have a biological "hard core," but also—to the extent that such understandings are adopted by those whom they describe—promotes a particularly rigid sort of identity politics. If our differences are understood to be rooted fundamentally in our bodies and in our genes, what possibilities are there of transcending those differences to find new commonalities or affinities? Friendly critics of identity politics have suggested a range of circumstances in which it can escape a narrow particularism—when identity is conceived of in a fluid and relational manner, when the presuppositions of identity-based claims are always up for debate, when agonistic forms of democratic negotiation lead to the emergence of new and larger collectivities that refuse to submerge difference.[65] Though it is impossible to be certain, I am skeptical that such forms of political action can flourish when the starting point is an assumption of primordial difference that is etched into our very bodies.

Analysts of so-called strategic essentialism quite rightly have pointed to the viability—indeed, the practical necessity—of adopting essentialist argumentation at certain moments in order to make political headway within institutions whose logic one cannot control.[66] However, essentialism is only truly strategic, and not merely reflexive or automatic, when its proponents are able to maintain a split consciousness—a constant awareness that essentialism is the game one is playing because one has to and not because it provides an accurate model of the nature of identity and difference. Otherwise, the risk is that "calling attention to [difference] in order to ameliorate inequality has the unintended effect of perpetuating the social divisions one wishes to eliminate."[67] I consider it highly debatable whether an opportunistic use of medical essentialism, rooted in the biological-differences frame, truly can be employed to serve the cause of justice in the domain of health.

Difference versus Disparity: How to Target Health Inequalities

In early 2005 U.S. President George W. Bush met with a group of African Americans to promote his plan to restructure and privatize Social Security. It was an opportunity both to build support for his proposal, which had come under heavy fire from critics, and to advance his party's agenda of convincing African Americans that their interests did not inevitably ally them to the Democrats. Bush informed his audience: "African-American males die sooner than other males do, which means the [Social Security] system is inherently unfair to a certain group of people." The implication was that members of this population would derive greater economic benefit should his alternative plan be put into place.[68] Thus, Bush took one of the most dramatic and enduring expressions of racial disparities in health outcomes in the United States—the gap in life expectancy between white and black Americans—and represented it as a simple fact of nature, built into the very order of things.[69] The possibility that features of the society he led might contribute to producing that gap, or that he, as president, might have some responsibility for finding ways to reduce it, appeared not to factor into his thinking. African American men were "destined" to die early, and the brute fact of difference—reified, naturalized, and severed from the social and political conditions that gave rise to it—could be presented as a baseline condition determining such men's objective interests.

The inclusion-and-difference paradigm offers inadequate intellectual resources to challenge such perceptions. Reformers who promoted inclusion pointed to health disparities—especially disparities by race—as part of the justification for changing biomedical research practices, but they did so typically without extended analysis of the complex array of conditions that might generate those disparities. Instead, they often fell back on a vaguer and less charged conception of group "difference," one that was more directly compatible with the biological-differences frame. To invoke disparities is to invoke a criterion of social justice; to refer to differences is to advance a somewhat more neutral understanding, one that lends itself to a wide array of uses. Differences do call out to be recognized, and to be responded to in a nonhomogenizing way. But disparities, by contrast, call out for their own elimination.[70]

During the Clinton administration, the president as well as the assistant secretary for health made eliminating health disparities an explicit policy aim, though not one that was successfully achieved. In recent years, many individual DHHS employees, working within agencies such as the NIH's National Center on Minority Health and Health Disparities, have worked hard pursuing this goal.[71] However, eliminating health disparities has received lip service more often than sustained attention from higher ranks within the DHHS and elsewhere in the federal government, while, as Nancy Krieger has described, allied conservative foundations have sought to portray that goal as so much "political correctness."[72]

The need for serious action could hardly be doubted: by the early years of the new millennium, a series of reports provided ample documentation of the extent of the continuing problem in the United States, particularly in the area of race and ethnicity.[73] According to the Institute of Medicine's lengthy report *Unequal Treatment*, "evidence of racial and ethnic disparities in healthcare is, with few exceptions, remarkably consistent across a range of illnesses and healthcare services."[74] One study, published in the *New England Journal of Medicine* in 2003, tracking the geographic patterns of utilization of a single procedure, knee arthroplasty, noted the complexity of the disparity in this case, given that the variation in use between blacks and non-Hispanic whites differed from that between non-Hispanic whites and Hispanics, and given that these ethnic disparities were crosscut by disparities by sex.[75] Risa Lavizzo-Mourey and James Knickman of the Robert Wood Johnson Foundation took the occasion to comment, in an accompanying editorial: "The root causes of these disparities in the health care sector are multifactorial. No simple, single explanation can be cited. The building of effective solutions requires an understanding of all the causes and the targeting of the right remedy."[76]

In 2002 Secretary of Health and Human Services Tommy Thompson declared: "Our goal is to eliminate disparities in health among all population groups by 2010."[77] The following year, the new Senate Republican majority leader, Bill Frist (himself a physician), said that "health care disparities, minority versus nonminority populations, is something I feel strongly about," and committed himself to reducing those disparities as evidence of his party's concern for the well-being of minorities.[78] Yet as much as politicians pledged to solve the problems that researchers continued to identify, critical observers had reason to be suspicious. In late 2003, when the DHHS released a 196-page *National Healthcare Disparities Report* that it had been required by law to prepare,[79] the public acquired an inside look at the administration's efforts to sanitize the problem. An unhappy DHHS staff member leaked the original draft, prepared in June of that year by researchers at the DHHS's Agency for Healthcare Research and Quality. As an investigative team commissioned by minority (Democratic) members of the House of Representatives Committee on Government Reform reported: The DHHS "substantially altered the conclusions of its scientists on healthcare disparities. In the June draft, the Department's scientists found 'significant inequality' in health care in the United States, called healthcare disparities 'national problems,' emphasized that these disparities are 'pervasive in our health care system,' and found that the disparities carry a significant 'personal and societal price.' The final version of the report, however, contains none of these conclusions." Indeed, the final version of the *National Healthcare Disparities Report* deleted most of the original draft's uses of the word *disparity*.[80] A few weeks later, the *New York Times* reported that an embarrassed DHHS Secretary Thompson was calling the revisions a "mistake" that would be rectified.[81] Thompson played down the issue by suggesting that "some individuals took it upon themselves" to provide a more upbeat tone.[82] However, an editorial in the *New England Journal of Medicine* by Gregg Bloche, who had served on the Institute of Medicine's committee on health disparities, cited DHHS sources and internal correspondence indicating that "Thompson's office twice refused to approve drafts by department researchers that emphasized detailed findings of racial disparity" and that "top officials within the offices of the assistant secretary for health and the assistant secretary for planning and evaluation asked for rewrites."[83]

Part of what was at stake in this confrontation was precisely the distinction between differences and disparities. The original draft presented the data on what it called "a broad array of differences related to access, use, and patient experience of care by racial, ethnic, socioeconomic and geographic groups, based on valid measures" and suggested it was reasonable to treat many of these as evidence of disparity. But the revised version instead stated: "Where we find variation among populations, this variation will simply be described as a 'difference.' By allowing the data to speak for themselves, there is no implication that these differences resulted in adverse health outcomes or imply prejudice in any way."[84] The risk here is that while the language of difference may provide an important opening for making claims about the need for group-tailored remedies, it fails to demand adequate attention to a crucial set of issues— specifically, the ways in which inequalities and power differentials in the broader society affects people's exposure to health risks, their capacity to access quality medical care, and the likelihood that they will be subject to conscious or unconscious discriminatory treatment by health care professionals.[85] To the extent that difference also is construed largely in biological terms, it becomes even less likely that these other issues will receive their due. It is certainly worthwhile to understand, for example, whether different groups of people respond differently at a biochemical level to pain medications. Yet it is also worth considering the implications of findings that pharmacies in heavily minority areas are far less likely than those in mainly white neighborhoods to stock pain medications on their shelves.[86]

The risk of reinterpreting disparity as difference is no idle concern; it has surfaced in a range of health-related contexts in recent years. For example, Sara Shostak has described how recent research in molecular genetics is transforming debates about the health risks that stem from exposures to toxins in the environment. While activists have framed the issue as one of "environmental justice"—pointing to the overwhelming tendency for toxic materials to be located in proximity to poor and heavily minority neighborhoods—some geneticists have focused on the extent to which individuals are genetically susceptible to cellular damage from toxins. The most obvious danger is that this reframing bypasses a social and political analysis of injustice by locating responsibility within individuals and their genes. But in addition, to the extent that the genetic variation in susceptibility is itself perceived to correlate with racial belonging, then members of racial minority groups are perceived to be at risk of illness not because of where they can afford to live but because of embodied aspects of their racial "essence."[87]

These considerations raise big and thorny questions. As Nancy Krieger has suggested, the pathways linking institutionalized racism to unequal

health outcomes may span the gamut from economic and social depriva-
tion, to increased exposure to toxic substances and hazardous conditions,
to socially inflicted trauma ranging "from verbal threats to violent acts,"
to "targeted marketing of commodities that can harm health, such as junk
food and psychoactive substances," to inappropriate or insufficient medical care.[88] These are enormous issues, and certainly not ones that biomedical institutions alone can address. If, for example, as David Williams and
Chiquita Collins have argued, racial residential segregation, mediated in
part by socioeconomic status, is a cause of racial disparities in health,[89]
then solutions demand a rather concerted marshalling of political will. In
the case of gender, as well, "a new approach . . . that focuses less on how
women are the same as or different from men and more on how women,
as a diverse group, are disadvantaged" (as Karen Baird has expressed the
goal) is, admittedly, a tall order.[90] But the bigger risk comes from simply
declining to ask the questions in the first place.

The attention to inclusion and difference described in preceding chapters is not irrelevant to these goals, but it is not sufficient, either, and
in some ways it is imperfectly fitted to them. As the National Cancer
Institute's Otis Brawley commented in 1996: "Everybody in Congress is
obsessing on a few more people in clinical trials, [while] thousands of
blacks are getting substandard care."[91] Moreover, to the extent that the
policies of the inclusion-and-difference paradigm focus attention on a
predetermined set of social categories, then they may actually get in the
way: they may obscure other aspects of social hierarchy that are highly
relevant to health, such as social class;[92] and they may disincline us from
recognizing that in many situations the practices one engages in, the networks within which one moves, and the resources one has on hand may
be much more immediately relevant to health risk than one's membership
in a categorical group.

However, at least one government attempt to specify medically relevant social categories may function somewhat better for these purposes—
what Congress, in the Minority Health and Health Disparities Research
and Education Act of 2000 (which created the National Center on Minority Health and Health Disparities), described as "health disparity populations." While the bureaucratic phrasing is less than elegant, the basic
idea behind "health disparity populations" is important: to designate all
those groups for which there "is a significant disparity in the overall
rate of disease incidence, prevalence, morbidity, mortality, or survival
rates in the population as compared to the health status of the general
population."[93] On one hand, this definition leaves open a wide range of
possible social groupings that might qualify; and on the other hand, there

is no suggestion that the causal processes that give rise to health disparity populations are strictly biological ones unfolding inside the bodies of those who are "different."

The point here is not to argue that to address health disparities we must talk about so-called social and political issues *rather than* biological ones. I have emphasized that this imagined dichotomy is meaningless in the domain of health (and elsewhere), where the goal instead is to understand how social structures are lived and experienced bodily and how embodied persons re-create or transform those structures.[94] Celia Roberts has argued, in relation to studies of women's bodies, that it is "inadequate (both theoretically and politically) . . . simply to reject the biological," and the goal must be "to find a more complex 'middle way' of approaching the biological in its powerful and historically specific instantiations . . . without being reductionist."[95] It follows, as a corollary, that for a number of important reasons we cannot simply rid ourselves of certain concepts because of their suspect biological connotations—for example, to expunge categories such as race from our critical vocabulary by suggesting they are "mere" social constructions. To quote Troy Duster: "To throw out the concept of race is to take the official approach to race and ethnicity pioneered and celebrated by the French government: 'We do not collect data on that topic. Therefore, it does not exist!' "[96] Addressing serious problems means having the capacity to track progress toward their solution, and that becomes impossible without recourse to the categories of everyday life. Certainly it would be impossible to measure the reduction of health disparities without monitoring and recording the health of various populations, and that means, inevitably, making use of the categories by which inequality is made meaningful in a given society.[97]

The invention of new ways of imaging the intertwining of the biological and the social is thus a prerequisite for addressing the crucial question: What does it mean to be a full biopolitical citizen of a robustly diverse society? Proponents of new policies calling for inclusion of groups in biomedical research put forward one part of the answer, by demanding that research institutions study women as well as men, people of color as well as whites, children and the elderly as well as middle-aged adults.[98] But eliminating health disparities presupposes a serious commitment to addressing the power differentials and access to social resources and rewards that actually give many of those "differences" their social meaning. It also requires the institution of some thoroughly universal measures— such as, in the United States, a social guarantee of universal access to health care, much as every other wealthy nation promises its citizens. The inclusionary policies are just one link in the chain of biopolitical citizenship that "connects discussions of rights, recognitions, and responsibilities to intimate, fundamental concerns about heritable identities, differential embodiment, and an ethics of care."[99] It is time to go beyond the basic idea of group difference to forge that chain in a way that will strengthen the just pursuit of the health of all.

1972   Tuskegee Syphilis Study "revealed" by reporter.

1974   National Research Act specifies new regulations to protect human subjects.

1977   FDA guideline excluding women of childbearing potential from drug testing for non-life threatening diseases.

1978   OMB issues Directive 15, "Race and Ethnic Standards for Federal Statistics and Administrative Reporting."

1979   FDA begins requiring pediatric information in product labels and package inserts.

1981   President Ronald Reagan takes office (Jan.).

Kinney et al. find evidence of underrepresentation of women in clinical trials for new drug development.

1983   NIMH establishes Office of Special Populations.

1985   Report of PHS Task Force on Women's Health Issues.

Report of HHS Task Force on Black and Minority Health.

DHHS establishes Office of Minority Health.

NIH establishes Advisory Committee on Women's Health Issues.

1986   New NIH policy urging inclusion of women (in NIH Guide for Grants and Contracts; Oct.).

1987   New NIH policy urging inclusion of minorities (in NIH Guide for Grants and Contracts; Sept. 25).

1988   FDA guideline calls for analyses of subpopulation differences (gender, age, race/ethnicity) in NDAs (Oct. 7).

CDC Office of the Associate Director for Minority Health created.

1989   President George H. W. Bush takes office (Jan.).

FDA guideline calls for inclusion of elderly patients in clinical trials.

Aspirin component of Physicians' Health Study published.

CCWI introduces Women's Health Equity Act Omnibus Bill, calls for GAO investigation.

1990   SAWHR founded (Feb.).

GAO issues report criticizing NIH (House subcommittee testimony, June 18).

NIH establishes ORWH and ORMH.

Bush administration announces intent to nominate Bernadine Healy as NIH director (Sept.).

NIH reiterates 1986 policy on inclusion of women and 1987 policy on inclusion of minorities in 1990 Guide for Grants and Contracts.

NIH Revitalization Act of 1990 dies in House.

FDA proposes in Federal Register to amend labeling regulation to require a "geriatric use" section (Nov. 1).

1991   Healy appointed; announces WHI.

Vivian Pinn appointed director of ORWH.

Office on Women's Health created within DHSS.

Congress passes NIH Revitalization Act of 1991.

1992   Bush vetoes NIH Revitalization Act of 1991 (June).

FDA proposes to amend regulation on drug labeling to include information on the use of drugs in children (Oct. 16).

GAO issues report on women in drug studies (Oct. 29).

1993   President Bill Clinton takes office (Jan.).

FDA lifts 1977 restriction on inclusion of women, calls for gender-related analysis (March 24).

Clinton signs NIH Revitalization Act (June 10).

FDA issues guideline calling for analysis of data by gender (July 22).

Clinton appoints Susan Blumenthal as first Deputy Assistant Secretary for Women's Health.

1994   NIH publishes guidelines implementing NIH Revitalization Act (March 9, revised March 24, affecting grants submitted on or after June 1).

CDC establishes Office of Women's Health.

FDA establishes Office of Women's Health.

FDA publishes rule requiring manufacturers of marketed drugs to determine if sufficient evidence exists to add pediatric use information to the labeling (Dec.).

1995   Republicans assume leadership in House and Senate, eliminate CCWI.

National Task Force on AIDS Drug Development calls for stronger FDA policy on inclusion of women and minorities (Jan. 19).

FDA calls for presentation of demographic data (age, gender, race) for all NDAs (Sept. 8).

CDC issues policy on inclusion of women and racial and ethnic minorities in externally awarded research (Sept. 15).

SAWHR holds first national meeting on "gender-based biology."

1996   House and Senate Appropriations Committee reports express concern to NIH about inadequate inclusion of children.

Canadian Health Minister requires inclusion of women in drug testing (Sept.).

1997   Revised "Uniform Requirements for Manuscripts Submitted to Biomedical Journals" calls for identification of "age, sex, and other important characteristics of the subjects."

NIH announces plan to develop policy for inclusion of children (Jan. 31).

President's Cancer Panel debates "meaning of race in science" (April).

Health Resources and Services Administration creates Office of Women's Health (May 20).

OWH launches National Centers of Excellence in Women's Health.

FDA proposes requiring pediatric data for NDAs (Aug. 13).

FDA issues final rule requiring labeling info on geriatric use of drugs (Aug. 27).

FDA proposes "clinical hold" policy for INDs if women or men are excluded (Sept. 24).

OMB publishes revised list of racial/ethnic categories in the Federal Register (Oct. 30).

Congress passes FDA Modernization Act, which provides an additional six months of patent protection to manufacturers who conduct studies of approved drugs in children (Nov.).

Health Canada publishes policy on inclusion of women.

1998   FDA issues final rule requiring tabulation of data by demographic subgroup (Feb. 11).

NIH announces policy on inclusion of children in clinical research (March 3).

Lead article in *American Journal of Public Health* calls for "abandoning 'race' as a variable in public health research" (Sept.).

Women's Health Research and Prevention Amendments signed into law, funding a research program on cardiovascular disease in women at the National Heart, Lung and Blood Institute (Oct.31).

FDA issues final rule requiring pediatric data for NDAs (Dec. 2).

FDA adopts ICH guidelines on "ethnic factors" in acceptability of foreign data.

1999   Institute of Medicine Committee on Cancer Research Among Minorities and the Medically Underserved issues report (Jan. 20).

2000   GAO issues second report on NIH.

Legislation introduced to create Office of Men's Health in DHHS.

Assistant Secretary of Health appoints DHHS interagency committee to consider possibility of an Office of Lesbian and Gay Health.

Congress passes Minority Health and Health Disparities Research and Education Act, creating new National Center on Minority Health and Health Disparities (signed into law Nov. 22).

Congress passes Children's Health Act (signed into law Oct. 17).

FDA issues final rule on clinical hold policy (June 1).

FDA pediatric rule is challenged in federal court (Dec.).

2001   President George W. Bush takes office (Jan.).

GAO issues second report on FDA.

DHHS revises regulations on participation of women and minorities.

New England Journal of Medicine publishes editorial blasting "racial profiling" in medicine (May 3).

AHRQ establishes Office of Priority Populations Research.

2002   Bush signs the Best Pharmaceuticals for Children Act, which reauthorizes the six-month patent extension until 2007 (Jan.).

In response to a lawsuit, the FDA announces it will suspend enforcement of the pediatric rule (March).

DHHS announces the FDA will continue to enforce the pediatric rule (April).

NHLBI creates Office of Minority Health Affairs (July 1).

Institute of Medicine publishes report on racial disparities (*Unequal Treatment*).

2003　AHRQ publishes new policy on inclusion and subgroup analyses for all "priority populations" (Feb. 27).

Smart Mom Act introduced in Congress: Would expand knowledge about safety and dosing of drugs to treat pregnant women (April 25).

NIH publishes guidelines for inclusion of women, minorities, and persons with disabilities in NIH-supported conference grants (Sept. 26).

Congress passes the Pediatric Research Equity Act, granting the FDA the authority to enforce the pediatric rule (Nov. 19).

Women's Health Office Act reintroduced in Congress.

2004　European Union issues guidance calling on researchers to indicate the numbers of subjects they intend to recruit, broken down by age and by gender.

Senate Appropriations Committee instructs NIH to incorporate sex-based biology in research.

FDA approves BiDil for use in African Americans (June).

2005　NIMH adopts policy requiring researchers to specify recruitment "milestones" in advance (July).

FDA issues guidance calling for the use of OMB racial and ethnic categories when collecting and reporting data to the agency (Sept.).

European Parliament passes law compelling companies to test new drugs in children.

INTERVIEWS

Note: The job titles indicated below were those held by the person at the time of the interview. In some cases, I conducted brief follow-up interviews (in person or by telephone or email). A few individuals whom I interviewed are not identified below because they asked to remain anonymous.

Alexander, Duane, M.D. Director of National Institute of Child Health and Human Development, NIH. Interviewed in Bethesda, MD, August 8, 2000.

Angell, Marcia, M.D. Executive Editor, *New England Journal of Medicine*. Interviewed in Boston, MA, April 27, 1999.

Baldwin, Wendy, Ph.D. Deputy Director for Extramural Research, NIH; and Belinda Seto, senior advisor to Dr. Baldwin. Interviewed in Bethesda, MD, March 23, 1998.

Bass, Marie. Bass and Howes (lobbying agency). Interviewed in Washington, DC, April 12, 1999.

Bates, Christopher. Senior Health Policy Analyst, Office of HIV/AIDS Policy, DHHS. Interviewed in Washington, DC, August 7, 2000.

Benet, Leslie, M.D. Department of Pharmacy, University of California, San Francisco. Interviewed in San Francisco, CA, May 15, 1998.

Brawley, Otis W., M.D. Director, Office of Special Populations Research, National Cancer Institute, NIH. Interviewed in Rockville, MD, March 18, 1998.

Bull, Jonca, M.D.. Acting Deputy Director, Office of Women's Health, FDA. Interviewed in Rockville, MD, April 12, 1999.

Buring, Julie, D.Sc. Brigham & Women's Hospital, Harvard Medical School, and Harvard School of Public Health. Interviewed in Boston, MA, April 28, 1999.

Chavkin, Wendy, M.D., Ph.D. Editor-in-Chief, *Journal of the American Medical Women's Association*. Interviewed in New York City, March 13, 1998.

Chlebowski, Rowan, M.D. Women's Health Initiative investigator, Harbor—UCLA Research and Education Institute. Interviewed in Torrance, CA, May 1, 1998.

Connor, James, M.D. Director of the San Diego Pediatric Pharmacology Research Unit for UCSD and Children's Hospital. Interviewed in La Jolla, CA, July 29, 1999.

Corbie-Smith, Giselle, M.D. Emory University. Interviewed in Atlanta, GA, March 29, 1998.

Cotton, Deborah, M.D. Director of the Office of Clinical Research at Boston University Medical Center. Interviewed in Boston, MA, April 27, 1999.

Dunn, Patricia. Policy Director, Gay and Lesbian Medical Association. Interviewed in San Francisco, CA, July 28, 2000.

Ellis, Gary, Ph.D. Office for Protection from Research Risks, NIH. Interviewed in Bethesda, MD, March 17, 1998.

El-Sadr, Wafaa, M.D. Harlem Hospital. Interviewed in New York City, March 12, 1998.

Faden, Ruth, Ph.D. Director of the Bioethics Institute at Johns Hopkins University. Interviewed in Baltimore, MD, April 21, 1999.

Federman, Daniel, M.D. Dean of Medical Education, Harvard Medical School. Interviewed in Boston, MA, April 26, 1999.

Foulkes, Mary, Ph.D. Statistics Collaborative. Interviewed in Washington, DC, March 19, 1998.

Gorelick, Philip, M.D. Rush-Presbyterian-St. Luke's Medical Center. Interviewed in Chicago, IL, April 5, 1999.

Haseltine, Florence, M.D., Ph.D. Center for Population Research at the National Institute of Child Health and Human Development, NIH. Interviewed in Rockville, MD, April 19, 1999.

Haynes, Suzanne, Ph.D. Senior Advisor for Science, Office of Women's Health, DHHS. Interviewed in Washington, DC, August 7, 2000.

Hayunga, Eugene, Ph.D. Office of Research on Women's Health, NIH. Interviewed in Bethesda, MD. March 23, 1998.

Howard, Barbara, M.D. Medlantic Research Institute. Interviewed in Washington, D.C., March 18, 1998.

Jackson, James S., Ph.D. Department of Psychology and Michigan Center for Urban African American Aging Research, University of Michigan. Interviewed in Ann Arbor, MI, April 9, 1999.

Jones, Wanda, Dr.P.H. Deputy Assistant Secretary for Health, DHHS. Interviewed in Washington, DC, April 13, 1999.

Katz, Ruth, J.D., M.P.H. Yale University School of Medicine (formerly counsel to Health and Environment Subcommittee, U.S. House of Representatives). Interviewed in New Haven, CT, April 21, 1999.

King, Patricia. Georgetown University Law Center. Interviewed in Washington, DC, April 20, 1999.

Klein, Richard. See Toigo, Teresa (below).

Koenig, Barbara, Ph.D. Executive Director, Stanford University Center for Biomedical Ethics. Interviewed in San Francisco, CA, May 15, 1998.

Kusek, John, M.D. National Institute of Diabetes and Digestive and Kidney Diseases, NIH. Interviewed in Bethesda, MD, March 23, 1998.

Langer, Robert, M.D. Department of Family and Preventive Medicine, University of California, San Diego. Interviewed in La Jolla, CA, May 25, 1999.

Lasser, Norman, M.D. University of Medicine and Dentistry of New Jersey. Interviewed in Newark, NJ, March 11, 1998.

Lenfant, Claude, M.D. Director of the National Heart, Lung, and Blood Institute, NIH (and Carl Roth, NHLBI). Interviewed in Bethesda, MD, April 14, 1999.

Levine, Robert J., M.D. Professor of Medicine and Lecturer in Pharmacology, Yale University School of Medicine. Interviewed in New Haven, CT, April 22, 1999.

Levy, Richard A., Ph.D. National Pharmaceutical Council. Interviewed in Reston, VA, March 29, 1998.

Lin, Keh-Ming, M.D. Director of the Research Center on the Psychobiology of Ethnicity, UCLA. Interviewed in Torrance, CA, November 9, 2000.

Lundberg, George, M.D. Northwestern University (former editor, *Journal of the American Medical Association*). Interviewed in Chicago, IL, April 5, 1999.

Manson, JoAnn, M.D. Harvard Medical School. Interviewed in Boston, MA, April 22, 1998.

Manson, Spero, M.D. Department of Psychiatry, University of Colorado Health Sciences Center. Interviewed in Denver, CO, June 29, 1999.

Marts, Sherry. Ph.D. Scientific Director of the Society for the Advancement of Women's Health Research. Interviewed in Washington, DC, April 20, 1999.

McGovern, Terry, J.D. HIV Law Project. Interviewed in New York, NY, May 10, 1998.

Meinert, Curtis, Ph.D. Department of Epidemiology, School of Hygiene and Public Health, Johns Hopkins University. Interviewed in Baltimore, MD, March 24, 1998.

Merkatz, Ruth, Ph.D., R.N. Pfizer (formerly with Office of Women's Health, FDA). Interviewed in New York, NY, March 9, 1998.

Nápoles-Springer, Anna, M.D., Resource Center for Minority Aging Research, UCSF. Interviewed in San Francisco, July 26, 2000.

Norsigian, Judy. Boston Women's Health Book Collective. Interviewed in Somerville, MA, April 20, 1998.

Parron, Delores. Deputy Assistant Secretary for Planning and Evaluation, Office of Program Assistance, DHHS. Interviewed in Washington, DC, August 8, 2000.

Pearson, Cynthia. Executive Director, National Women's Health Network. Interviewed in Washington, DC, March 19, 1998.

Piantadosi, Steven, M.D., Ph.D. Johns Hopkins University Oncology Center. Interviewed in Baltimore, MD, March 24, 1998.

Pinn, Vivian, M.D. Director, Office of Research on Women's Health, NIH (and Marietta Anthony). Interviewed in Bethesda, MD, April 14, 1999.

Raub, William, M.D. U.S. Department of Health and Human Services (formerly Acting Director of NIH). Interviewed in Washington, DC, April 13, 1999.

Rofes, Eric, Ph.D. Activist, writer, and professor at Humboldt State University. Interviewed in Washington, DC, August 11, 2000. Died June 26, 2006.

Saunders, Elijah, M.D. University of Maryland School of Medicine. Interviewed in Baltimore, MD, April 18, 1999.

Schmucker, Douglas, M.D. UCSF and VA Medical Center. Interviewed in San Francisco, CA, July 26, 2000.

Schroeder, Patricia. Former U.S. Representative (D-Colorado). Interviewed in Washington, DC, March 18, 1998.

Schultz, Marjorie. Professor of Law, UC Berkeley School of Law. Interviewed in Berkeley, CA, May 14, 1998.

Scott, Julia R., R.N. President, National Black Women's Health Project. Interviewed in Washington, DC, March 19, 1998.

Sherman, Sherry, M.D. National Center on Aging, NIH. Interviewed in Bethesda, MD, March 16, 1998.

Smoller, Sylvia, M.D. Albert Einstein College of Medicine of Yeshiva University. Interviewed in New York City, March 11, 1998.

Stellman, Jeanne, Ph.D. Editor of *Women & Health*, Columbia University School of Public Health. Interviewed in New York City, February 8, 1999.

Stokes, Louis. Former member of U.S. Congress. Interviewed in Washington, DC, August 16, 2000.

Streeter, Oscar, M.D. University of Southern California. Interviewed in Los Angeles, CA, May 1, 1998.

Szefler, Stanley, M.D. National Jewish Medical Research Center. Interviewed in Denver, CO, June 29, 1999.

Temple, Robert J., M.D. Associate Director for Medical Policy, Center for Drug Evaluation and Research, FDA. Interviewed in Rockville, MD, August 11, 2000.

Toigo, Teresa, R.Ph., M.B.A. Office of Special Health Issues, FDA (and Richard Klein). Interviewed in Rockville, MD, April 12, 1999.

Wittes, Janet, Ph.D. Statistics Collaborative. Interviewed in Washington, DC, March 19, 1998.

Wood, Susan, Ph.D. Associate Director for Policy, Office on Women's Health, DHHS. Interviewed in Washington, DC, April 13, 1999.

Woosley, Raymond, M.D. Chair of Pharmacology, Georgetown University Medical Center (and Marietta Anthony). Interviewed in Washington, DC, August 9, 2000.

Yaffe, Sumner, M.D. Special Assistant to the Director, National Institute of Child Health and Human Development, NIH. Interviewed in Rockville, Maryland, August 9, 2000.

NOTES

INTRODUCTION

1. Throughout this book, I use the terms *biomedical* and *biomedicine* in the manner suggested by Peter Keating and Alberto Cambrosio, who note that "biology and medicine are now such tightly intertwined research enterprises that practitioners of the activity known as biomedicine can no longer say beforehand whether a particular research project, clinical investigation, or even clinical intervention will result in biological or in medical facts." Peter Keating and Alberto Cambrosio, "From Screening to Clinical Research: The Cure of Leukemia and the Early Development of the Cooperative Oncology Groups, 1955–1966," *Bulletin of History of Medicine* 76, no. 2 (2002): 300. Adele Clarke and coauthors observe that the prefix *bio-* before *medicine* connotes "the transformations of both the human and nonhuman made possible by such technoscientific innovations as molecular biology, biotechnologies, genomization, transplant medicine, and new medical technologies." Adele E. Clarke et al., "Biomedicalization: Technoscientific Transformations of Health, Illness, and U.S. Biomedicine," *American Sociological Review* 68 (April 2003): 162.

2. Terms such as *sex, gender, race,* and *ethnicity* have no simple definitions, and it is important to the arguments of this book to note that they are used in many different ways in academic and professional discourse, bureaucratic language, and everyday life. I discuss my own use of terminology at the end of chapter 1.

3. Doug Bowles, "A Radical Idea: Men and Women Are Different," *Cardiovascular Research* 61, no. 1 (January 1, 2004): 5–6; Robert Pear, "Research Neglects Women, Studies Find: Reports Say Health Trials Often Disregard Differences in the Sexes," *New York Times*, April 30, 2000, A14.

4. News segment, ABC, November 4, 2002, 5:45 pm. Jennings's source was a recent article in the journal *Pediatrics*.

5. Holly Auer, "Clinical Trials Seek More Minorities," *Charleston Post and Courier*, April 25, 2005, 1.

6. Anne L. Taylor et al., "Combination of Isosorbide Dinitrate and Hydralazine in Blacks with Heart Failure," *New England Journal of Medicine* 351, no. 20 (November 11, 2004): 2049–57.

7. These figures are from 2002, which is the most recent data reported in the 2005 version of the National Center for Health Statistics's annual report, *Health, United States*

(data from www.cdc.gov/nchs/data/hus/hus05.pdf; for the most up-to-date figures, see www.cdc.gov/nchs/hus.htm).

8. Ibid.

9. Kathleen Phalen Tomaselli, "Most in U.S. See Disparities in Care of Minority Patients," amednews.com, October 20, 2003,

www.ama-assn.org/sci-pubs/amnews/pick_03/hlsc1020.htm.

10. David R. Williams and Chiquita Collins, "U.S. Socioeconomic and Racial Differences in Health: Patterns and Explanations," *Annual Review of Sociology* 21 (1995): 349–86; Judith Lorber, *Gender and the Social Construction of Illness* (Thousand Oaks, CA: Sage, 1997); Brian D. Smedley, Adrienne Y. Stith, and Alan R. Nelson, eds., *Unequal Treatment: Confronting Racial and Ethnic Disparities in Health Care* (Washington, DC: National Academy Press, 2003); Thomas A. LaVeist, *Minority Populations and Health: An Introduction to Health Disparities in the United States* (San Francisco: Jossey-Bass, 2005); H. Jack Geiger, "Health Disparities: What Do We Know? What Do We Need to Know? What Should We Do?" in *Gender, Race, Class, and Health: Intersectional Approaches*, ed. Amy J. Schulz and Leith Mullings, 261–88 (San Francisco: Jossey-Bass, 2006). On the global dimensions of health inequalities, see Paul Farmer, *Pathologies of Power: Health, Human Rights, and the New War on the Poor* (Berkeley: University of California Press, 2004).

11. It is by no means new for the meaning of health disparities to be a politically contested issue. For historical perspective on this issue, see David S. Jones, *Rationalizing Epidemics: Meanings and Uses of American Indian Mortality since 1600* (Cambridge, MA: Harvard University Press, 2004), esp. 5–6.

12. According to the U.S. National Center for Health Statistics, 40.6 million Americans under the age of 65 lacked health insurance in 2002 (the last year for which data were available as of 2006). This constitutes nearly 17 percent of the population; however, the percentage uninsured varies substantially by race and ethnic group (data from www.cdc.gov/nchs/data/hus/hus05.pdf; for the most up-to-date figures, see www.cdc.gov/nchs/hus.htm). Nongovernmental sources typically provide higher figures. Moreover, statistics on the uninsured leave out the substantial numbers who are underinsured or are uninsured for less than the entire year. Popular critiques of pharmaceutical company drug development and marketing practices have become ubiquitous in recent years; see, for example, Marcia Angell, *The Truth about the Drug Companies: How They Deceive Us and What to Do about It* (New York: Random House, 2004). Similarly, quite a few critiques of managed care and of the corporatization of U.S. health care delivery have been published recently; see, for example, Donald L. Bartlett and James B. Steele, *Critical Condition: How Health Care in American Became Big Business—and Bad Medicine* (New York: Doubleday, 2004).

13. In addition to "differences," and "disparities," there is also a third language for approaching the question of difference in health, one which has grown in visibility in recent years: that of "culturally competent" care. (See, for example, the June 2003 special issue of *Academic Medicine*, which is devoted to the theme of cultural competence with particular attention to medical education.) While influential within medical schools and in certain policy arenas, the idea that practitioners should be culturally competent in relation to the communities that they treat has been far less likely than the approach to difference analyzed in this book to take root in the form of enforceable policies. Also, it has been less present in the particular biomedical domain that is the focus of this book, namely, clinical

research—although ideas about cultural competence intersect with new conceptions of outreach to communities by researchers who hope to study them, the topic of chapter 9.

14. "Science Meets Reality: Recruitment and Retention of Women in Clinical Studies, and the Critical Role of Relevance," conference summary made available online by the NIH Office of Research on Women's Health in 2003 and subsequently removed. A slightly different version of Healy's remarks appears in the final report from the conference. Bernadine Healy, "Challenging Sameness: Women in Clinical Trials," in *Science Meets Reality: Recruitment and Retention of Women in Clinical Studies, and the Critical Role of Relevance* (Rockville, MD: NIH, Office of Research on Women's Health, NIH, January 6–9, 2003), http://orwh.od.nih.gov/pubs/SMR_Final.pdf, 16.

15. In this book I use the terms *clinical research* and *clinical studies* interchangeably to refer to medical experiments or studies conducted with human subjects. These include randomized clinical trials (where subjects are randomly assigned to different treatments) as well as nonrandomized research such as observational studies.

16. Pat Schroeder, *24 Years of House Work . . . and the Place Is Still a Mess: My Life in Politics* (Kansas City: Andrew McNeel, 1998), 77.

17. Hamilton Moses III et al., "Financial Anatomy of Biomedical Research," *Journal of the American Medical Association* 294, no. 11 (September 21, 2005): 1336. This includes funding for both basic and clinical research.

18. A list of frequently used abbreviations appears at the front of the book, following the acknowledgments. A chronology of key events described in these pages appears at the back of the book, before the notes.

19. Ibid., 1335 (this includes all types of research). According to this study, the NIH accounts for 28 percent of spending; other federal, state, and local government agencies, another 12 percent; pharmaceutical, biotechnology, and medical device firms, 58 percent; and foundations and charities, 3 percent. From 1994 to 2004 these proportions remained roughly constant, even while total spending on biomedical research doubled (after adjusting for inflation).

20. Debra A. DeBruin, "Justice and the Inclusion of Women in Clinical Studies: A Conceptual Framework," in *Women and Health Research: Ethical and Legal Issues of Including Women in Clinical Studies*, ed. Anna C. Mastroianni, Ruth Faden, and Daniel Federman (Washington, DC: National Academy Press, 1994), 2:127–50; Tracy Johnson and Elizabeth Fee, "Women's Participation in Clinical Research: From Protectionism to Access," in *Women and Health Research*, ed. Mastroianni, Faden, and Federman, 2:1–10; Sue V. Rosser, *Women's Health—Missing from U.S. Medicine* (Bloomington: Indiana University Press, 1994); Judith D. Auerbach and Anne E. Figert, "Women's Health Research: Public Policy and Sociology," *Journal of Health and Social Behavior* 35, extra issue (1995): 115–31; Jean A. Hamilton, "Women and Health Policy: On the Inclusion of Females in Clinical Trials," in *Gender and Health*, ed. Carolyn F. Sargent and Caroline Brettell, 292–325 (Englewood Cliffs, NJ: Prentice-Hall, 1996); Deborah Narrigan et al., "Research to Improve Women's Health: An Agenda for Equity," in *Women's Health: Complexities and Differences*, ed. Sheryl Burt Ruzek, Virginia L. Olesen, and Adele E. Clarke, 551–79 (Columbus: Ohio State University Press, 1997); Lesley Primmer, "Women's Health Research: Congressional Action and Legislative Gains: 1990–1994," in *Women's Health Research: A Medical and Policy Primer*, ed. Florence B. Haseltine and Beverly Greenberg Jacobson, 301–30 (Washington, DC: Health Press International, 1997); Anne K. Eckman, "Beyond 'the Yentl Syndrome':

Making Women Visible in Post-1990 Women's Health Discourse," in *The Visible Woman: Imaging Technologies, Gender, and Science*, ed. Paula A. Treichler, Lisa Cartwright, and Constance Penley, 130–68 (New York: New York University Press, 1998); Carol S. Weisman, *Women's Health Care: Activist Traditions and Institutional Change* (Baltimore: Johns Hopkins University Press, 1998); Karen L. Baird, "The New NIH and FDA Medical Research Policies: Targeting Gender, Promoting Justice," *Journal of Health Politics, Policy and Law* 24, no. 3 (1999): 531–65; Lisa Eckenwiler, "Pursuing Reform in Clinical Research: Lessons from Women's Experience," *Journal of Law, Medicine and Ethics* 27, no. 2 (1999): 158–88; Londa Schiebinger, *Has Feminism Changed Science?* (Cambridge, MA: Harvard University Press, 1999), 14–15, 107–25; Carol S. Weisman, "Breast Cancer Policymaking," in *Breast Cancer: Society Shapes an Epidemic*, ed. Anne S. Kasper and Susan J. Ferguson, 213–43 (New York: St. Martin's, 2000); Oonagh P. Corrigan, " 'First in Man': The Politics and Ethics of Women in Clinical Drug Trials," *Feminist Review* 72 (2002): 40–52; Donna J. Haraway, *Modest_Witness@Second_Millenium.Femaleman© _Meets OncoMouse™* (New York: Routledge, 1997), chap. 6.

21. See Troy Duster, *Backdoor to Eugenics* (New York: Routledge, 1990); Sandra G. Harding, *The "Racial" Economy of Science: Toward a Democratic Future* (Bloomington: Indiana University Press, 1993); Margaret Lock, "The Concept of Race: An Ideological Construct," *Transcultural Psychiatric Research Review* 30 (1993): 203–27; Jonathan Marks, *Human Biodiversity: Genes, Race, and History* (New York: Aldine de Gruyter, 1995); Evelynn Hammonds, "New Technologies of Race," in *Processed Lives: Gender and Technology in Everyday Life*, ed. Jennifer Terry and Melodie Calvert, 107–21 (London: Routledge, 1997); Keith Wailoo, *Drawing Blood: Technology and Disease Identity in Twentieth-Century America* (Baltimore: Johns Hopkins University Press, 1997); David R. Williams, "Race and Health: Basic Questions, Emerging Directions," *Annals of Epidemiology* 7, no. 5 (July 1997); Melbourne Tapper, *In the Blood: Sickle Cell Anemia and the Politics of Race* (Philadelphia: University of Pennsylvania Press, 1999); Janet K. Shim, "Bio-Power and Racial, Class, and Gender Formation in Biomedical Knowledge Production," *Research in the Sociology of Health Care* 17 (2000): 173–95; Joseph L. Graves, *The Emperor's New Clothes: Biological Theories of Race at the Millennium* (New Brunswick, NJ: Rutgers University Press, 2001); Sandra Soo-Jin Lee, Joanna Mountain, and Barbara A. Koenig, "The Meanings of 'Race' in the New Genomics: Implications for Health Disparities Research," *Yale Journal of Health Policy, Law and Ethics* 1 (spring 2001): 33–75; Michael Root, "The Problem of Race in Medicine," *Philosophy of the Social Sciences* 31, no. 1 (March 2001): 20–39; Lundy Braun, "Race, Ethnicity, and Health: Can Genetics Explain Disparities?" *Perspectives in Biology and Medicine* 45, no. 2 (spring 2002); Pamela Sankar and Mildred Cho, "Toward a New Vocabulary of Human Genetic Variation," *Science* 298 (November 15, 2002): 1337–38; Richard S. Cooper, Jay S. Kaufman, and Ryk Ward, "Race and Genomics," *New England Journal of Medicine* 348, no. 12 (March 20, 2003); Troy Duster, "Buried Alive: The Concept of Race in Science," in *Genetic Nature/Culture: Anthropology and Science beyond the Two-Culture Divide*, ed. Alan H. Goodman, Deborah Heath, and M. Susan Lindee, 258–77 (Berkeley: University of California Press, 2003); Jay S. Kaufman and Susan A. Hall, "The Slavery Hypertension Hypothesis: Dissemination and Appeal of a Modern Race Theory," *Epidemiology* 14, no. 1 (January 2003); Alan R. Templeton, "Human Races in the Context of Recent Human Evolution: A Molecular Genetic Perspective," in *Genetic Nature/Culture: Anthropology and Science beyond the Two-Culture Divide*, ed. Goodman, Heath, and Lindee,

234–57; Keith Wailoo, "Inventing the Heterozygote: Molecular Biology, Racial Identity, and the Narratives of Sickle Cell Disease, Tay-Sachs, and Cystic Fibrosis," in *Race, Nature, and the Politics of Difference*, ed. Donald D. Moore, Jake Kosek, and Anand Pandian, 235–53 (Durham, NC: Duke University Press, 2003); Anne Fausto-Sterling, "Refashioning Race: DNA and the Politics of Health Care," *differences: A Journal of Feminist Cultural Studies* 15, no. 3 (2004): 1–37; Jonathan Kahn, "How a Drug Becomes 'Ethnic': Law, Commerce, and the Production of Racial Categories in Medicine," *Yale Journal of Health Policy, Law and Ethics* 4, no. 1 (2004): 1–46; Alan Goodman, "Two Questions about Race," April 20, 2005, in *Is Race Real*, Web forum organized by the Social Science Research Council, http://raceandgenomics.ssrc.org/Goodman/; Jennifer Reardon, *Race to the Finish: Identity and Governance in an Age of Genomics* (Princeton, NJ: Princeton University Press, 2005); Alexandra E. Shields et al., "The Use of Race Variables in Genetic Studies of Complex Traits and the Goal of Reducing Health Disparities: A Transdisciplinary Perspective," *American Psychologist* 60, no. 1 (January 2005): 77–103; Janet K. Shim, "Constructing 'Race' across the Science-Lay Divide: Racial Formation in the Epidemiology and Experience of Cardiovascular Disease," *Social Studies of Science* 35, no. 3 (June 2005): 405–36. On the history of the science of race, see also Nancy Stepan, *The Idea of Race in Science: Great Britain, 1800–1960* (London: Macmillan, 1982); Robert N. Proctor, *Racial Hygiene: Medicine under the Nazis* (Cambridge, MA: Harvard University Press, 1988); Elazar Barkan, *The Retreat of Scientific Racism: Changing Concepts of Race in Britain and the United States between the World Wars* (Cambridge: Cambridge University Press, 1992).

22. The exception is that the focus by the DHHS on specific social identities has received attention from ideological opponents of this emphasis, such as Sally Satel, who criticize what they term the intrusion of "political correctness" into medicine. Sally Satel, *P.C., M.D.: How Political Correctness Is Corrupting Medicine* (New York: Basic, 2000). More generally, and from a very different perspective, Barbara Hanson also has studied the biomedical emphasis on categories of gender, race, and age. Barbara Hanson, *Social Assumptions, Medical Categories* (Greenwich, CT: JAI Press, 1997).

23. I discuss my use of the term *paradigm* in chapter 1.

24. Clarke et al., "Biomedicalization." See also Margaret Lock, Allan Young, and Alberto Cambrosio, eds., *Living and Working with the New Medical Technologies: Intersections of Inquiry* (Cambridge: Cambridge University Press, 2000); Sarah Franklin and Margaret Lock, eds., *Remaking Life and Death: Toward an Anthropology of the Biosciences* (Santa Fe, NM: School of American Research Press, 2003); Peter Keating and Alberto Cambrosio, *Biomedical Platforms: Realigning the Normal and the Pathological in Late-Twentieth-Century Medicine* (Cambridge, MA: MIT Press, 2003); Sheila M. Rothman and David J. Rothman, *The Pursuit of Perfection: The Promise and Perils of Medical Enhancement* (New York: Pantheon Books, 2003); Stefan Timmermans and Marc Berg, *The Gold Standard: The Challenge of Evidence-Based Medicine and Standardization in Health Care* (Philadelphia: Temple University Press, 2003); Andrew Lakoff, *Pharmaceutical Reason: Knowledge and Value in Global Psychiatry* (New York: Cambridge University Press, 2005); Peter Conrad, *The Medicalization of Society* (Baltimore: Johns Hopkins University Press, 2006); Adriana Petryna, Andrew Lakoff, and Arthur Kleinman, eds., *Global Pharmaceuticals: Ethics, Markets, Practices* (Durham, NC: Duke University Press, 2006).

25. On the nation-state's "continuing influence in the realm of forces and connections" even within global processes, see Michael Burawoy, "Introduction: Reading for the Global,"

in *Global Ethnography: Forces, Connections, and Imaginations in a Postmodern World*, ed. Michael Burawoy et al. (Berkeley: University of California Press, 2000), 35. For a recent strong argument in favor of keeping the nation-state central when we study culturally distinctive "ways of knowing" (or "civic epistemologies"), see Sheila Jasanoff, *Designs on Nature: Science and Democracy in Europe and the United States* (Princeton, NJ: Princeton University Press, 2005).

26. Moses et al., "Financial Anatomy of Biomedical Research," 1333.

27. John David Skrentny, *The Minority Rights Revolution* (Cambridge, MA: Harvard University Press, 2002).

28. Jeffrey C. Alexander and Neil J. Smelser, "Introduction: The Ideological Discourse of Cultural Discontent," in *Diversity and Its Discontents: Cultural Conflict and Common Ground in Contemporary American Society*, ed. Neil J. Smelser and Jeffrey C. Alexander (Princeton, NJ: Princeton University Press, 1999), 3–21; Skrentny, *Minority Rights Revolution*.

29. Much has been written on identity politics. For an excellent recent overview, see Mary Bernstein, "Identity Politics," *Annual Review of Sociology* 31, no. 1 (2005): 47–74.

30. Frank De Zwart, "The Dilemma of Recognition: Administrative Categories and Cultural Diversity," *Theory and Society* 34, no. 2 (April 2005): 137–69.

31. My thanks to Long Bui for suggesting this term.

32. On evidence-based medicine and standardization in biomedicine, see Timmermans and Berg, *Gold Standard*. On efforts to "harmonize" drug regulation, see Arthur A. Daemmrich, *Pharmacopolitics: Drug Regulation in the United States and Germany* (Chapel Hill: University of North Carolina Press, 2004), 157–60, 219.

33. Adam Hedgecoe, *The Politics of Personalized Medicine: Pharmacogenetics in the Clinic* (Cambridge: Cambridge University Press, 2004).

34. J. Marks, *Human Biodiversity*, 112, 133, 162–67. To be sure, the fact that humans are astonishingly similar at the genetic level has not preempted scientific interest in studying the small degree to which they differ. I return to this issue in chapter 10.

35. Iris Marion Young, *Justice and the Politics of Difference* (Princeton, NJ: Princeton University Press, 1990); Will Kymlicka, *Multicultural Citizenship: A Liberal Theory of Minority Rights* (Oxford: Clarendon Press, 1995); Iris Marion Young, "Polity and Group Difference: A Critique of the Ideal of Universal Citizenship," in *The Citizenship Debates: A Reader*, ed. Gershon Shafir, 263–90 (Minneapolis: University of Minnesota Press, 1998). For applications of Young's work to the case of inclusion of women in research, see DeBruin, "Justice and the Inclusion of Women"; Eckenwiler, "Pursuing Reform in Clinical Research."

36. Sandra Harding, *The Science Question in Feminism* (Ithaca, NY: Cornell University Press, 1986); Donna J. Haraway, *Simians, Cyborgs, and Women: The Reinvention of Nature* (New York: Routledge, 1991), chap. 9; Steven Epstein, *Impure Science: AIDS, Activism, and the Politics of Knowledge* (Berkeley: University of California Press, 1996); Steven Epstein, "Patient Groups and Health Movements," in *New Handbook of Science and Technology Studies*, ed. Edward J. Hackett et al. (Cambridge, MA: MIT Press, 2007). For a recent rethinking of the notion of "standpoint" in epistemic politics, see Alison Wylie, "Why Standpoint Matters," in *Science and Other Cultures*, ed. Robert Figueroa and Sandra Harding, 26–48 (New York: Routledge, 2003).

37. Natalie Angier and Kenneth Chang, "Gray Matter and the Sexes: Still a Scientific Gray Area," *New York Times*, January 24, 2005, A1, A15.

38. Richard J. Herrnstein and Charles A. Murray, *The Bell Curve: Intelligence and Class*

Structure in American Life (New York: Free Press, 1994). For a careful critique, see Claude S. Fischer et al., *Inequality by Design: Cracking the Bell Curve Myth* (Princeton, NJ: Princeton University Press, 1996).

39. On the tension between formal and substantive rationality in medical ethics, and the tendency for preoccupation with the former to swamp consideration of the latter, see also John Hyde Evans, *Playing God? Human Genetic Engineering and the Rationalization of Public Bioethical Debate* (Chicago: University of Chicago Press, 2002).

40. A list of those interviewed appears at the back of the book, before the notes.

41. For an explanation of the logic of studying encounters across "social worlds," see Adele Clarke, "A Social Worlds Adventure: The Case of Reproductive Science," in *Theories of Science in Society*, ed. Susan E. Cozzens and Thomas F. Gieryn, 15–42 (Bloomington: Indiana University Press, 1990).

42. While chapter 1 is critical for an understanding of the theoretical questions at the heart of this book and the theoretical resources that I bring to bear in my analysis, some readers with less interest in these matters may prefer to proceed directly to chapter 2.

43. On "boundary work" in science—the practices and rhetoric by which "science" is defined and distinguished from other things, such as "politics" and "religion," and by which the professional autonomy of scientists is defended—see Thomas F. Gieryn, "Boundary Work and the Demarcation of Science from Non-Science: Strains and Interests in Professional Ideologies of Scientists," *American Sociological Review* 48 (December 1983): 781–95; Thomas F. Gieryn, "Boundaries of Science," in *Handbook of Science and Technology Studies*, ed. Sheila Jasanoff et al. (Thousand Oaks, CA: Sage, 1995), 393–443; Thomas F. Gieryn, *Cultural Boundaries of Science: Credibility on the Line* (Chicago: University of Chicago Press, 1999). See also Sheila Jasanoff, *The Fifth Branch: Science Advisers as Policymakers* (Cambridge, MA: Harvard University Press, 1990); Kelly Moore, "Organizing Integrity: American Science and the Creation of Public Interest Organizations, 1955–1975," *American Journal of Sociology* 101 (1996): 1592–627; David H. Guston, *Between Science and Politics: Assuring the Integrity and Productivity of Research* (New York: Cambridge University Press, 2000).

44. My thanks to Stefan Timmermans for suggesting this term.

45. James H. Jones, *Bad Blood: The Tuskegee Syphilis Experiment* (New York: Free Press, 1981).

CHAPTER ONE

1. Thomas S. Kuhn, *The Structure of Scientific Revolutions* (Chicago: University of Chicago Press, 1970).

2. For somewhat similar reasons, inclusion-and-difference would not precisely qualify as what Joan Fujimura calls a "bandwagon," what Peter Keating and Alberto Cambrosio call a "platform," or what Scott Frickel and Neil Gross call a "scientific/intellectual movement." However, it may overlap with all of these, as well as with what Sheila Jasanoff calls a "civic epistemology." See Joan H. Fujimura, "The Molecular Biological Bandwagon in Cancer Research: Where Social Worlds Meet," *Social Problems* 35, no. 3 (1988): 261–83; Keating and Cambrosio, *Biomedical Platforms*; Scott Frickel and Neil Gross, "A General Theory of Scientific/Intellectual Movements," *American Sociological Review* 70, no. 2 (April 2005): 204–32; Jasanoff, *Designs on Nature*.

3. Hall introduced the concept of the policy paradigm to describe how the intentions and actions of state policymakers achieve coherence. According to Hall, a policy paradigm is "a framework of ideas and standards that specifies not only the goals of policy and the kinds of instruments that can be used to attain them, but also the very nature of the problems they are meant to be addressing." Peter A. Hall, "Policy Paradigms, Social Learning, and the State: The Case of Economic Policymaking in Britain," *Comparative Politics* 25 (April 1993): 279. While the Kuhnian notion of paradigm suffers from a cognitivist bias, in Hall's terms a paradigm is not just a way of thinking but also a way of doing: it describes and orients the everyday activities of people within institutions, often operating below the level of conscious awareness or shared understandings.

4. Foucault used the term *biopolitics* to refer to the increasing concern by modern states with human biological life processes. As Foucault described it, governments in recent centuries have become preoccupied with matters of health, reproduction, and demography and have understood these matters to be central to their administration of peoples and territories. Michel Foucault, *The History of Sexuality*, vol. 1, *An Introduction* (New York: Vintage, 1980), 135–59.

5. The resulting configuration is similar to what Tania Murray Li has called an "assemblage." As Li has observed, "Rather than emerging fully formed from a single source, many improvement schemes are formed through an assemblage of objectives, knowledges, techniques, and practices of diverse provenance." While an assemblage may develop in a somewhat haphazard way, once stabilized it "supplies a complex of knowledge and practice in terms of which certain kinds of problems and solutions become thinkable whereas others are submerged, at least for a time." Tania Murray Li, "Beyond 'the State' and Failed Schemes," *American Anthropologist* 107, no. 3 (2005): 386. On assemblages, see also Aihwa Ong and Stephen J. Collier, eds., *Global Assemblages: Technology, Politics, and Ethics as Anthropological Problems* (Malden, MA: Blackwell, 2005).

6. For introductions to the field, see Sheila Jasanoff et al., eds., *Handbook of Science and Technology Studies* (Thousand Oaks, CA: Sage, 1995); Edward J. Hackett et al., eds., *New Handbook of Science and Technology Studies* (Cambridge, MA: MIT Press, 2007).

7. This project is especially in conversation with the substantial body of work at the intersection of science studies with historical, sociological, and anthropological studies of medical practice and biomedical research. On the emergence and development of this arena of intersection, see Adele E. Clarke and Joan H. Fujimura, eds., *The Right Tools for the Job: At Work in Twentieth-Century Life Sciences* (Princeton, NJ: Princeton University Press, 1992); Monica J. Casper and Marc Berg, "Constructivist Perspectives on Medical Work: Medical Practices and Science and Technology Studies," *Science, Technology, and Human Values* 20, no. 4 (1995): 395–407; Mary Ann Elston, ed., *The Sociology of Medical Science and Technology* (Oxford: Blackwell, 1997); Lock, Young, and Cambrosio, *Living and Working with the New Medical Technologies*.

8. There is an increasing amount of work on modern biomedicine and bodies. See, for example, Stefan Hirschauer, "The Manufacture of Bodies in Surgery," *Social Studies of Science* 21, no. 2 (May 1991): 279–319; Nelly Oudshoorn, *Beyond the Natural Body: An Archeology of Sex Hormones* (London: Routledge, 1994); Catherine Waldby, *AIDS and the Body Politic: Biomedicine and Sexual Difference* (London: Routledge, 1996); Sarah Franklin, *Embodied Progress: A Cultural Account of Assisted Conception* (London: Routledge, 1997); Margaret Lock, "Decentering the Natural Body: Making Difference Matter," *Configurations* 5 (1997): 267–92; Margaret Lock, "Anomalous Ageing: Managing the Postmenopausal

Body," *Body and Society* 4, no. 1 (1998): 35–61; Annemarie Mol, *The Body Multiple: Ontology in Medical Practice* (Durham, NC: Duke University Press, 2002); Charis Thompson, *Making Parents: The Ontological Choreography of Reproductive Technologies* (Cambridge, MA: MIT Press, 2005).

9. Scott Frickel and Kelly Moore, eds., *The New Political Sociology of Science: Institutions, Networks, and Power* (Madison: University of Wisconsin Press, 2006).

10. Sheila Jasanoff, "The Idiom of Co-Production," in *States of Knowledge: The Co-Production of Science and Social Order*, ed. Sheila Jasanoff (London: Sage, 2004), 2. See also the other essays in the same volume.

11. Karin Knorr Cetina, *Epistemic Cultures: How the Sciences Make Knowledge* (Cambridge, MA: Harvard University Press, 1999).

12. For overviews of this broad literature, see Epstein, "Patient Groups and Health Movements"; David Hess et al., "Science, Technology, and Social Movements," in *New Handbook of Science and Technology Studies*, ed. Edward J. Hackett et al. (Cambridge, MA: MIT Press, 2007). On "concerned groups," see Michel Callon, "The Increasing Involvement of Concerned Groups in R&D Policies: What Lessons for Public Powers?" in *Science and Innovation: Rethinking the Rationales for Funding and Governance*, ed. Aldo Geuna, Ammon J. Salter, and W. Edward Steinmueller, 30–68 (Cheltenham, UK: Edward Elgar, 2003).

13. On new modes of scientific, technological, biological, genetic, or biomedical citizenship, see Madeleine Akrich, "The De-Scription of Technical Objects," in *Shaping Technology/Building Society: Studies in Sociotechnical Change*, ed. Weibe E. Bijker and John Law (Cambridge, MA: MIT Press, 1992), 214–15; Alan Irwin, "Constructing the Scientific Citizen: Science and Democracy in the Biosciences," *Public Understanding of Science* 10 (2001): 1–18; Nayan Shah, *Contagious Divides: Epidemics and Race in San Francisco's Chinatown* (Berkeley: University of California Press, 2001), 7; Alan Petersen and Robin Bunton, *The New Genetics and the Public Health* (London: Routledge, 2002), 180–207; Adriana Petryna, *Life Exposed: Biological Citizens after Chernobyl* (Princeton, NJ: Princeton University Press, 2002); Charles L. Briggs and Clara Mantini-Briggs, *Stories in Times of Cholera: Racial Profiling during a Medical Nightmare* (Berkeley: University of California Press, 2003); Alan Irwin and Mike Michael, *Science, Social Theory, and Public Knowledge* (Maidenhead, PA: Open University Press, 2003), esp. 123–35; Dale Rose and Stuart Blume, "Citizens as Users of Technology: An Exploratory Study of Vaccines and Vaccination," in *How Users Matter: The Co-Construction of Users and Technology*, ed. Nelly Oudshoorn and Trevor Pinch, 103–31 (Cambridge, MA: MIT Press, 2003); Deborah Heath, Rayna Rapp, and Karen-Sue Taussig, "Genetic Citizenship," in *A Companion to the Anthropology of Politics*, ed. David Nugent and Joan Vincent, 152–167 (London: Blackwell, 2004); Vinh-Kim Nguyen, "Antiretroviral Globalism, Biopolitics, and Therapeutic Citizenship," in *Global Assemblages: Technology, Politics, and Ethics as Anthropological Problems*, ed. Aihwa Ong and Stephen J. Collier, 124–44 (Malden, MA: Blackwell, 2005); Nikolas Rose and Carlos Novas, "Biological Citizenship," in *Global Assemblages*, ed. Ong and Collier, 439–63; Natalia Molina, *Fit to Be Citizens? Public Health and Race in Los Angeles, 1879–1939* (Berkeley: University of California Press, 2006); Vololona Rabeharisoa, "From Representation to Mediation: The Shaping of Collective Mobilization on Muscular Dystrophy in France," *Social Science and Medicine* 62, no. 3 (February 2006): 564–76.

14. Scott Frickel and Kelly Moore, "Prospects and Challenges for a New Political Sociology of Science," in *New Political Sociology of Science*, ed. Frickel and Moore, 7.

15. The point is not to deny that social structures, organizational interests, and social

identities are all themselves constructed in particular historical circumstances (as many science studies scholars have been at pains to insist). However, as Daniel Kleinman has put it, "at any given time, these phenomena have an established character, and this configuration has effects" on the ways in which knowledge and technology are produced. Daniel Lee Kleinman, *Impure Cultures: University Biology and the World of Commerce* (Madison: University of Wisconsin Press, 2003), 62.

16. Diane Vaughan, *The Challenger Launch Decision: Risky Technology, Culture, and Deviance at NASA* (Chicago: University of Chicago Press, 1996); Diane Vaughan, "The Rôle of the Organization in the Production of Techno-Scientific Knowledge," *Social Studies of Science* 29, no. 6 (December 1999): 913-43.

17. Vaughan, "Rôle of the Organization," 931. Vaughan borrows the phrase "machineries of knowing" from Knorr Cetina, *Epistemic Cultures*, 10.

18. Frickel and Moore, "Prospects and Challenges," 7.

19. Elisabeth S. Clemens and James M. Cook, "Politics and Institutionalism: Explaining Durability and Change," *Annual Review of Sociology* 25, no. 1 (1999): 443, 461. To be sure, the goal of avoiding the reification of "the state" is not new; see Philip Abrams, "Notes on the Difficulty of Studying the State (1977)," *Journal of Historical Sociology* 1, no. 1 (March 1988): 58-89. On this point, see also Timothy Mitchell, "Society, Economy, and the State Effect," in *Culture: State-Formation after the Cultural Turn*, ed. George Steinmetz, 76-97 (Ithaca, NY: Cornell University Press, 1999); Li, "Beyond 'the State' and Failed Schemes," 383-94. For useful reviews of approaches to studying the state, see also Karen Barkey and Sunita Parikh, "Comparative Perspectives on the State," *Annual Review of Sociology* 17 (1991): 523-49; George Steinmetz, "Introduction: Culture and the State," in *Culture: State-Formation after the Cultural Turn*, ed. George Steinmetz (Ithaca, NY: Cornell University Press, 1999), 1-49.

20. Steven Shapin and Simon Schaffer, *Leviathan and the Air-Pump: Hobbes, Boyle and the Experimental Life* (Princeton, NJ: Princeton University Press, 1985); Chandra Mukerji, *A Fragile Power: Scientists and the State* (Princeton, NJ: Princeton University Press, 1989); Yaron Ezrahi, *The Descent of Icarus: Science and the Transformation of Contemporary Democracy* (Cambridge, MA: Harvard University Press, 1990); Ian Hacking, *The Taming of Chance* (Cambridge: Cambridge University Press, 1990); Jasanoff, *Fifth Branch*; Bruno Latour, *We Have Never Been Modern* (Cambridge, MA: Harvard University Press, 1993); Chandra Mukerji, "Toward a Sociology of Material Culture: Science Studies, Cultural Studies and the Meanings of Things," in *The Sociology of Culture: Emerging Theoretical Perspectives*, ed. Diana Crane (Oxford: Blackwell, 1994), 143-62; Susan E. Cozzens and Edward J. Woodhouse, "Science, Government and the Politics of Knowledge," in *Handbook of Science and Technology Studies*, ed. Sheila Jasanoff et al. (Thousand Oaks, CA: Sage, 1995), 533-53; Theodore M. Porter, *Trust in Numbers: The Pursuit of Objectivity in Science and Public Life* (Princeton, NJ: Princeton University Press, 1995); Alain Desrosières, *The Politics of Large Numbers: A History of Statistical Reasoning* (Cambridge, MA: Harvard University Press, 1998); Jasanoff, *Designs on Nature*; Patrick Carroll, *Science, Culture, and Modern State Formation* (Berkeley: University of California Press, 2006).

21. Mark Wolfson, *The Fight against Big Tobacco: The Movement, the State, and the Public's Health* (New York: Aldine de Gruyter, 2001); Skrentny, *Minority Rights Revolution*, 5; Jack A. Goldstone, "Introduction: Bridging Institutionalized and Noninstitutionalized Politics," in *States, Parties, and Social Movements*, ed. Jack A. Goldstone, 1-24 (Cambridge: Cambridge University Press, 2003); David S. Meyer, Valerie Jenness, and Helen M. Ingram,

eds., *Routing the Opposition: Social Movements, Public Policy, and Democracy* (Minneapolis: University of Minnesota Press, 2005).

22. Kelly Moore, "Political Protest and Institutional Change: The Anti-Vietnam War Movement and American Science," in *How Social Movements Matter*, ed. Marco Giugni, Doug McAdam, and Charles Tilly, 97–118 (Minneapolis: University of Minnesota Press, 1999); Elizabeth Armstrong and Mary Bernstein, "Culture, Power, and Institutions: A Multi-Institutional Politics Approach to Social Movements" (unpublished article, Indiana University and University of Connecticut, 2004); Francesca Polletta, "Culture in and Outside Institutions," in *Research in Social Movements, Conflicts and Change*, vol. 25, *Authority in Contention*, ed. Daniel J. Myers and Daniel M. Cress (Amsterdam: Elsevier, 2004), 162–63; Nella Van Dyke, Sarah A. Soule, and Verta A. Taylor, "The Targets of Social Movements: Beyond a Focus on the State," in *Research in Social Movements, Conflicts and Change*, vol. 25, *Authority in Contention*, ed. Daniel J. Myers and Daniel M. Cress (Amsterdam: Elsevier, 2004).

23. Hayagreeva Rao, Calvin Morrill, and Mayer N. Zald, "Power Plays: How Social Movements and Collective Action Create New Organizational Forms," *Research in Organizational Behavior* 22 (2000): 237–81; Elizabeth A. Armstrong, *Forging Gay Identities: Organizing Sexuality in San Francisco, 1950–1994* (Chicago: University of Chicago Press, 2002); Doug McAdam and W. Richard Scott, "Organizations and Movements," in *Social Movements and Organization Theory*, ed. Gerald F. Davis et al., 4–40 (Cambridge: Cambridge University Press, 2005); Mayer N. Zald, Calvin Morrill, and Hayagreeva Rao, "The Impact of Social Movements on Organizations," in *Social Movements and Organization Theory*, ed. Gerald F. Davis et al., 253–79 (Cambridge: Cambridge University Press, 2005).

24. Nikolas Rose, "The Politics of Life Itself," *Theory, Culture and Society* 18, no. 6 (2001): 1–30.

25. Epstein, *Impure Science*; Rebecca Dresser, *When Science Offers Salvation: Patient Advocacy and Research Ethics* (Oxford: Oxford University Press, 2001). There is a burgeoning literature on the politics of relations between experts and laypeople in the health field; for an overview, see Epstein, "Patient Groups and Health Movements." On the relation between science and technology and democratic processes more generally, see Jasanoff, *Designs on Nature*.

26. On the expansion of the concept of citizenship and "the diversity of arenas in which citizenship is being claimed and contested today," see Stuart Hall and David Held, "Citizens and Citizenship," in *New Times: The Changing Face of Politics in the 1990s*, ed. Stuart Hall and Martin Jacques, 173–88 (London: Verso, 1990). There is, of course, a huge literature on citizenship; for a summary of some of the recent debates surrounding the concept, see Gershon Shafir, ed., *The Citizenship Debates: A Reader* (Minneapolis: University of Minnesota Press, 1998).

27. See the references in n. 13.

28. Petryna, *Life Exposed*, 5.

29. Paul Rabinow, *Essays on the Anthropology of Reason* (Princeton, NJ: Princeton University Press, 1996), 91–111.

30. Aihwa Ong, "Making the Biopolitical Subject: Cambodian Immigrants, Refugee Medicine and Cultural Citizenship in California," *Social Science and Medicine* 40, no. 9 (1995): 1243–57; Aihwa Ong, "Cultural Citizenship as Subject-Making: Immigrants Negotiate Racial and Cultural Boundaries in the United States," *Current Anthropology* 37, no.

5 (December 1996): 737–62; Shah, *Contagious Divides*, esp. 7; Charles L. Briggs, "Why Nation-States and Journalists Can't Teach People to Be Healthy: Power and Pragmatic Miscalculation in Public Discourses on Health," *Medical Anthropology Quarterly* 17, no. 3 (September 2003): 287–321, esp. 288; Briggs and Mantini-Briggs, *Stories in Times of Cholera*; Molina, *Fit to Be Citizens*.

31. I already have hinted at a fourth process that also is important to my analysis: *representing*. I return to questions of representation in chapter 4.

32. Geoffrey C. Bowker and Susan Leigh Star, *Sorting Things Out: Classification and Its Consequences* (Cambridge, MA: MIT Press, 1999). On classification, see also Michel Foucault, *The Order of Things: An Archaeology of the Human Sciences* (New York: Vintage, 1973); Mary Douglas, *Purity and Danger* (New York: Routledge & Kegan Paul, 1979); Pierre Bourdieu, "The Social Space and the Genesis of Groups," *Theory and Society* 14, no. 6 (1985): 723–44; Paul Starr, "Social Categories and Claims in the Liberal State," in *How Classification Works: Nelson Goodman among the Social Sciences*, ed. Mary Douglas and David Hull, 159–74 (Edinburgh: Edinburgh University Press, 1992); John Dupré, *The Disorder of Things: Metaphysical Foundations of the Disunity of Science* (Cambridge, MA: Harvard University Press, 1993); Eviatar Zerubavel, "Lumping and Splitting: Notes on Social Classification," *Sociological Forum* 11, no. 3 (1996): 421–33; Amâde M'charek, "Technologies of Population: Forensic DNA Testing Practices and the Making of Differences and Similarities," *Configurations* 8 (2000): 121–58; Michèle Lamont and Virág Molnár, "The Study of Boundaries in the Social Sciences," *Annual Review of Sociology* 28 (2002): 167–95; Edward E. Telles, *Race in Another America: The Significance of Skin Color in Brazil* (Princeton, NJ: Princeton University Press, 2004), 78–106.

33. Starr, "Social Categories and Claims," 154, 160.

34. Seyla Benhabib, "Civil Society and the Politics of Identity and Difference in a Global Context," in *Diversity and Its Discontents: Cultural Conflict and Common Ground in Contemporary American Society*, ed. Neil J. Smelser and Jeffrey C. Alexander (Princeton, NJ: Princeton University Press, 1999), 298.

35. Starr, "Social Categories and Claims," 160–161. See also Yen Le Espiritu, *Asian American Panethnicity: Bridging Institutions and Identities* (Philadelphia: Temple University Press, 1992); Joane Nagel, "American Indian Ethnic Renewal: Politics and the Resurgence of Identity," *American Sociological Review* 60 (1995): 947–65; Porter, *Trust in Numbers*; Benhabib, "Civil Society and the Politics of Identity and Difference," 293–312; Skrentny, *Minority Rights Revolution*, esp. 85–142; Telles, *Race in Another America*, 78–106; De Zwart, "Dilemma of Recognition."

36. Bourdieu, "Social Space and the Genesis of Groups," 729.

37. Pierre Bourdieu, *Practical Reason: On the Theory of Action* (Stanford, CA: Stanford University Press, 1998), 35, 45.

38. Rogers Brubaker and Frederick Cooper, "Beyond 'Identity,'" *Theory and Society* 29 (2000): 16.

39. Alberto Melucci, *Nomads of the Present: Social Movements and Individual Needs in Contemporary Society* (Philadelphia: Temple University Press, 1989); Aldon D. Morris and Carol McClurg Mueller, eds., *Frontiers in Social Movement Theory* (New Haven, CT: Yale University Press, 1992); Hank Johnston, Enrique Laraña, and Joseph R. Gusfield, "Identities, Grievances, and New Social Movements," in *New Social Movements: From Ideology to*

Identity, ed. Enrique Laraña, Hank Johnston, and Joseph R. Gusfield, 3–35 (Philadelphia: Temple University Press, 1994).

40. Lamont and Molnár, "Study of Boundaries in the Social Sciences," 187. On the performing of difference, see also Judith Butler, *Gender Trouble: Feminism and the Subversion of Identity*, *Thinking Gender* (New York: Routledge, 1990); Candace West and Sarah Fenstermaker, "Doing Difference," *Gender and Society* 9, no. 1 (February 1995): 8–37.

41. Ian Hacking, *The Social Construction of What?* (Cambridge, MA: Harvard University Press, 1999), 104. For an example, see Matthew Waites, "The Fixity of Sexual Identities in the Public Sphere: Biomedical Knowledge, Liberalism and the Heterosexual/Homosexual Binary in Late Modernity," *Sexualities* 8, no. 5 (2005): 539–69.

42. See, for example, Harry Collins, "The Seven Sexes: A Study in the Sociology of a Phenomenon, or the Replication of Experiments in Physics," *Sociology* 9 (1975): 205–24; Shapin and Schaffer, *Leviathan and the Air-Pump*; Thomas F. Gieryn and Anne E. Figert, "Ingredients for a Theory of Science in Society: O-Rings, Ice Water, C-Clamp, Richard Feynman, and the Press," in *Theories of Science in Society*, ed. Susan E. Cozzens and Thomas F. Gieryn, 67–97 (Bloomington: Indiana University Press, 1990); Donald A. MacKenzie, *Inventing Accuracy: A Historical Sociology of Nuclear Missile Guidance* (Cambridge, MA: MIT Press, 1990); Trevor Pinch, " 'Testing—One, Two Three . . . Testing!': Toward a Sociology of Testing," *Science, Technology, and Human Values* 18, no. 1 (winter 1993): 25–51; Steven Shapin, "Cordelia's Love: Credibility and the Social Studies of Science," *Perspectives on Science* 3, no. 3 (1995): 76–96; Benjamin Sims, "Concrete Practices: Testing in an Earthquake-Engineering Laboratory," *Social Studies of Science* 29, no. 4 (August 1999): 485–518.

43. Bruno Latour, "Give Me a Laboratory and I Will Raise the World," in *Science Observed: Perspectives on the Social Study of Science*, ed. Karin D. Knorr-Cetina and Michael Mulkay, 141–70 (London: Sage, 1983).

44. On generalizability in biomedical research specifically, see Ruth Bleier, "Social and Political Bias in Science: An Examination of Animal Studies and Their Generalizations to Human Behaviors and Evolution," in *Genes and Gender II: Pitfalls in Research on Sex and Gender*, ed. Ruth Hubbard and Marian Lowe, 49–69 (New York: Gordian Press, 1979); Adele E. Clarke, "Human Materials as Contested Objects: Problematics of Subjects Who Speak" (unpublished manuscript, University of California, San Francisco, 1995); Ilana Löwy and Jean-Paul Gaudillière, "Disciplining Cancer: Mice and the Practice of Genetic Purity," in *The Invisible Industrialist: Manufactures and the Production of Scientific Knowledge*, ed. Jean-Paul Gaudillière and Ilana Löwy, 209–49 (Houndsmills, UK: Macmillan, 1998); Lawrence Busch, Keiko Tanaka, and Valerie J. Gunter, "Who Cares If the Rat Dies? Rodents, Risks, and Humans in the Science of Food Safety," in *Illness and the Environment: A Reader in Contested Medicine*, ed. Steve Kroll-Smith, Phil Brown, and Valerie J. Gunter, 108–19 (New York: New York University Press, 2000). On the particular difficulties of credibly establishing success in experiments on human, see Steven Epstein, "Activism, Drug Regulation, and the Politics of Therapeutic Evaluation in the AIDS Era: A Case Study of ddC and the 'Surrogate Markers' Debate," *Social Studies of Science* 27, no. 5 (October 1997): 691–726.

45. William H. Sewell, "A Theory of Structure: Duality, Agency, and Transformation," *American Journal of Sociology* 98, no. 1 (July 1992): 17, 17 n. 9. On cultural schemas and their relationship to social institutions, see also Mary Blair-Loy, *Competing Devotions: Career*

and Family among Women Executives (Cambridge, MA: Harvard University Press, 2003); Polletta, "Culture in and Outside Institutions," 161–83.

46. Valerie Jenness, "Social Movement Growth, Domain Expansion, and Framing Processes: The Case of Violence against Gays and Lesbians as a Social Problem," *Social Problems* 42, no. 1 (February 1995): 145–70; Mary Fainsod Katzenstein and Judith Reppy, "Introduction: Rethinking Military Culture," in *Beyond Zero Tolerance: Discrimination in Military Culture*, ed. Mary Fainsod Katzenstein and Judith Reppy, 1–21 (Lanham, MD: Rowman & Littlefield, 1999); Valerie Jenness and Ryken Grattet, *Making Hate a Crime: From Social Movement to Law Enforcement* (New York: Russell Sage Foundation, 2001); Skrentny, *Minority Rights Revolution*.

47. David S. Meyer and Nancy Whittier, "Social Movement Spillover," *Social Problems* 41, no. 2 (1994): 277–98; Doug McAdam, " 'Initiator' and 'Spin-Off' Movements: Diffusion Processes in Protest Cycles," in *Repertoires and Cycles of Collective Action*, ed. Mark Traugott, 217–39 (Durham, NC: Duke University Press, 1995).

48. Stephen Hilgartner and Charles L. Bosk, "The Rise and Fall of Social Problems: A Public Arenas Model," *American Journal of Sociology* 94, no. 1 (July 1988): 72.

49. This is an adaptation of Bowker and Star's definition. They also note that standards span more than one "community of practice" or activity site; that they make things work together over distance or heterogeneous metrics; and that they are backed up by bodies such as professional organizations, manufacturers' associations, or the state. See Bowker and Star, *Sorting Things Out*, 13–14.

50. On standardization in general, see ibid.; Nils Brunsson and Bengt Jacobsson, *A World of Standards* (Oxford: Oxford University Press, 2000); Lawrence Busch, "The Moral Economy of Grades and Standards," *Journal of Rural Studies* 16 (2000); Martha Lampland and Susan Leigh Star, eds., "Formalizing Practices: Reckoning with Standards, Numbers, and Models in Science and Everyday Life" (book manuscript, University of California, San Diego, and Santa Clara University). Work specifically on standardization and science has been proliferating; see Robert E. Kohler, *Lords of the Fly: Drosophila Genetics and the Experimental Life* (Chicago: University of Chicago Press, 1994); Linda F. Hogle, "Standardization across Non-Standard Domains: The Case of Organ Procurement," *Science, Technology, and Human Values* 20, no. 4 (1995): 482–500; Porter, *Trust in Numbers*; Monica J. Casper and Adele E. Clarke, "Making the Pap Smear into the 'Right Tool' for the Job: Cervical Cancer Screening in the USA, circa 1940–95," *Social Studies of Science* 28, no. 2 (April 1998): 255–90; Wendy Nelson Espeland and Mitchell L. Stevens, "Commensuration as a Social Process," *Annual Review of Sociology* 24 (1998): 313–43; Kathleen Jordan and Michael Lynch, "The Dissemination, Standardization and Routinization of a Molecular Biological Technique," *Social Studies of Science* 28, nos. 5–6 (October–December 1998): 773–800; Ken Alder, *The Measure of All Things: The Seven-Year Odyssey and Hidden Error That Transformed the World* (New York: Free Press, 2002); Keating and Cambrosio, *Biomedical Platforms*; Timmermans and Berg, *Gold Standard*; Andrew Lakoff, "Diagnostic Liquidity: Mental Illness and the Global Trade in DNA," *Theory and Society* 34, no. 1 (February 2005): 63–92.

51. Brunsson and Jacobsson, *World of Standards*, 1.

52. Bowker and Star, *Sorting Things Out*; Susan Leigh Star, "The Ethnography of Infrastructure," *American Behavioral Scientist* 43, no. 3 (November/December 1999): 377–91.

53. Michael Mann, *The Sources of Social Power*, vol. 2, *The Rise of Classes and Nation*

States, 1760–1914 (Cambridge: Cambridge University Press, 1993), 59. I am grateful to Catherine Lee for pointing out the relevance of Mann's work to my concerns.

54. Bowker and Star, *Sorting Things Out*, 14.

55. John W. Kingdon, *Agendas, Alternatives, and Public Policies* (Boston: Little, Brown, 1984), 201.

56. Margaret Weir, *Politics and Jobs: The Boundaries of Employment Policy in the United States* (Princeton, NJ: Princeton University Press, 1992), 19. See also Theda Skocpol and Edwin Amenta, "States and Social Policies," *Annual Review of Sociology* 12 (1986): 131–57; Margaret Weir, Ann Shola Orloff, and Theda Skocpol, "Introduction: Understanding American Social Politics," in *The Politics of Social Policy in the United States*, ed. Margaret Weir, Ann Shola Orloff, and Theda Skocpol, 3–27 (Princeton, NJ: Princeton University Press, 1988); Paul Burstein, "Policy Domains: Organization, Culture, and Policy Outcomes," *Annual Review of Sociology* 17 (1991): 327–50; Frank Dobbin, *Forging Industrial Policy: The United States, Britain, and France in the Railway Age* (Cambridge: Cambridge University Press, 1994); Skrentny, *Minority Rights Revolution*.

57. In his classic essay on bureaucracy, Max Weber considered the "leveling" function of the modern bureaucratic state to be essentially inconsistent with notions of individualized treatment; see H. H. Gerth and C. Wright Mills, eds., *From Max Weber*, 196–244 (New York: Oxford University Press, 1946). For a recent revisiting of similar issues, see James C. Scott, *Seeing Like a State: How Certain Schemes to Improve the Human Condition Have Failed* (New Haven, CT: Yale University Press, 1998). On the movement within biomedicine away from one-size-fits-all technologies and toward customization and niche marketing, see Clarke et al., "Biomedicalization," 169.

58. Of course, within the inclusion-and-difference paradigm, the ability of the new standards to coerce behavior is backed up by federal laws and by the rules and guidelines issued by regulatory agencies. Peter Keating and Alberto Cambrosio's broad concept of "regulation" is helpful for conceptualizing this mix of coercive powers that "include, in addition to state intervention, de facto, informal, and even tacit agreements, standards, and guidelines"—though I am probably doing some violence to the authors' concept by wresting it out of the context in which they define it, that of the biomedical platform. Keating and Cambrosio, *Biomedical Platforms*, 258.

59. Key works include Sandra Harding and Jean F. O'Barr, eds., *Sex and Scientific Inquiry*, 2nd ed. (Chicago: University of Chicago Press, 1987); Harding, *Science Question in Feminism*; Thomas Lacquer, "Orgasm, Generation, and the Politics of Reproductive Biology," in *The Making of the Modern Body: Sexuality and Society in the Nineteenth Century*, ed. Catherine Gallagher and Thomas Lacquer, 1–41 (Berkeley: University of California Press, 1987); Londa Schiebinger, "Skeletons in the Closet: The First Illustrations of the Female Skeleton in Eighteenth-Century Anatomy," in *Making of the Modern Body*, ed. Gallagher and Lacquer, 42–82; Ludmilla Jordanova, *Sexual Visions: Images of Gender in Science and Medicine between the Eighteenth and Twentieth Centuries* (Madison: University of Wisconsin Press, 1989); Haraway, *Simians, Cyborgs, and Women*, 132–36; Anne Fausto-Sterling, "The Five Sexes: Why Male and Female Are Not Enough," *Sciences* 33, no. 2 (March–April 1993): 20–26; Oudshoorn, *Beyond the Natural Body*; Emily Martin, "The Egg and the Sperm: How Science Has Constructed a Romance Based on Stereotypical Male-Female Roles," in *Gender and Health*, ed. Sargent and Brettell, 29–43; Marianne van den Wijngaard, *Reinventing the Sexes: The Biomedical Construction of Femininity and Masculinity* (Bloomington: Indiana University

Press, 1997); Adele Clarke, *Disciplining Reproduction: Modernity, American Life Sciences, and "the Problems of Sex"* (Berkeley: University of California Press, 1998); Stefan Hirschauer, "Performing Sexes and Genders in Medical Practices," in *Differences in Medicine: Unraveling Practices, Techniques, and Bodies*, ed. Marc Berg and Annemarie Mol, 13–27 (Durham, NC: Duke University Press, 1998); Suzanne J. Kessler, *Lessons from the Intersexed* (New Brunswick, NJ: Rutgers University Press, 1998); Michelle Murphy, "Liberation through Control in the Body Politics of U.S. Radical Feminism," in *The Moral Authority of Nature*, ed. Lorraine Daston and Fernando Vidal, 331–55 (Chicago: University of Chicago Press, 2004).

60. See the references in the introduction, n. 21.

61. Of course, much the same can be said of other social categories, such as sexual identity (see n. 70 below) and social class.

62. Michael Omi and Howard Winant, *Racial Formation in the United States: From the 1960's to the 1980's* (New York: Routledge & Kegan Paul, 1986), 68; see also Howard Winant, "Race and Race Theory," *Annual Review of Sociology* 26 (2000): 169–85. To underscore the contingent and constructed nature of these attributes, some analysts decline to use terms such as *race* unless they are safely contained within quotation marks (what are sometimes called "scare quotes"). I appreciate the sentiment but object to the practice—not only on aesthetic grounds, but also because there is no limit, in principle, to the number of ordinary English words that might be seen as in need of such tagging.

63. Charles L. Briggs, "Communicability, Racial Discourse, and Disease," *Annual Review of Anthropology* 34 (2005): 269–91.

64. Omi and Winant, *Racial Formation in the United States*; R. W. Connell, "The State, Gender, and Sexual Politics," *Theory and Society* 19, no. 5 (October 1990): 507–44; Wendy Brown, "Finding the Man in the State," *Feminist Studies* 18, no. 1 (spring 1992): 7–34; Kristin Luker, "Sex, Social Hygiene, and the State: The Double-Edged Sword of Social Reform," *Theory and Society* 27, no. 5 (October 1998): 601–34; David Theo Goldberg, *The Racial State* (Malden, MA: Blackwell, 2002).

65. Joan Wallach Scott, *Gender and the Politics of History* (New York: Columbia University Press, 1988), 42–44.

66. West and Fenstermaker, "Doing Difference," 8–37. For a different approach to the performance of difference, see J. Butler, *Gender Trouble*.

67. Kimberlé Williams Crenshaw, "Mapping the Margins: Intersectionality, Identity Politics, and Violence against Women of Color," in *The Public Nature of Private Violence*, ed. Martha Albertson Feineman and Rixanne Mykitiuk, 93–118 (New York: Routledge, 1994). On the implications of these intersections for health, see Amy J. Schulz and Leith Mullings, eds., *Gender, Race, Class, and Health: Intersectional Approaches* (San Francisco: Jossey-Bass, 2006).

68. For a related and influential formulation, see Gayle Rubin's definition of the "sex/gender system." Gayle Rubin, "The Traffic in Women: Notes on the 'Political Economy' of Sex," in *Toward an Anthropology of Women*, ed. Rayna Rapp Reiter, 157–210 (New York: Monthly Review Press, 1975).

69. Examples of work articulating this new understanding of the relationship between sex and gender include those in n. 59 above, as well as J. Butler, *Gender Trouble*, 1–13; Stefan Hirschauer and Annemarie Mol, "Shifting Sexes, Moving Stories: Feminist/Constructivist Dialogues," *Science, Technology, and Human Values* 20, no. 3 (summer 1995): 368–85; Celia

Roberts, "Biological Sex? Hormones, Psychology, and Sex," *NWSA Journal* 12, no. 3 (2000): 1–20; Laura Severin and Mary Wyer, "The Science and Politics of the Search for Sex Differences," *NWSA Journal* 12, no. 3 (2000): vii–xvi; Joanne J. Meyerowitz, *How Sex Changed: A History of Transsexuality in the United States* (Cambridge, MA: Harvard University Press, 2002).

70. It is also worth noting that both sex and gender (as defined here) are implicated in the construction of sexuality and sexual identity (an important topic of chapter 12). However, sexual identity cannot be reduced to either sex or gender and must be treated as a relatively autonomous domain of social stratification and identity formation. Gayle Rubin, "Thinking Sex: Notes for a Radical Theory of the Politics of Sexuality," in *Pleasure and Danger: Exploring Female Sexuality*, ed. Carole S. Vance (New York: Routledge, 1984), 27–34.

71. Mindy Thompson Fullilove, "Comment: Abandoning 'Race' as a Variable in Public Health Research—An Idea Whose Time Has Come," *American Journal of Public Health* 88, no. 9 (1998): 1297–98.

72. Matthew Frye Jacobson, *Whiteness of a Different Color: European Immigrants and the Alchemy of Race* (Cambridge MA: Harvard University Press, 1998).

73. Stephen Cornell and Douglas Hartmann, *Ethnicity and Race: Making Identities in a Changing World* (Thousand Oaks, CA: Pine Forge Press, 1998), xvii, 24.

74. Ibid., 19. This is the authors' quotation from a definition by Richard A. Schemerhorn (which is itself, the authors note, an adaptation of the work of Max Weber).

75. Judith Treas, "Age as a Standard and Standards for Age: The Institutionalization of Chronological Age as Biographical Necessity," in "Formalizing Practices," ed. Lampland and Star (manuscript).

76. Philippe Ariès, *Centuries of Childhood: A Social History of Family Life* (New York: Vintage, 1962); Lock, "Anomalous Ageing"; Claudia Castañeda, *Figurations: Child, Bodies, Worlds* (Durham, NC: Duke University Press, 2002).

77. This useful terminology is from Rogers Brubaker and Frederick Cooper, who cite Bourdieu as an influence. Brubaker and Cooper note that, as a term, "categories of practice" is preferable to more familiar notions such as "folk" categories, "for while the latter imply a relatively sharp distinction between 'native' or 'folk' or 'lay' concepts on one hand and 'scientific' categories on the other, such concepts as 'race,' 'ethnicity,' or 'nation' are marked by close reciprocal connection and mutual influence among their practical and analytical uses." Brubaker and Cooper, "Beyond 'Identity,' " 4. An alternative and common formulation of this same distinction is that between "actors' categories" and "analysts' categories."

78. There remain two last points of clarification regarding my own uses of identifying terms. First, it is sometimes difficult to select the most appropriate term for a group, because competing names may exist and possess different political valences. The sometimes fraught choice between "Hispanic" and "Latino" is one example; the different associations that adhere to "black" as opposed to "African American" or "Afro-Caribbean" is another; and the relation between "American Indian" and "Native American" is yet a third. My practice will be to use the terms that seem most appropriate in a given context, with the hope that those who disapprove of my choices will at least concede that there is no terminological solution that satisfies everyone. Second, I have given some thought to my practice of capitalization in the naming of groups. To my mind, the use of capital letters and lowercase letters are both problematic, though for different reasons: capitalization because

it promotes the reification of identities, and lowercase because it may inadvertently suggest a lack of respect. My approach is mainly to follow grammatical convention. Therefore, racial and ethnic group names are capitalized if they are derived from locations or terms that are capitalized in English (*Asians, Latinos, African Americans*, etc.) and otherwise are not capitalized (*whites, minorities, people of color*, etc.). Readers should draw no assumptions about the implied importance or authenticity of a group based on my use of capitalization.

CHAPTER TWO

1. See Eileen Nechas and Denise Foley, *Unequal Treatment: What You Don't Know about How Women Are Mistreated by the Medical Community* (New York: Simon & Schuster, 1994); Rosser, *Women's Health*. For a more complicated analysis of the "paradoxes of visibility" in biomedicine, see Paula A. Treichler, Lisa Cartwright, and Constance Penley, "Introduction: Paradoxes of Visibility," in *The Visible Woman: Imaging Technologies, Gender, and Science*, ed. Paula A. Treichler, Lisa Cartwright, and Constance Penley, 1–17 (New York: New York University Press, 1998).

2. Healy, "Challenging Sameness."

3. NIH, "Outreach Notebook for the Inclusion, Recruitment and Retention of Women and Minority Subjects in Clinical Research: Principal Investigators' Notebook," NIH Publication no. 03-7036, December 2002, 55.

4. For a strong argument advancing the latter position, see Nancy Krieger and Elizabeth Fee, "Man-Made Medicine and Women's Health: The Biopolitics of Sex/Gender and Race/Ethnicity," in *Man-Made Medicine: Women's Health, Public Policy, and Reform*, ed. Kary L. Moss (Durham, NC: Duke University Press, 1996), 21. Krieger and Fee note that to imagine that medical researchers took white men as the norm (and hence representative of other groups) is to misread how medicine privileged white men as a *distinct* group and stigmatized others for being different from them.

5. For an incisive consideration of how concepts such as these informed medical experimentation in the eighteenth century, see Londa Schiebinger, "Human Experimentation in the Eighteenth Century: Natural Boundaries and Valid Testing," in *Moral Authority of Nature*, ed. Daston and Vidal, 384–408.

6. I present some of those recent numbers on inclusion in chapter 8.

7. The phrase "working objects" is from Lorraine Daston and Peter Galison, "The Image of Objectivity," *Representations* 40 (fall 1992): 85. See also Bruno Latour, *Science in Action: How to Follow Scientists and Engineers through Society* (Cambridge, MA: Harvard University Press, 1987); Clarke and Fujimura, *Right Tools for the Job*; Porter, *Trust in Numbers*, 29–32; Jordan and Lynch, "Dissemination, Standardization and Routinization."

8. Daston and Galison, "Image of Objectivity," 85.

9. Kohler, *Lords of the Fly*.

10. Löwy and Gaudillière, "Disciplining Cancer."

11. Porter, *Trust in Numbers*, 29.

12. Busch, Tanaka, and Gunter, "Who Cares If the Rat Dies?" 108–19. See also Donna J. Haraway, *Primate Visions: Gender, Race, and Nature in the World of Modern Science* (New York: Routledge, 1989); Haraway, *Simians, Cyborgs, and Women*, 7–20; Clarke, "Human Materials as Contested Objects."

13. Schiebinger, "Skeletons in the Closet," 46.

14. Lacquer, "Orgasm, Generation, and the Politics of Reproductive Biology," 5.

15. Ibid., 18.

16. Schiebinger, "Skeletons in the Closet," 51. See also Londa Schiebinger, *Nature's Body: Gender in the Making of Modern Science* (Boston: Beacon Press, 1993).

17. Barbara Ehrenreich and Deirdre English, *For Her Own Good: 150 Years of the Experts' Advice to Women* (New York: Anchor Books, 1978), 120 (emphasis in the original).

18. Schiebinger, "Skeletons in the Closet," 51, 63. See also Jordanova, *Sexual Visions*.

19. Weisman, *Women's Health Care*, 33–34.

20. Steven Jay Gould, *The Mismeasure of Man* (New York: Norton, 1981).

21. Quotations from William H. Tucker, *The Science and Politics of Racial Research* (Urbana: University of Illinois Press, 1994), 13–14; see also Todd L. Savitt, *Medicine and Slavery: The Diseases and Health Care of Blacks in Antebellum Virginia* (Urbana: University of Illinois Press, 1978).

22. Gerald N. Grob, *Mental Institutions in America: Social Policy to 1875* (New York: Free Press, 1973), 243 n. 38.

23. Stephen M. Stowe, *Doctoring the South* (Chapel Hill: University of North Carolina Press, 2004), 208–18, quotation from 214.

24. John Harley Warner, *The Therapeutic Perspective: Medical Practice, Knowledge, and Identity in America, 1820–1885* (Cambridge, MA: Harvard University Press, 1986), 58–59.

25. David McBride, *From TB to AIDS: Epidemics among Urban Blacks since 1900* (Albany: State University of New York Press, 1991), 16, 18.

26. Seale Harris, "Tuberculosis in the Negro," in *Germs Have No Color Line: Blacks and American Medicine, 1900–1940*, ed. Vanessa Northington Gamble (New York: Garland, 1989), 2–3; reprinted from *JAMA* 41 (1903): 834–38. While blacks were thus considered to be at special risk of contracting tuberculosis, Jews, by contrast, were considered by some physicians to be peculiarly resistant; see Bass Hödl, "The Black Body and the Jewish Body: A Comparison of Medical Images," *Patterns of Prejudice* 36, no. 1 (2002): 24–25.

27. Allan M. Brandt, "Racism and Research: The Case of the Tuskegee Syphilis Experiment," in *Tuskegee's Truths: Rethinking the Tuskegee Syphilis Study*, ed. Susan M. Reverby (Chapel Hill: University of North Carolina Press, 2000), 16.

28. J. Jones, *Bad Blood*, esp. 16–29.

29. Quoted in Vanessa Northington Gamble, introduction to *Germs Have No Color Line: Blacks and American Medicine, 1900–1940*, ed. Vanessa Northington Gamble (New York: Garland, 1989), n.p.

30. Ibid.

31. Joan Trauner, "The Chinese as Medical Scapegoats in San Francisco, 1870–1905," *California History*, spring 1978, 70–87. See also Shah, *Contagious Divides*, 45–76.

32. Tucker, *Science and Politics of Racial Research*, 37–137. On eugenics and racial science, see also Daniel J. Kevles, *In the Name of Eugenics: Genetics and the Uses of Human Heredity* (New York: Knopf, 1985); Proctor, *Racial Hygiene*.

33. Wailoo, *Drawing Blood*, 134–61; Tapper, *In the Blood*.

34. On the formation of this consensus concerning the science of race, see Barkan, *Retreat of Scientific Racism*; and for a critical review, see Reardon, *Race to the Finish*.

35. On Nazi claims about the racial specificity of disease, including notions that "measles . . . was rare among Mongols and Negroes; myopia and difficulties associated with giving birth were more common among civilized than among primitive peoples . . . [and]

that Jews suffered more from diabetes, flat feet, staggers (*Torsiondystonie*), hemophilia, xeroderma pigmentosum, deafness, and nervous disorders than non-Jews," see Proctor, *Racial Hygiene*, 196–97.

36. Barkan, *Retreat of Scientific Racism*, 334.

37. John W. Dower, *War without Mercy: Race and Power in the Pacific War* (New York: Pantheon, 1986), 175, 348 n. 40. Dower's quotation is from Congressman John Rankin of Mississippi.

38. For the Medical Subject Headings (MeSH), see www.nlm.nih.gov/mesh/meshhome .html, and for the 2002 coding instructions for medical librarians, see www.nlm.nih.gov/ mesh/indman/chapter_30.html. I conducted the literature search in August 2002 using the National Library of Medicine's "PubMed" database (www.pubmed.org). On the 2004 changes in the MeSH categories, see Stuart J. Nelson, "Reply to 'MEDLINE Definitions of Race and Ethnicity and Their Application to Genetic Research,'" *Nature Genetics* 34, no. 2 (2003). Nelson's letter came in response to a critique by Pamela Sankar. Pamela Sankar, "MEDLINE Definitions of Race and Ethnicity and Their Application to Genetic Research," *Nature Genetics* 34, no. 2 (June 2003): 119.

39. David J. Rothman, *Strangers at the Bedside* (New York: Basic, 1991), 19–20.

40. Lawrence K. Altman, *Who Goes First? The Story of Self-Experimentation in Medicine* (New York: Random House, 1987).

41. Schiebinger, "Human Experimentation," 386, 393, 405.

42. Vanessa Northington Gamble, "Under the Shadow of Tuskegee: African Americans and Health Care," *American Journal of Public Health* 87, no. 11 (November 1997): 1773.

43. Deborah Kuhn McGregor, *Sexual Surgery and the Origins of Gynecology: J. Marion Sims, His Hospital, and His Patients* (New York: Garland, 1989), 58–62. For another graphic example, concerning experimentation on a slave to test remedies for heatstroke, see Gamble, "Under the Shadow of Tuskegee," 1774. On the tendency of Southern physicians to experiment on poor people in general and slaves in particular, see also Savitt, *Medicine and Slavery*, 281–307. On medical claims about racial differences in the nineteenth century, see also Nancy Krieger, "Shades of Difference: Theoretical Underpinnings of the Medical Controversy on Black/White Differences in the United States 1830–1870," *International Journal of Health Services* 17, no. 2 (1987): 259–78.

44. Quoted in Gamble, "Under the Shadow of Tuskegee," 1773.

45. Robert L. Blakely and Judith M. Harrington, "Grave Consequences: The Opportunistic Procurement of Cadavers at the Medical College of Georgia," in *Bones in the Basement: Postmortem Racism in 19th Century Medical Training*, ed. Robert L. Blakely and Judith M. Harrington (Washington, DC: Smithsonian Institution Press, 1997), 163.

46. On clinical trials of the Pill, see Laura Briggs, *Reproducing Empire: Race, Sex, Science, and U.S. Imperialism in Puerto Rico* (Berkeley: University of California Press, 2002), 135–40. On geneticists' interests in studying African Americans, see Jennifer Reardon, "Affirmative Action Genomics? Struggles over the Meaning of Democratic Participation in a Genomic Age" (paper presented at the Annual Meeting of the Society for Social Studies of Science, Atlanta, GA, October 16, 2003).

47. Heather Munro Prescott, "Using the Student Body: College and University Students as Research Subjects in the United States during the Twentieth Century," *Journal of the History of Medicine* 57 (January 2002): 5, 16, 19–20, 37–38.

48. Jordan Goodman, Anthony McElligott, and Lara Marks, eds., *Useful Bodies: Hu-*

mans in the Service of Medical Science in the Twentieth Century (Baltimore: Johns Hopkins University Press, 2003).

49. Rothman, *Strangers at the Bedside*, 51.

50. Ibid., 16–17, 70–84.

51. J. Jones, *Bad Blood*.

52. A third implication of the Tuskegee study will be considered in chapter 9: its repercussions for the ability of medical researchers to recruit African Americans for clinical studies.

53. J. Jones, *Bad Blood*, 10.

54. Patricia A. King, "The Dangers of Difference," *Hastings Center Report* 22, no. 6 (1992): 35–38.

55. On radiation, see Ruth R. Faden, "Human-Subjects Research Today: Final Report of the Advisory Committee on Human Radiation Experiments," *Academic Medicine* 71, no. 5 (May 1996): 482–83. For an extended discussion of one prewar psychiatric horror story that, as its author notes, we should not "dismiss . . . as a momentary aberration in the march of psychiatric progress," see Andrew Scull, *Madhouse: A Tragic Tale of Megalomania and Modern Medicine* (New Haven, CT: Yale University Press, 2005), quotation from 273.

56. Sydney A. Halpern, *Lesser Harms: The Morality of Risk in Medical Research* (Chicago: University of Chicago Press, 2004), 9. For recent scholarly evaluations of the Tuskegee study and its impact, see also Susan M. Reverby, ed., *Tuskegee's Truths: Rethinking the Tuskegee Syphilis Study* (Chapel Hill: University of North Carolina Press, 2000).

57. Halpern, *Lesser Harms*.

58. National Commission for the Protection of Human Subjects of Biomedical and Behavioral Research, "The Belmont Report: Ethical Principles and Guidelines for the Protections of Human Subjects of Research" (Washington, DC: U.S. Department of Health, Education and Welfare, April 18, 1979).

59. Ibid.; Rothman, *Strangers at the Bedside*; Jeffrey P. Kahn, Anna C. Mastroianni, and Jeremy Sugarman, eds., *Beyond Consent: Seeking Justice in Research* (New York: Oxford University Press, 1998).

60. Anna C. Mastroianni, Ruth Faden, and Daniel Federman, *Women and Health Research: Ethical and Legal Issues of Including Women in Clinical Studies* (Washington, DC: National Academy Press, 1994), 1:40–41.

61. Gerd Gigerenzer et al., *The Empire of Chance: How Probability Changed Science and Everyday Life* (Cambridge: Cambridge University Press, 1989), 41.

62. J. Warner, *Therapeutic Perspective*, 248–49.

63. See, for example, Marc Berg, *Rationalizing Medical Work: Decision-Support Techniques and Medical Practices* (Cambridge, MA: MIT Press, 1997); Harry M. Marks, *The Progress of Experiment: Science and Therapeutic Reform in the United States, 1900–1990* (Cambridge: Cambridge University Press, 1997); William G. Rothstein, *Public Health and the Risk Factor: A History of an Uneven Medical Revolution* (Rochester, NY: University of Rochester Press, 2003); Timmermans and Berg, *Gold Standard*.

64. Peggy Wallace, "Following the Threads of an Innovation: The History of Standardized Patients in Medical Education," *Caduceus* 13, no. 2 (fall 1997): 5–28; Perry Garfinkel, "Medical Students Get Taste of Real-Life Doctoring," *New York Times*, October 23, 2001, D-7.

65. Ericka Johnson, "The Ghost of Anatomies Past: Simulating the One-Sex Body in Modern Medical Training," *Feminist Theory* 6, no. 2 (August 2005): 141–59, esp. 146.

66. Alan Petersen, "Sexing the Body: Representations of Sex Differences in Gray's *Anatomy*, 1858 to the Present," *Body and Society* 4, no. 1 (1998): 1–3. For another study of gender representations in anatomy textbooks over a long period, see Susan C. Lawrence and Kae Bendixen, "His and Hers: Male and Female Anatomy in Anatomy Texts for U.S. Medical Students, 1890–1989," *Social Science and Medicine* 35, no. 7 (October 1992). For an extensive study of recent textbooks, see Kathleen D. Mendelsohn et al., "Sex and Gender Bias in Anatomy and Physical Diagnosis Text Illustrations," *Journal of the American Medical Association* 272, no. 16 (October 26, 1994): 1267–70; and for critical commentary, see the letters section of the April 26, 1995, issue of the journal.

67. E. Johnson, "Ghost of Anatomies Past," 154. The tendency for women to be conceived of as "special objects" rather than "normal subjects" of medicine is also suggested by the subject headings of a key medical index from 1880 to 1932; see Diana E. Long, "Hidden Persuaders: Medical Indexing and the Gendered Professionalism of American Medicine, 1880–1932," *Osiris* 12 (1997): 100–120.

68. As Robert Aronowitz has observed, the idea of the risk factor is consistent with the ethos of individualism: "If [the belief is that] we are all individually responsible for our own health and illness, then we need a road map to tell us where our fateful choices lie." Robert A. Aronowitz, *Making Sense of Illness: Science, Society, and Disease* (Cambridge: Cambridge University Press, 1998), 111–44, quotation from 130. On the rise of the risk factor and its significance in modern medicine, see also Rose, "Politics of Life Itself," 6–11; W. Rothstein, *Public Health and the Risk Factor*; Colin Talley, Howard I. Kushner, and Claire E. Sterk, "Lung Cancer, Chronic Disease Epidemiology, and Medicine, 1948–1964," *Journal of the History of Medicine* 59, no. 3 (July 2004): 329–74.

69. Thomas Royle Dawber, *The Framingham Study: The Epidemiology of Atherosclerotic Disease* (Cambridge, MA: Harvard University Press, 1980), 16–17, 222–29; W. Rothstein, *Public Health and the Risk Factor*, 279–85. See also www.nhlbi.nih.gov/about/framingham/.

70. Dawber, *Framingham Study*, 22.

71. Bernadine Healy, *A New Prescription for Women's Health* (New York: Viking, 1995), 333.

72. Jennifer Fosket gives another example of a risk assessment tool that presents itself as applicable to everyone even when its design is based on a racially unrepresentative population; see Jennifer Fosket, "Constructing 'High-Risk Women': The Development and Standardization of a Breast Cancer Risk Assessment Tool," *Science, Technology, and Human Values* 29, no. 3 (summer 2004): 291–313.

73. H. Marks, *Progress of Experiment*.

74. William A. Silverman, *Human Experimentation: A Guided Step into the Unknown* (Oxford: Oxford University Press, 1985), 48–50; Curtis L. Meinert and Susan Tonascia, *Clinical Trials: Design, Conduct, and Analysis* (New York: Oxford University Press, 1986); Bert Spilker, *Guide to Clinical Trials* (New York: Raven Press, 1991), 69–70.

75. However, in trials with fewer than fifty subjects per arm, if a patient characteristic is known to influence an outcome, investigators sometimes "stratify" their subject population into different strata prior to randomization, in order to ensure that the characteristic is equally distributed across arms. For example, if the outcome being tested is known to differ by sex, then an investigator might separate men from women and then, within each stratum, randomly assign each individual to the treatment arm or the control arm. In trials with more than fifty subjects per arm, experts generally consider stratification prior to randomization to be unnecessary. See Meinert and Tonascia, *Clinical Trials*, 93–95.

76. Spilker, *Guide to Clinical Trials*, 147–48.

77. Alvan R. Feinstein, "An Additional Basic Science for Clinical Medicine: II. The Limitations of Randomized Trials," *Annals of Internal Medicine* 99, no. 4 (October 1983): 544–50. On the more general problem in science of credibly extrapolating findings from contrived experimental situations, see the references in chap. 1, nn. 42–44.

78. Steven Piantadosi, *Clinical Trials: A Methodological Perspective* (New York: Wiley, 1997), 197–98. Recently, clinical researchers have expressed the hope of using the techniques of the new field of pharmacogenomics to put together homogenous subject populations, for example, by screening out those whom genetic tests reveal to be likely nonresponders. Andrew Lakoff, *Pharmaceutical Reason*, 173–77.

79. Indeed, we lack a full-fledged history of human experimentation that puts the subjects of those experiments front and center. As Harry Marks acknowledges in his history of modern clinical research, scholarly attention to experimenters has greatly outpaced investigation of those experimented upon, largely because of the dearth of sources describing the latter. H. Marks, *Progress of Experiment*, 13.

CHAPTER THREE

1. I draw generally from the scholarship on social movements in understanding these developments. On the kinds of political opportunities that foster the development of activism, see H. P Kitschelt, "Political Opportunity Structures and Political Protest: Anti-Nuclear Movements in Four Democracies," *British Journal of Political Science* 16 (1986): 57–85. On the "external relational fields" that structure movement action and shape possibilities for success, see Jack A. Goldstone, "More Social Movements or Fewer? Beyond Political Opportunity Structures to Relational Fields," *Theory and Society* 33, nos. 3–4 (June 2004): 333–65. On how movements mobilize, see John D. McCarthy and Mayer N. Zald, "Resource Mobilization and Social Movements: A Partial Theory," *American Journal of Sociology* 82, no. 6 (1977): 1212–41; Bert Klandermans and Sidney Tarrow, "Mobilization into Social Movements: Synthesizing European and American Approaches," *International Social Movement Research* 1 (1988): 1–38. On the development of perceptions that change is possible ("cognitive liberation"), see Doug McAdam, *Political Process and the Development of Black Insurgency, 1930–1970* (Chicago: University of Chicago Press, 1982), 48–51. On social movement success, see William A. Gamson, *The Strategy of Social Protest* (Belmont, CA: Wadsworth, 1990); Marco Giugni, Doug McAdam, and Charles Tilly, eds., *How Social Movements Matter* (Minneapolis: University of Minnesota Press, 1999).

2. It typically has been argued that the politics of funding for health and medical research in the United States is unique in its disease-specific, "squeaky-wheel-gets-the-grease" character. In the traditional incarnation of these politics, sufferers of a disease form a national association to represent their interests, lobby sympathetic members of Congress (ideally, ones who have the disease themselves or who have a family member with the disease), and, before long, a new institute is funded within the NIH, focusing on that specific disease. See Stephen P. Strickland, *Politics, Science, and Dread Disease: A Short History of United States Medical Research Policy* (Cambridge, MA: Harvard University Press, 1972). In the more recent, radical variant of these politics, an activist group, such as ACT UP or one of those inspired by it, engages in highly visible and confrontational direct action protest until Congress agrees to increase NIH funding to study that disease. See Epstein, *Impure Science*. But this disease-specific approach to transforming health research

coexists and intertwines with a different kind of political claims-making that is identity-group specific, rather than just disease-specific. For a review of recent thinking on this issue, see Epstein, "Patient Groups and Health Movements."

3. Controversy thus unfolded in the sort of space that Michel Callon has called a "hybrid forum," one in which "groups and the spokespersons who claim to represent them are heterogeneous—consisting of experts, politicians, technicians and lay people who consider themselves to be concerned." Callon, "Increasing Involvement of Concerned Groups," 59.

4. Ann Swidler, "Cultural Power and Social Movements," in *Social Movements and Culture*, ed. Hank Johnston and Bert Klandermans (Minneapolis: University of Minnesota Press, 1995), 39. On the production of "isomorphism," see also Paul J. DiMaggio and Walter W. Powell, "The Iron Cage Revisited: Institutional Isomorphism and Collective Rationality in Organizational Fields," *American Sociological Review* 48 (April 1983): 147–60.

5. I discuss these issues of "domain expansion" and "policy legacies" in much greater detail in chapters 7 and 12. On domain expansion, see the references in chap. 1, n. 46. On policy legacies, see the references in chap. 1, n. 56.

6. Primmer, "Women's Health Research," 307–9.

7. Weisman, *Women's Health Care*, 2.

8. The following discussion borrows the accepted understandings of distinctions between radical feminism, socialist feminism, and liberal feminism in the 1970s and afterward. See, for example, Alice Echols, *Daring to Be Bad: Radical Feminism in America, 1967–1975* (Minneapolis: University of Minnesota Press, 1989).

9. For introductions to the feminist women's health movement in the United States, see Sheryl Burt Ruzek, *Feminist Alternatives to Medical Control* (New York: Praeger, 1978); Auerbach and Figert, "Women's Health Research"; Byllye Y. Avery, "Breathing Life into Ourselves: The Evolution of the National Black Women's Health Project," in *Perspectives in Medical Sociology*, ed. Phil Brown, 761–76 (Prospect Heights, IL: Waveland Press, 1996); Paula A. Treichler, Lisa Cartwright, and Constance Penley, eds., *The Visible Woman: Imaging Technologies, Gender and Science* (New York: New York University Press, 1998); Weisman, *Women's Health Care*; Adele E. Clarke and Virginia L. Olesen, eds., *Revisioning Women, Health, and Healing: Feminist, Cultural and Technoscience Perspectives* (New York: Routledge, 1999); Deborah R. Grayson, "'Necessity Was the Midwife of Our Politics': Black Women's Health Activism in the 'Post'—Civil Rights Era (1980–1996)," in *Still Lifting, Still Climbing: Contemporary African American Women's Activism*, ed. Kimberly Springer, 131–48 (New York: New York University Press, 1999); Sandra Morgen, *Into Our Own Hands: The Women's Health Movement in the United States, 1969–1990* (New Brunswick, NJ: Rutgers University Press, 2002); M. Murphy, "Liberation through Control."

10. Boston Women's Health Book Collective, *Our Bodies, Ourselves: A Book by and for Women* (New York: Simon & Schuster, 1979), 337.

11. Kay Weiss, "What Medical Students Learn about Women," in *Seizing Our Bodies: The Politics of Women's Health*, ed. Claudia Dreifus (New York: Vintage, 1978), 212, 214.

12. On the role of educated, middle-class women in recent health advocacy, see also Patricia A. Kaufert, "Women, Resistance and the Breast Cancer Movement," in *Pragmatic Women and Body Politics*, ed. Margaret Lock and Patricia A. Kaufert (Cambridge: Cambridge University Press, 1998), 303.

13. Cynthia Pearson, interviewed by author; Healy, *New Prescription for Women's Health*,

6; Sherry Sherman, interviewed by author. A list of those interviewed for this book, along with their job titles at the time of interview and the date and location of each interview, appears at the back of the book before the notes.

14. Morgen, *Into Our Own Hands*, 153.

15. In this chapter and the next, I benefit from a number of analyses that trace the politics of women's health research during the 1980s and 1990s; these are cited in the introduction, n. 20. By contrast, next to nothing has been written about the efforts of other groups to gain inclusion within research populations.

16. Wilbur H. Watson, *Blacks in the Profession of Medicine in the United States: Against the Odds* (New Brunswick, NJ: Transaction, 1999), 154. On the history of the NMA, see also Alondra Nelson, "Black Power, Biomedicine, and the Politics of Knowledge" (Ph.D. dissertation, New York University, 2003).

17. See the references in chap. 1, n. 46.

18. David A Snow and Robert D. Benford, "Ideology, Frame Resonance, and Participant Mobilization," *International Social Movement Research* 1 (1988): 198. See also David A. Snow et al., "Frame Alignment Processes: Micromobilization and Movement Participation," *American Sociological Review* 51 (1986): 464–81; William A Gamson, "Constructing Social Protest," in *Social Movements and Culture*, ed. Hank Johnston and Bert Klandermans, 85–106 (Minneapolis: University of Minnesota Press, 1995); Robert D. Benford and David A. Snow, "Framing Processes and Social Movements: An Overview and Assessment," *Annual Review of Sociology* 26 (2000): 611–39.

19. Polletta, "Culture in and Outside Institutions," 162. It has become common to criticize the social movement framing literature for its overemphasis on the strategic dimensions of collective belief. However, the approach remains useful in describing aspects of the everyday work of persuading in which political actors often engage.

20. Skrentny, *Minority Rights Revolution*, 351; Jerome Karabel, *The Chosen: The Hidden History of Admission and Exclusion at Harvard, Yale, and Princeton* (Boston: Houghton Mifflin, 2005).

21. Both Valerie Jenness and John Skrentny have emphasized the importance of analogies to the process of "domain expansion" by which old solutions are applied to new problems or extended to new groups. Valerie Jenness, "Managing Differences and Making Legislation: Social Movements and the Racialization, Sexualization, and Gendering of Federal Hate Crime Law in the U.S., 1985–1998," *Social Problems* 46, no. 4 (1999): 548–71; Skrentny, *Minority Rights Revolution*. See also Kingdon, *Agendas, Alternatives, and Public Policies*, 202–3; David A. J. Richards, *Identity and the Case for Gay Rights: Race, Gender, Religion as Analogies* (Chicago: University of Chicago Press, 1999).

22. Karabel, *Chosen*.

23. Evlin L. Kinney et al., "Underrepresentation of Women in New Drug Trials: Ramifications and Remedies," *Annals of Internal Medicine* 95 (1981): 496. Many of the studies considered by Kinney and coauthors simply did not report data on the gender of subjects, so it cannot be concluded that there were no women in the remaining thirty-four studies.

24. Barbara A. Levey, "Bridging the Gender Gap in Research," *Clinical Pharmacology and Therapeutics* 50, no. 6 (1991): 643; Douglas L. Schmucker and Elliot S. Vesell, "Underrepresentation of Women in Clinical Drug Trials," *Clinical Pharmacology and Therapeutics* 54 (1993): 11–15.

25. Claude Lenfant, "Heart Disease Research in Women: A Look Back and a View to

the Future" (keynote address, "Beyond Hunt Valley" conference, Bethesda, MD, November 1998); Claude Lenfant, interviewed by author.

26. Normal Lasser, interviewed by author.

27. Lenfant, "Heart Disease Research in Women."

28. Lori Mosca et al., "Cardiovascular Disease in Women: A Statement for Healthcare Professionals from the American Heart Association," *Circulation* 96 (October 7, 1997): 2468–82.

29. Craig K. Svensson, "Representation of American Blacks in Clinical Trials of New Drugs," *Journal of the American Medical Association* 261, no. 2 (January 13, 1989): 263–64; Camara Phyllis Jones, Thomas A. LaVeist, and Marsha Lillie-Blanton, "'Race' in the Epidemiologic Literature: An Examination of the *American Journal of Epidemiology*, 1921–1990," *American Journal of Epidemiology* 134, no. 10 (1991): 1082.

30. The phrase "therapeutic orphan" was coined by Dr. Harry Shirkey; see Lawrence Bachorik, "Why FDA Is Encouraging Drug Testing in Children," *FDA Consumer* 25, no. 6 (July–August 1991): 14–17. On the effects of the FDA's 1979 policy, see Ross E. McKinney Jr., "Congress, the FDA, and the Fair Development of New Medications for Children," *Pediatrics* 112, no. 3 (September 2003): 669. Yaffe reported his findings in Sumner J. Yaffe, "Problems of Drug Testing in Children in the United States," *Pediatric Pharmacology* 3 (1983): 339.

31. Robert Steinbrook, "AIDS Trials Shortchange Minorities and Drug Users," *Los Angeles Times*, September 25, 1989, 1; J. E. D'Eramo, "Women and Minorities Have Less Access to AIDS Drug Trials" (paper presented at the seventh International Conference on AIDS, Florence, June 16–21, 1991). See also Epstein, *Impure Science*, 258–62.

32. Nechas and Foley, *Unequal Treatment*, 14.

33. On the role of VA hospital studies in contributing to underrepresentation, see Douglas L. Schmucker, M. Sinead O'Mahony, and Elliot Vesell, "Women in Clinical Drug Trials: An Update," *Clinical Pharmacokinetics* 27, no. 6 (1994): 415. (Many of those I interviewed identified this factor as significant, including George Lundberg, former editor of *JAMA*.) On single-city studies, see my discussion of the Framingham Study in the preceding chapter.

34. See my discussion in chapter 9 of African Americans' suspicions of medical research.

35. Steinbrook, "AIDS Trials," 1. Of course it is debatable whether this factor is purely "circumstantial": it would make sense to ask *why* the federal AIDS research program had not become established in those cities.

36. Harold Edgar and David J. Rothman, "New Rules for New Drugs: The Challenge of AIDS to the Regulatory Process," *Milbank Quarterly* 68, suppl. 1 (1990): 121. See also Andrew Feenberg, "On Being a Human Subject: Interest and Obligation in the Experimental Treatment of Incurable Disease," *Philosophical Forum* 23, no. 3 (spring 1992); Epstein, *Impure Science*, 208–64.

37. Jim Eigo et al., "FDA Action Handbook" (New York: ACT UP/New York, September 21, 1988), 29 (emphasis in the original). See also Epstein, *Impure Science*, 208–64.

38. The delay was due, in part, to slowness on the part of the manufacturer, Burroughs Wellcome, in filing with the FDA; see Gina Kolata, "Hundreds of Children with AIDS Are Unable to Obtain AZT," *New York Times*, September 23, 1989, A8.

39. Vanessa Merton, "The Exclusion of Pregnant, Pregnable, and Once-Pregnable People (a.k.a. Women) from Biomedical Research," *American Journal of Law and Medicine* 19, no. 4 (1993): 369–451.

40. Janice K. Bush, "The Industry Perspective on the Inclusion of Women in Clinical Trials," *Academic Medicine* 69, no. 9 (1994): 708–15; Theresa McGovern, interviewed by author.

41. Jeanne Mager Stellman, *Women's Work, Women's Health: Myths and Realities* (New York: Pantheon, 1977), 170–73; Elaine Draper, "Fetal Exclusion Policies and Gendered Constructions of Suitable Work," *Social Problems* 40, no. 1 (February 1993): 90–107; Cynthia R. Daniels, "Between Fathers and Fetuses: The Social Construction of Male Reproduction and the Politics of Fetal Harm," *Signs* 22, no. 3 (spring 1997): 579–616.

42. Pearson, interview.

43. Edgar and Rothman, "New Rules," 111–42; Anna C. Mastroianni and Jeffrey Kahn, "Swinging on the Pendulum: Shifting Views of Justice in Human Subjects Research," *Hastings Center Report*, May–June 2001, 21–28.

44. Gary Ellis, interviewed by author.

45. Richard Klein, interviewed by author.

46. DeBruin, "Justice and the Inclusion of Women," 132.

47. Schmucker, O'Mahony, and Vesell, "Women in Clinical Drug Trials: An Update," 415.

48. T. Johnson and Fee, "Women's Participation in Clinical Research," 6; Mastroianni, Faden, and Federman, *Women and Health Research*, 1:80.

49. By contrast, other experts on clinical trials argued that homogeneity is not necessary in a properly randomized trial and that overly restrictive inclusion/exclusion criteria risked lessening the generalizability of research results. See, for example, Salim Yusuf et al., "Selection of Patients for Randomized Controlled Trials: Implications of Wide or Narrow Eligibility Criteria," *Statistics in Medicine* 9, nos. 1–2 (1990): 77.

50. Rebecca Dresser, "Wanted: Single White Male for Medical Research," *Hastings Center Report*, January–February 1992, 28.

51. See, for example, Catherine A. MacKinnon, *Toward a Feminist Theory of the State* (Cambridge, MA: Harvard University Press, 1989).

52. Lawrence and Bendixen, "His and Hers: Male and Female Anatomy," 930. On the gender of the researcher, see Margaret F. Jensvold, Jean A. Hamilton, and Billie Mackey, "Including Women in Clinical Trials: How about the Women Scientists?" *Journal of the American Medical Women's Association* 49, no. 4 (July/August 1994): 110–12.

53. Paul Cotton, "Is There Still Too Much Extrapolation from Data on Middle-Aged White Men?" *Journal of the American Medical Association* 263, no. 8 (February 23, 1990): 1049–50.

54. This is a restatement of the so-called equality versus difference debate in feminism; see David L. Kirp, Mark G. Yudof, and Marlene Strong Franks, *Gender Justice* (Chicago: University of Chicago Press, 1986); Ruth Milkman, "Women's History and the Sears Case," *Feminist Studies* 12, no. 2 (summer 1986): 375–400; Joan Scott, *Gender and the Politics of History*, esp. 172–76; Martha Minow, *Making All the Difference: Inclusion, Exclusion and American Law* (Ithaca, NY: Cornell University Press, 1990); Lisa Vogel, *Mothers on the Job: Maternity Policy in the U.S. Workplace* (New Brunswick, NJ: Rutgers University Press, 1993); Lisa Vogel, *Woman Questions: Essays for a Materialist Feminism* (New York: Routledge, 1995); I. Young, "Polity and Group Difference, 281–82.

55. Leigh Thompson, "Dose-Utility Relationships in Diverse Populations: Ethnic, Age, Gender and Cultural Factors in Efficacy and Safety," in *The Relevance of Ethnic Factors in*

the Clinical Evaluation of Medicines, ed. Stuart Walker, Cyndy Lumley, and Neil McAuslane (Dordrecht: Kluwer Academic Publishers, 1994), 219, 222.

56. Raymond Williams, *Keywords* (New York: Oxford University Press, 1983), 298.

57. For further discussion of this issue, see Steven Epstein, "Beyond the Standard Human?" in "Formalizing Practices," ed. Lampland and Star (manuscript).

58. A "typological" standard human therefore differs from a "statistical" one, who might be defined in terms of means and standard deviations. See my discussion in ibid.

59. For summaries, see the introduction, n. 10.

60. It should be noted that this six-year gap was still in place in 2000, even though the life expectancy for both groups had lengthened by a few years in the interim. Life expectancy at birth by year, sex, and race is available from the CDC's National Center for Health Statistics at www.cdc.gov/nchs/data/dvs/nvsr51_03t12.pdf.

61. Margaret M. Heckler, "Report of the Secretary's Task Force on Black and Minority Health" (Washington, DC: U.S. Department of Health and Human Services, August 1985), x.

62. Todd Benson, "Race, Health, and Power: The Federal Government and American Indian Health, 1909–1955" (PhD dissertation, Stanford University, 1994).

63. Frans C. Goble, "Sex as a Factor in Metabolism, Toxicity, and Efficacy of Pharmacodynamic and Chemotherapeutic Agents," in *Advances in Pharmacology and Chemotherapy*, ed. Silvio Garattini et al. (New York: Academic Press, 1975), 174.

64. In chapters 10 and 11, I describe how reports of medically relevant biological differences by sex and race have further multiplied in recent years, in large measure as a consequence of the new sensibilities and policies that reformers succeeded in promoting.

65. W. Kalow, "Race and Therapeutic Drug Response," *New England Journal of Medicine* 329, no. 9 (March 2, 1989): 589; Paul Cotton, "Examples Abound of Gaps in Medical Knowledge Because of Groups Excluded from Scientific Study," *Journal of the American Medical Association* 263, no. 8 (February 23, 1990): 1051, 1055. See also Keh-Ming Lin et al., "Pharmacokinetic and Other Related Factors Affecting Psychotropic Responses in Asians," *Psychopharmacology Bulletin* 27, no. 4 (1991): 427–39; Richard A. Levy, *Ethnic and Racial Differences in Responses to Medicines: Preserving Individualized Therapy in Managed Pharmaceutical Programs* (Reston, VA: National Pharmaceutical Council, 1993).

66. Leslie Z. Benet, "Health Consequences of Exclusion or Underrepresentation of Women in Clinical Studies(II)," in *Women and Health Research*, ed. Mastroianni, Faden, and Federman, 2:41–44.

67. Schmucker, O'Mahony, and Vesell, "Women in Clinical Drug Trials: An Update," 413. For recent critiques of how pharmaceutical testing and approval practices may contribute to adverse drug reactions, see Jay S. Cohen, *Overdose: The Case against the Drug Companies* (New York: Penguin Putnam, 2001); Oonagh P. Corrigan, "A Risky Business: The Detection of Adverse Drug Reactions in Clinical Trials and Post-Marketing Exercises," *Social Science and Medicine* 55 (2002): 497–507.

68. Jan Howard and Gary Tiedeman, "The Relative Effectiveness of Antihypertensive Drugs in Caucasians and Negroes," *Clinical Pharmacology and Therapeutics* 8, no. 4 (July–August 1966): 502–20; Elijah Saunders, "Tailoring Treatment to Minority Patients," *American Journal of Medicine* 88, suppl. 3B (12 March 1990): 21S–23S; Levy, *Ethnic and Racial Differences*; Marvin Moser, "Black-White Differences in Response to Antihypertensive Medication," *Journal of the National Medical Association* 87, suppl. (1995): 612–13. In

recent years, the question of whether there are meaningful racial differences in the effects of antihypertensive drugs has become more controversial. I return to this topic in chapter 10.

69. Cotton, "Is There Still Too Much Extrapolation," 1049.

70. Richard A. Meckel, *Save the Babies: American Public Health Reform and the Prevention of Infant Mortality, 1850–1929* (Baltimore: Johns Hopkins University Press, 1990), 46–47.

71. Sumner J. Yaffe, ed., *Pediatric Pharmacology: Therapeutic Principles in Practice* (New York: Grune & Stratton, 1980).

72. Elizabeth Fox and Frank M. Balis, "Drug Therapy in Neonates and Pediatric Patients," in *Principles of Clinical Pharmacology*, ed. Arthur J. Atkinson et al. (San Diego: Academic Press, 2001), 294–94.

73. Douglas L. Schmucker, "Drug Disposition in the Elderly: A Review of the Critical Factors," *Journal of the American Geriatric Society* 32, no. 2 (1984): 144–49.

74. These are my calculations using the National Library of Medicine's "PubMed" database at www.pubmed.org.

75. Gena Corea, *The Invisible Epidemic: The Story of Women and AIDS* (New York: Harper Collins, 1992), 49; Epstein, *Impure Science*, 258–62.

76. Steinbrook, "AIDS Trials," 1.

77. Mark D. Smith, "Zidovudine: Does It Work for Everyone?" *Journal of the American Medical Association* 266, no. 19 (20 November 1991): 2750–51.

78. Robert N. Proctor, *Cancer Wars: How Politics Shapes What We Know and Don't Know about Cancer* (New York: Basic, 1995), 8.

79. On recent trends toward the understanding of differences in biological or genetic terms, see, for example, Carol Tavris, *The Mismeasure of Woman* (New York: Simon & Schuster, 1992); Dorothy Nelkin and M. Susan Lindee, *The DNA Mystique: The Gene as a Cultural Icon* (New York: Freeman, 1995); Krieger and Fee, "Man-Made Medicine and Women's Health"; Jennifer Terry, *An American Obsession: Science, Medicine, and Homosexuality in Modern Society* (Chicago: University of Chicago Press, 1999); Troy Duster, "Race and Reification in Science," *Science* 307, no. 5712 (February 18, 2005): 1050–51; Waites, "Fixity of Sexual Identities in the Public Sphere."

80. By the mid 1990s, however, a contrast could be distinguished between the case of sex or gender differences, where there continued to be little controversy about the wisdom of calling attention to differences, and the case of racial differences, which provoked sometimes heated debate about the dangers of "racial profiling." I discuss this contrast in chapter 11.

81. Levy, *Ethnic and Racial Differences*, iii–v.

CHAPTER FOUR

1. Kelly Moore has described the relative feasibility, for social movements, of challenging the state as opposed to other social institutions; see Moore, "Political Protest and Institutional Change."

2. Myrna E. Watanabe, "From Internal Guidelines to the Law," *Scientist*, March 6, 1995.

3. Delores Parron, interviewed by author.

4. Watanabe, "From Internal Guidelines to the Law."

5. Public Health Service Task Force on Women's Health Issues, "Women's Health:

Report of the Public Health Service Task Force on Women's Health Issues: Volume 1," *Public Health Reports* 100, no. 1 (January–February 1985): 76, 78.

6. Auerbach and Figert, "Women's Health Research," 117.

7. Parron, interview; Watanabe, "From Internal Guidelines to the Law."

8. Gary Ellis, interviewed by author.

9. Florence B. Haseltine and Beverly Greenberg Jacobson, eds., *Women's Health Research: A Medical and Policy Primer* (Washington, DC: Health Press International, 1997), xiv.

10. Florence Haseltine, interviewed by author.

11. Marie Bass, interviewed by author; Society for the Advancement of Women's Health Research, "Women's Health Research: Prescription for Change" (Washington, DC: Society for the Advancement of Women's Health Research, January 1991); Weisman, *Women's Health Care*, 81. The society was later renamed the Society for Women's Health Research.

12. Weisman, *Women's Health Care*; Weisman, "Breast Cancer Policymaking," 213–43.

13. Patricia Schroeder, interviewed by author.

14. Haseltine, interview.

15. Ruth Katz, interviewed by author.

16. Primmer, "Women's Health Research," 303.

17. Mark V. Nadel, General Accounting Office (GAO), "Statement of Mark V. Nadel before the Subcommittee on Health and the Environment, Committee on Energy and Commerce" (Washington, DC: House of Representatives, GAO, June 18, 1990), 1, 5.

18. Gina Kolata, "N.I.H. Neglects Women, Study Says," *New York Times*, June 19, 1990, C6.

19. Weisman, *Women's Health Care*, 83.

20. Katz, interview; William Raub, interviewed by author.

21. Joseph Palca, "Women Left out at NIH," *Science* 248 (June 29, 1990): 1601.

22. Nadel, "Statement of Mark V. Nadel," 2. I discuss the logic of selecting male subjects for this study in chapter 5. A complementary study by many of the same investigators, called the Women's Health Study, eventually did find differences between men and women in terms of the preventive benefits of aspirin, and I discuss these findings in chapter 11.

23. Scott Jaschik, "Report Says NIH Ignores Own Rules on Including Women in Its Research," *Chronicle of Higher Education*, June 27, 1990, A27.

24. Malcolm Gladwell, "Women's Health Research to Be New Priority at NIH," *Washington Post*, September 11, 1990, A17.

25. Schroeder, interview.

26. Primmer, "Women's Health Research," 305. Using alternative terminology drawn from political science, Weisman noted that the need for reauthorization opened up a "policy window" for consideration of women's health issues at the agency. Weisman, "Breast Cancer Policymaking," 215.

27. Louis Stokes, interviewed by author; Susan E. Cozzens and Shana Solomon, "Women and Minorities in Biomedical Politics: Case Studies in Democracy?" (paper presented at the Annual Meeting of the American Sociological Association, Los Angeles, August 1994). On Congressional attention to minority health, see Drew Halfmann, Jesse Rude, and Kim Ebert, "The Biomedical Legacy in Minority Health Policy-Making, 1975–2002," *Research in the Sociology of Health Care* 23 (2005): 245–75.

28. Schroeder, interview.

29. Katz, interview.

30. On the history of the NIH Revitalization Act and the Women's Health Equity Act, see Auerbach and Figert, "Women's Health Research"; Narrigan et al., "Research to Improve Women's Health"; Primmer, "Women's Health Research," 301–30; Weisman, *Women's Health Care*, 77–89; Weisman, "Breast Cancer Policymaking," 220–22.

31. Weisman, "Breast Cancer Policymaking," 214–17.

32. Ibid., 213.

33. Primmer, "Women's Health Research," 302–4.

34. "NIH Director Selected after Yearlong Search," *CQ Almanac* (1990): 602. Biographies of all past directors of the NIH appear at www.nih.gov/about/almanac/historical/directors.htm.

35. Primmer, "Women's Health Research," 301.

36. Bernadine Healy, "The Yentl Syndrome," *New England Journal of Medicine* 325, no. 4 (1991): 275.

37. Malcolm Gladwell, "New Face for Science," *Washington Post Magazine*, June 21, 1992, 24.

38. Stephen Burd, "NIH Chief Angers Advocates of Bill for Research on Women's Health," *Chronicle of Higher Education*, June 10, 1992, A21; Traci Watson, "Affirmative Action for Clinical Trials," *Science* 260, no. 5109 (May 7, 1993): 746.

39. Susan Wood, interviewed by author. Wood later became director of the FDA's Office of Women's Health and the FDA's assistant commissioner for women's health. She resigned in 2005 to protest the FDA Commissioner's decision to delay approval of over-the-counter sales of the "Plan B" morning-after pill. Gardiner Harris, "Official Quits on Pill Delay at the F.D.A.," *New York Times*, September 1, 2005, A12.

40. "National Institutes of Health Revitalization Act of 1993," Public Law 103–43 (S. 1), 103rd Congress, June 10, 1993.

41. Ibid.

42. Baird, "New NIH and FDA Medical Research Policies," 562.

43. Ruth Merkatz, interviewed by author; Robert Temple, interviewed by author; Theresa Toigo and Richard Klein, interviewed by author.

44. Mark V. Nadel, GAO, "Women's Health: FDA Needs to Ensure More Study of Gender Differences in Prescription Drug Testing" (Washington, DC: GAO, October 1992), 1–3.

45. Wood, interview.

46. Ruth B. Merkatz et al., "Women in Clinical Trials of New Drugs: A Change in Food and Drug Administration Policy," *New England Journal of Medicine* 329, no. 4 (July 22, 1993): 294; U.S. Department of Health & Human Services, Food and Drug Administration (hereafter FDA), "Guidelines for the Study and Evaluation of Gender Differences in the Clinical Evaluation of Drugs," *Federal Register* 58, no. 139 (July 22, 1993): 39407; Merkatz, interview; Temple, interview.

47. "FDA Debunks Myth of Too-Few-Women-in-Clinical-Trials," *PMA Newsletter*, October 19, 1992, 2–3.

48. Bonnie J. Goldmann, "A Drug Company Report: What Is the Same and What Is Changing with Respect to Inclusion/Exclusion of Women in Clinical Trials," *Food and Drug Law Journal* 48 (1993): 174.

49. Rick DelVecchio, "500 Protesters Block Market Street Traffic," *San Francisco Chronicle*, June 23, 1990, A11.

50. International AIDS Conference, San Francisco, CA, June 23, 1990 (author's field notes).

51. Mary-Rose Mueller, "'Women and Minorities' in Federal Research for AIDS," *Race, Gender and Class* 5, no. 2 (1998): 79–98. Mueller shows that, cumulatively, by the end of 1995, 28 percent of the participants in AIDS Clinical Trial Group studies were female and 52 percent were members of racial and ethnic minority groups.

52. Theresa McGovern, interviewed by author.

53. Lisa Auer, "Developing a Clinical Research Agenda for Women," *PI Perspectives* 9 (October 9, 1990).

54. Theresa M. McGovern, Martha S. Davis, and Alma M. Gomez, "Citizen Petition" (New York: HIV Law Project of the AIDS Service Center, December 15, 1992), 15.

55. Ibid., 25. For an analysis of sex-based protections and the "consequences of paternalism," see Kirp, Yudof, and Franks, *Gender Justice*, 29–45.

56. Merkatz, interview; Temple, interview; Toigo and Klein, interview.

57. FDA, "Guidelines for the Study and Evaluation of Gender Differences," 34906–16.

58. Ibid., 39406, 39408–9.

59. Merkatz et al., "Women in Clinical Trials of New Drugs," 292–96.

60. Eckman, "Beyond 'the Yentl Syndrome,'" 133.

61. "Unequal Treatment," news segment, ABC, April 13, 1994; news segment, ABC, May 22, 1994.

62. Chris Bull, "Seizing Control of the FDA," *Gay Community News*, October 16–22, 1988, 3.

63. Florence Haseltine, interviewed by author.

64. Moore, "Political Protest and Institutional Change," 104; see also Polletta, "Culture in and Outside Institutions," 162–63. Moore and Polletta provide a number of examples of studies showing the significance of insiders or mediators, including my own work on AIDS activism and the role of gay physicians; Mary Katzenstein's analysis of priests in the Catholic Church; Verta Taylor's discussion of women doctors and nurses who became involved in struggles around postpartum depression; and Amy Binder's analysis of educators who pressed for Afrocentric curricula. See Epstein, *Impure Science*; Mary Fainsod Katzenstein, "The Spectacle of Life and Death: Feminist and Lesbian/Gay Politics in the Military," in *Gay Rights, Military Wrongs: Political Perspectives on Lesbians and Gays in the Military*, ed. Craig A. Rimmerman (New York: Garland Publishing, 1996), 229–47; Verta Taylor, *Rock-a-by Baby: Feminism, Self-Help, and Postpartum Depression* (New York: Routledge, 1996); Amy Binder, *Contentious Curricula: Afrocentrism and Creationism in American Public Schools* (Princeton, NJ: Princeton University Press, 2002).

65. Goldstone, "Bridging Institutionalized and Noninstitutionalized Politics," 2; Skrentny, *Minority Rights Revolution*, 7. See also Jenness, "Managing Differences and Making Legislation"; Meyer, Jenness, and Ingram, *Routing the Opposition*.

66. Wolfson, *Fight against Big Tobacco*, 7, 144–45. For another example of an "interpenetrated" movement, see my analysis of AIDS treatment activism in Epstein, *Impure Science*.

67. On a theoretical level, the politics of representation or delegation in this sense has been discussed most thoroughly by Pierre Bourdieu, who noted that "the speech of the *spokesperson* owes part of its 'illocutionary force' to the force (the number) of the group that he helps to produce as such by the act of symbolization or representation." Pierre

Bourdieu, *Language and Symbolic Power* (Cambridge, MA: Harvard University Press, 1991), 191 (emphasis in the original). However, as Bourdieu points out, the notion that the representative in some sense brings the represented into being through acts of representation is one that goes back to Thomas Hobbes. Bourdieu, *Language and Symbolic Power*, 208. I am grateful to Jeff Weintraub for discussion of this issue. For an analysis of invocations by social movements of abstract notions of the group represented (such as "women"), see Leila Rupp and Verta Taylor, "Forging Feminist Identity in an International Movement: A Collective Identity Approach to Twentieth-Century Feminism," *Signs* 24, no. 2 (1999): 363–86.

68. Reardon, *Race to the Finish*.

69. By the late 1980s, as the social critic Naomi Klein has observed, identity politics in the United States had increasingly become preoccupied with just this issue of symbolic representation. For example, by calling attention to how oppressed groups were depicted (in movies, on television, in the literary canon, and so on), activists hoped to transform the political imaginations of both dominant and subordinate groups. Naomi Klein, *No Logo* (New York: Picador, 2002), 107–8.

70. For two different approaches to understanding the relation between, on one hand, representation in terms of how the natural and the social are depicted and, on the other, representation in the sense of "speaking on behalf of," see Shapin and Schaffer, *Leviathan and the Air-Pump*; and Latour, *We Have Never Been Modern*, 27–29. For a critical review of uses of the concept of "representation" in science studies, see Michael Lynch, "Representation Is Overrated: Some Critical Remarks about the Use of the Concept of Representation in Science Studies," *Configurations* 2, no. 1 (winter 1994): 137–49. On the various meanings collapsed into the English word *representation*, see also Gayatri Chakravorty Spivak, "Can the Subaltern Speak?" in *Marxism and the Interpretation of Culture*, ed. Cary Nelson and Lawrence Grossberg (Urbana: University of Illinois Press, 1988), 275–80.

71. My case study thereby joins a growing body of scholarship that demonstrates how science and technology in general, and biomedicine in particular, have become increasingly central to the modern constitution of citizenship and public identity. See the references in chap. 1, n. 13.

72. On classification in science and society, see the references in chap. 1, n. 32.

73. See chap. 1, n. 35.

74. Brubaker and Cooper, "Beyond 'Identity,'" 16.

75. Bowker and Star, *Sorting Things Out*, 197–210.

76. Bourdieu, "Social Space and the Genesis of Groups," 731–732 (emphasis in the original). Bourdieu argued, moreover, that it is the state that will tend to be victorious in such struggles; see Bourdieu, *Practical Reason*, 35–63.

77. Indeed, the fact that, at any given moment, important social classifications, such as racial terms, have a hybrid or syncretic character (a complex mixing of expert and lay meanings) itself reflects a past history of both categorical competition and categorical alignment.

78. Susan Leigh Star and James R. Griesemer, "Institutional Ecology, 'Translations' and Boundary Objects: Amateurs and Professionals in Berkeley's Museum of Vertebrate Zoology, 1907–39," *Social Studies of Science* 19 (1989): 393.

79. My emphasis on alignment also builds on Joan Fujimura's analysis of the alignment of work as an important component of scientific activity. Joan Fujimura, "Constructing

'Do-Able' Problems in Cancer Research: Articulating Alignments," *Social Studies of Science* 17 (1987): 257–93.

80. On identity politics as a "politics of recognition," see Nancy Fraser, "From Re-distribution to Recognition? Dilemmas of Justice in a 'Post-Socialist' Age," in *Feminism and Politics*, ed. Anne Phillips, 430–60 (Oxford: Oxford University Press, 1998). On the strategic "deployment" of identity, see Mary Bernstein, "Celebration and Suppression: The Strategic Uses of Identity by the Lesbian and Gay Movement," *American Journal of Sociology* 103, no. 3 (1997): 531–65.

81. I return to the questions of alternative political framings in chapter 7 and alternative scientific framings in chapters 10 and 11.

82. Lock, "Decentering the Natural Body," 284.

CHAPTER FIVE

1. Otis W. Brawley, "Response to 'Inclusion of Women and Minorities in Clinical Trials and the NIH Revitalization Act of 1993—the Perspective of NIH Clinical Trialists,'" *Controlled Clinical Trials* 16, no. 5 (October 1995): 295. At a conference in 2003, Brawley indicated that his criticism of the inclusionary policies has lessened somewhat as he learned about their implementation. However, he remained worried that African American patients may get the "hard sell." "Questions and Answers from 'Point and Counterpoint,'" in *Science Meets Reality*, 35.

2. Brawley, "Response to 'Inclusion of Women and Minorities,'" 293.

3. Andrew G. Kadar, "The Sex-Bias Myth in Medicine," *Atlantic Monthly*, August 1994, 66–70.

4. Baird, "New NIH and FDA Medical Research Policies"; O. Corrigan, "First in Man."

5. Mary McGrae McDermott et al., "Changes in Study Design, Gender Issues, and Other Characteristics of Clinical Research Published in Three Major Medical Journals from 1971 to 1991," *Journal of General Internal Medicine* 10, no. 1 (January 1995): 13–18.

6. Elaine Larson, "Exclusion of Certain Groups from Clinical Research," *Image: Journal of Nursing Scholarship* 26, no. 3 (fall 1994): 185–90.

7. Heriberto A. Tejeda et al., "Representation of African-Americans, Hispanics, and Whites in National Cancer Institute Cancer Treatment Trials," *Journal of the National Cancer Institute* 88, no. 12 (June 19, 1996): 812–16. This overall close correspondence in the racial breakdowns was somewhat less evident when investigators disaggregated the different kinds of cancer.

8. Otis Brawley, quoted in Myrna E. Watanabe, "Amid Criticism, NCI Tries to Boost Minority Clinical Trial Recruitment," *Scientist*, April 1, 1996, 4–5.

9. Otis Brawley, quoted in "Deadly Diseases and People of Color: Are Clinical Trials an Option?" (online summary of proceedings for the Deadly Diseases and People of Color: Are Clinical Trials an Option? symposium, Washington, DC, October 25, 1996, presented by the FDA), www.fda.gov/oashi/patrep/howard.html.

10. Curtis Meinert, interviewed by author; Curtis L. Meinert and Adele Kaplan Gilpin, "Estimation of Gender Bias in Clinical Trials," *Statistics in Medicine* 20 (2001): 1153–64.

11. Mastroianni, Faden, and Federman, *Women and Health Research*, 1:vi.

12. Ruth Faden, interviewed by author; Daniel Federman, interviewed by author.

13. Mastroianni, Faden, and Federman, *Women and Health Research*, 1:50–63.

14. Ibid., 1:49.

15. Chloe E. Bird, "Women's Representation as Subjects in Clinical Studies: A Pilot Study of Research Published in JAMA in 1990 and 1992," in *Women and Health Research*, ed. Mastroianni, Faden, and Federman, 2:151–73. Subsequent unpublished research by Bird and collaborators, examining a larger sample, has supported the trends described here.

16. Curtis L. Meinert et al., "Gender Representation in Trials," *Controlled Clinical Trials* 21 (2000): 462–75; Meinert and Gilpin, "Estimation of Gender Bias," 1153–64.

17. Lila Guterman, "Clinical Trials on Women Outpace Those on Men, Study Finds," *Chronicle of Higher Education*, May 1, 2001.

18. Meinert et al., "Gender Representation," 468, 473.

19. Steering Committee of the Physicians' Health Study Research Group, "Final Report on the Aspirin Component of the Ongoing Physicians' Health Study," *New England Journal of Medicine* 321, no. 3 (July 20, 1989): 129–35.

20. Julie Buring, interviewed by author.

21. Buring, interview.

22. Julie E. Buring and Charles H. Hennekens, "Aspirin and Migraine: What about Women (Reply)," *Journal of the American Medical Association* 265, no. 4 (January 23/30, 1991): 461. For a more extensive discussion, see also Julie E. Buring, "Women in Clinical Trials—a Portfolio for Success," *New England Journal of Medicine* 343, no. 7 (August 17, 2000): 505–6.

23. The study of aspirin in women, called the Women's Health Study, was completed in 2005 and in fact reported important differences between the sexes. Paul M. Ridker et al., "A Randomized Trial of Low-Dose Aspirin in the Primary Prevention of Cardiovascular Disease in Women," *New England Journal of Medicine* 352, no. 13 (March 31, 2005): 1293–1304. I discuss the Women's Health Study's findings in chapter 11.

24. Mastroianni, Faden, and Federman, *Women and Health Research*, 1:99–100.

25. Satel, *P.C., M.D.*, 118–22.

26. Mastroianni, Faden, and Federman, *Women and Health Research*, 1:5.

27. Curtis Meinert, "The Inclusion of Women in Clinical Trials," *Science* 269, no. 5225 (August 11, 1995): 796.

28. Sally L. Satel, "Science by Quota: P.C. Medicine," *New Republic*, February 27, 1995, 14–15.

29. "NIH Reauthorization Stalled in Senate," *CQ Almanac* (1991): 347; House of Representatives, "National Institutes of Health Revitalization Amendments of 1992—Veto Message from the President of the United States (H. Doc. No. 102–349)," *Congressional Record*, June 24, 1992, H5084–89.

30. House Committee on Energy and Commerce, "National Institutes of Health Revitalization Amendments of 1990" (101–869), October 15, 1990, 144–45.

31. "NIH Reauthorization Stalled," 347.

32. House of Representatives, "National Institutes of Health Revitalization Amendments of 1992—Veto Message from the President of the United States (H. Doc. No. 102–349)," H5084–89.

33. Steven Piantadosi, interviewed by author; Meinert, interview.

34. Benjamin Wittes and Janet Wittes, "Group Therapy," *New Republic*, April 5, 1993, 16 (emphasis in the original). For an expression of the same argument in more formal

statistical terms, see Steven Piantadosi and Janet Wittes, letter to the editor, "Politically Correct Clinical Trials," *Controlled Clinical Trials* 14, no. 6 (1993): 564.

35. Wittes and Wittes, "Group Therapy," 16.

36. Patricia Schroeder, interviewed by author; Schmucker, O'Mahony, and Vesell, "Women in Clinical Drug Trials: An Update," 412; Marcia Angell, editorial, "Caring for Women's Health: What Is the Problem?" *New England Journal of Medicine* 329, no. 4 (July 22, 1993): 272.

37. News segment, ABC, May 25, 1994; Bush, "Industry Perspective on the Inclusion of Women," 712–13.

38. Piantadosi and Wittes, "Politically Correct Clinical Trials," 562, 565.

39. "Petition Regarding the 103rd Congressional Mandate Regarding Clinical Trials Society for Clinical Trials May 24–27, 1993," *Controlled Clinical Trials* 14, no. 6 (December 1993): 558.

40. Meinert, interview; Wittes, interview; Piantadosi, interview.

41. See the references in chap. 1, nn. 42–44.

42. See the discussion in chapter 2.

43. Epstein, *Impure Science*; Epstein, "Activism, Drug Regulation."

44. For example, volunteers may be more health conscious than others, as well as more likely to comply with the experimental protocol. See Kent R. Bailey, "Generalizing the Results of Randomized Clinical Trials," *Controlled Clinical Trials* 15 (1994): 20.

45. Wittes, interview; Meinert, interview. See also Meinert, "Inclusion of Women," 795.

46. Meinert, "Inclusion of Women," 795.

47. Meinert, interview.

48. Meinert, "Inclusion of Women," 796.

49. Ibid.

50. Buring, interview.

51. ISIS-2 Collaborative Group, "Randomised Trial of Intravenous Streptokinase, Oral Aspirin, Both, or Neither among 17,187 Cases of Suspected Acute Myocardial Infarction: ISIS-2," *Lancet* 332, no. 8607 (August 13, 1988): 356; Salim Yusuf et al., "Analysis and Interpretation of Treatment Effects in Subgroups of Patients in Randomized Clinical Trials," *Journal of the American Medical Association* 266, no. 1 (July 3, 1991): 94. On this point, see also Silverman, *Human Experimentation*, 134. In chapter 10 I return to this issue of "data mining" in subgroup analyses and argue that it is indeed a legitimate concern.

52. Mastroianni, Faden, and Federman, *Women and Health Research*, 1:6–7, 104.

53. Meinert, interview; Wittes, interview.

54. Sylvia Smoller, interviewed by author.

55. On the relation between formal knowledge and "work-arounds," see Susan Leigh Star, "The Politics of Formal Representations: Wizards, Gurus, and Organizational Complexity," in *Ecologies of Knowledge: Work and Politics in Science and Technology*, ed. Susan Leigh Star (Albany: State University of New York Press, 1995), 100–104, 111.

56. Gieryn, "Boundaries of Science," 405. On boundary work, see also the references in the introduction, n. 43.

57. *National Institutes of Health Revitalization Act of 1993*, Public Law 103–43 (S. 1), 103rd Congress, June 10, 1993.

58. Susan Halebsky Dimock, "Demanding Disease Dollars: How Activism and Institutions Shaped Medical Research Funding for Breast and Prostate Cancer" (Ph.D. disser-

tation, University of California, San Diego, 2003), 206–10, quotation from 210. See also Strickland, *Politics, Science, and Dread Disease.*

59. Susan Wood, interviewed by author.

60. Wendy Baldwin and Belinda Seto, interviewed by author.

61. Laurence S. Freedman et al., "Response to Discussants' Letters," *Controlled Clinical Trials* 16, no. 5 (October 1995): 312.

62. NIH, "NIH Guidelines on the Inclusion of Women and Minorities as Subjects in Clinical Research: Notice," *Federal Register* 59, no. 59 (1994): 14511.

63. On the implicit distinction in the guidelines between issues of "effectiveness" and "efficacy" (and hence between external and internal validity), see Ann A. Hohmann and Delores L. Parron, "How the New NIH Guidelines on Inclusion of Women and Minorities Apply: Efficacy Trials, Effectiveness Trials, and Validity," *Journal of Consulting and Clinical Psychology* 64, no. 5 (1996): 853.

64. For a clear account of what the new NIH policy did and did not require, see also ibid., 851–55.

65. NIH, "NIH Guidelines on the Inclusion of Women and Minorities," 14509–11; Laurence S. Freedman et al., "Inclusion of Women and Minorities in Clinical Trials and the NIH Revitalization Act of 1993: The Perspective of NIH Clinical Trialists," *Controlled Clinical Trials* 16 (1995): 277–85.

66. NIH, "NIH Guidelines on the Inclusion of Women and Minorities," 14509.

67. Baldwin and Seto, interview; Eugene Hayunga, interviewed by author.

68. Steven Piantadosi, "Commentary Regarding 'Inclusion of Women and Minorities in Clinical Trials and the NIH Revitalization Act of 1993—the Perspective of NIH Clinical Trialists,'" *Controlled Clinical Trials* 16, no. 5 (October 1995): 307; Curtis L. Meinert, "Comments on NIH Clinical Trials Valid Analysis Requirement," *Controlled Clinical Trials* 16, no. 5 (October 1995): 304.

69. The self-protective boundary work of DHHS officials suggests that federal health agencies are similar to other public agencies in wanting to defend their turf: especially as they develop their own cultures of professionalism, they will resist political influence by outsiders. See Terry M. Moe, "Interests, Institutions, and Positive Theory: The Politics of the NLRB," in *Studies in American Political Development: An Annual*, vol. 2, ed. Karen Orren and Stephen Skowronek, 236–99 (New Haven, CT: Yale University Press, 1987).

CHAPTER SIX

1. See my discussion of the concept of biopolitical paradigms in chapter 1. While my definition focuses on biomedical and state institutions, in this case the paradigm also extends into the realm of market institutions such as pharmaceutical companies.

2. Latour, *Science in Action.*

3. See the chronology preceding the notes for a detailed list of policies and offices.

4. DiMaggio and Powell, "Iron Cage Revisited," 147. On the diffusion of practices, see also David Strang and Sarah A. Soule, "Diffusion in Organizations and Social Movements: From Hybrid Corn to Poison Pills," *Annual Review of Sociology* 24 (1998): 265–81; Isin Guler, Mauro Guillen, and John Muir Macpherson, "Global Competition, Institutions, and the Diffusion of Organizational Practices: The International Spread of ISO 9000 Quality Certificates," *Administrative Science Quarterly* 47, no. 2 (2002): 207–35.

5. Margaret Weir, *Politics and Jobs*, 19.

6. Dobbin, *Forging Industrial Policy*, 227.

7. Weir, Orloff, and Skocpol, "Understanding American Social Politics," 25. On policy legacies, see also the references in chap. 1, n. 56.

8. On the ethics of research in children, see Robert N. Nelson, "Children as Research Subjects," in *Beyond Consent*, ed. Kahn, Mastroianni, and Sugarman, 47–66.

9. Nicola Kay Beisel, *Imperiled Innocents: Anthony Comstock and Family Reproduction in Victorian America* (Princeton, NJ: Princeton University Press, 1997). See also Viviana A. Zelizer, *Pricing the Priceless Child: The Changing Social Value of Children* (New York: Basic, 1985); Judith Levine, *Harmful to Minors: The Perils of Protecting Children from Sex* (Minneapolis: University of Minnesota Press, 2002).

10. Sydney A. Halpern, *American Pediatrics: The Social Dynamics of Professionalism, 1880–1980* (Berkeley: University of California Press, 1988), 9–10.

11. Howard S. Becker, *Outsiders: Studies in the Sociology of Deviance* (New York: Free Press, 1963), 147–63.

12. Sumner Yaffe, interviewed by author; Duane Alexander, interviewed by author.

13. NIH, "NIH Policy and Guidelines on the Inclusion of Children as Participants in Research Involving Human Subjects," *NIH Guide for Grants and Contracts*, March 6, 1998.

14. Dimock, "Demanding Disease Dollars," 24.

15. Bachorik, "Why FDA Is Encouraging Drug Testing in Children," 14–17.

16. FDA, "Regulations Requiring Manufacturers to Assess the Safety and Effectiveness of New Drugs and Biological Products in Pediatric Patients: Final Rule," *Federal Register* 63, no. 231 (December 2, 1998): 66632.

17. Alexander, interview.

18. Alexander, interview.

19. NIH, "NIH Policy and Guidelines on the Inclusion of Children."

20. *Food and Drug Administration Modernization Act of 1997*, Public Law 105-115 (S. 830), 105th Congress, November 21, 1997.

21. The normal period of market exclusivity guaranteed by a drug patent is twenty years, but this includes the time required to test a drug and bring it to market, which may be a decade or more.

22. *Best Pharmaceuticals for Children Act*, Public Law 107-109, 107th Congress, January 4, 2002. Meanwhile, Congress also demonstrated its general commitment to children's health research by passing the Children's Health Act of 2000, which funded a wide range of children's health activities within the NIH. *Children's Health Act of 2000*, Public Law 106–310, 106th Congress, October 17, 2000.

23. FDA, "Regulations Requiring Manufacturers," 66632.

24. Ibid., 66631–72.

25. FDA, "FDA Proposes to Require Pediatric Data Prior to Drug and Biologic Product Approvals," August 13, 1997.

26. Robert Pear, "Drug Makers Face Order for New Pediatric Studies," *New York Times*, August 13, 1997, A14.

27. Marc Kaufman and Ceci Connolly, "U.S. Backs Pediatric Tests in Reversal on Drug Safety," *Washington Post*, April 20, 2002, A3; Robert Pear, "Judge Voids Rules on Pharmaceutical Tests," *New York Times*, October 19, 2002, A9.

28. Pear, "Judge Voids Rules on Pharmaceutical Tests," A9; McKinney, "Congress, the FDA, and the Fair Development," 669–70.

29. News segment, ABC, November 4, 2002, 5:45 p.m.

30. "Statement by Tommy G. Thompson, Secretary of Health and Human Services, and Mark B. McClellan, M.D., Ph.D., Commission of Food and Drugs, Regarding Passage of S. 650, the Pediatric Research Equity Act of 2003" (Washington, DC: U.S. Department of Health and Human Services, July 24, 2003).

31. I return to this issue in chapter 12.

32. Douglas L. Schmucker and Elliot S. Vesell, "Are the Elderly Underrepresented in Clinical Drug Trials?" *Journal of Clinical Pharmacology* 38 (1999): 1105.

33. Ibid.; Robert Temple, interviewed by author.

34. FDA, "Specific Requirements on Content and Format of Labeling for Human Prescription Drugs; Addition of 'Geriatric Use' Subsection in the Labeling," *Federal Register* 62, no. 166 (August 27, 1997): 45313.

35. FDA, "Investigational New Drug Applications and New Drug Applications," *Federal Register* 63, no. 28 (February 11, 1998): 6854–55.

36. Maxine Wolfe, Mary Beth Caschetta, and Linda Meredith, "What's Wrong with the Food and Drug Administration's 'Proposed Guidelines for the Study and Evaluation of Gender Differences in the Clinical Evaluation of Drugs' " (New York: ACT UP/New York, July 22, 1993).

37. Terry McGovern, interviewed by author.

38. FDA, "Investigational New Drug Applications; Amendment to Clinical Hold Regulations for Products Intended for Life-Threatening Diseases and Conditions," *Federal Register* 65, no. 106 (June 2000): 34963–71.

39. Karen Birmingham, "Women in Trials: Clinical Hold or Stranglehold?" *Nature Medicine*, November 1997, 1179.

40. Inclusion was mandated for extramural research (research funded by the CDC but conducted by outside investigators) in 1995 and intramural research (research conducted by CDC scientists) in 1996. Wanda K. Jones, Dixie E. Snider, and Rueben C. Warren, "Deciphering the Data: Race, Ethnicity, and Gender as Critical Variables," *Journal of the American Medical Women's Association* 51, no. 4 (1996): 137–38.

41. Agency for Healthcare Research and Quality, U.S. Department of Health and Human Services, *AHRQ Policy on the Inclusion of Priority Populations in Research*, Notice #NOT-HS-03-010, February 27, 2003, http://grants.nih.gov/grants/guide/notice-files/NOT-HS-03-010.html.

42. NIH, "Guidelines for Inclusion of Women, Minorities, and Persons with Disabilities in NIH-Supported Conference Grants," Notice NOT-OD-03-066, September 26, 2003.

43. "Eliminating Racial and Ethnic Disparities in Health: Response to the Presidential Initiative on Race," *Public Health Reports* 113, no. 4 (July–August 1998): 372–75; Janet Hook, "Clinton Offers Plan to Close Racial Health Gap," *Los Angeles Times*, February 22, 1998.

44. "Eliminating Racial and Ethnic Disparities," 372–75.

45. Weisman, *Women's Health Care*, 87.

46. Gwen Mayes, "Policies of Importance to Women's Health Vary Considerably among States," *Medscape Ob/Gyn and Women's Health* 8, no. 2 (November 11, 2003).

47. See John Skrentny's analysis in the context of government affirmative action programs, in Skrentny, *Minority Rights Revolution*, and Chris Bonastia's discussion of the "institutional homes" of social policies, in Chris Bonastia, "Why Did Affirmative Action in Housing Fail during the Nixon Era? Exploring the 'Institutional Homes' of Social Policies," *Social Problems* 47, no. 4 (November 2000): 523–42.

48. Susan Wood, interviewed by author; National Cancer Institute, "Final Report for the 108th Congress, 2004: Women's Health," www3.cancer.gov/legis/final04/womenshealth.html.

49. Temple, interview.

50. Jeffrey Brainard, "Debate over Improving Minority Health Pits NIH Director against Black Leaders," *Chronicle of Higher Education*, September 10, 1999.

51. President Bill Clinton, "Statement by the President," November 22, 2000 (Office of the Press Secretary, White House); *Minority Health and Health Disparities Research and Education Act of 2000*, P.L. 106-525, 108th Congress, 2nd session, November 22, 2000.

52. As part of their definition, Bowker and Star further note that standards span more than one "community of practice" or activity site; that they make things work together over distance or heterogeneous metrics; and that they are backed up by bodies such as professional organizations, manufacturers' associations, or the state. Bowker and Star, *Sorting Things Out*, 13–14. On standardization, see also the references in chap. 1, n. 50.

53. Michael Mann, *Sources of Social Power*, 2:59.

54. Brunsson and Jacobsson, *World of Standards*, 2, 31–36. Theodore Porter makes an analogous point about how practices of quantification (on which standardization often relies) often arise as a solution to organizational weakness. Porter, *Trust in Numbers*, esp. 230–31.

55. Timmermans and Berg, *Gold Standard*, 24–25. Alternatively, Brunsson and Jacobsson distinguish three types of standards: "standards about being something, about doing something, or about having something." See Brunsson and Jacobsson, *World of Standards*, 4.

56. Kingdon, *Agendas, Alternatives, and Public Policies*, 201. On the stabilizing effect of standards, see also Bowker and Star, *Sorting Things Out*.

57. James Morone, *The Democratic Wish: Popular Participation and the Limits of American Government* (New York: Basic, 1990).

58. Center for Drug Evaluation and Research, FDA, "Guideline for the Format and Content of the Clinical and Statistical Sections of New Drug Applications," July 1988, 17.

59. The congressional mandate to develop this database was described by Susan Wood, then the director of the FDA's Office of Women's Health, in a presentation at the "Science Meets Reality" workshop. Susan F. Wood, "Gender, Race, and Regulation: An FDA Perspective," in *Science Meets Reality*, 109.

60. Center for Drug Evaluation and Research, "Guideline for the Format and Content."

61. Daemmrich, *Pharmacopolitics*, 138.

62. Center for Drug Evaluation and Research, "Guideline for the Format and Content."

63. Public Health Service, "PHS 2590 Non-Competing Grant Progress Report," May 2001, http://grants1.nih.gov/grants/funding/2590/2590.htm.

64. NIH, *U.S. Public Health Service, Grant Application Instructions (PHS 398)*, 1998 www.nih.gov/grants/funding/phs398/phs398.html. The term *sex/gender* replaced *gender* in the PHS 398 form in 2000.

65. NIH, "NIH Instructions to Reviewers for Evaluating Research Involving Human Subjects in Grant and Cooperative Agreement Applications," April 25, 2001.

66. Eugene Hayunga, interviewed by author.

67. Wendy Baldwin and Belindo Seto, interviewed by author; Hayunga, interview; Eugene G. Hayunga and Vivian W. Pinn, "Implementing the 1994 NIH Guidelines," *Applied Clinical Trials*, October 1996, 35–40.

68. Hayunga, interview; Eugene G. Hayunga and Vivian W. Pinn, "NIH Response to Researchers' Concerns," *Applied Clinical Trials*, November 1996, 61.

69. Gary Ellis, interviewed by author. In 2000, NIH's OPRR was disbanded and its functions were assumed by the DHHS Office for Human Research Protections.

70. Instructions available online at http://irb.ucsd.edu/SBSApplication.pdf (emphasis in the original).

71. It is worth noting that IRBs themselves are now subject to federal regulations intended to promote diversity in their membership. In 1994, when informing IRBs of the NIH inclusion policy, Gary Ellis, the director of the OPRR, advised IRBs that gender and racial diversity in their own internal composition would be a salutary step (Ellis, interview). Since 1998, the DHHS has required that IRBs make "every nondiscriminatory effort" to ensure that both women and men sit on these boards, and the agency expects race, gender, and cultural background all to be considered in the selection of a diverse and qualified board. FDA, "Institutional Review Boards, Food and Drug Administration, Department of Health and Human Services Code of Federal Regulations" (Washington, DC: U.S. Government Printing Office, April 1, 1998), 257–58.

CHAPTER SEVEN

1. See the discussion of these historical developments in chapter 2.

2. Gerth and Mills, *From Max Weber*, 215, 226; James Scott, *Seeing Like a State*, 346.

3. On technologies of individuation, see John C. Torpey, *The Invention of the Passport: Surveillance, Citizenship, and the State* (Cambridge: Cambridge University Press, 2000); Jane Caplan and John C. Torpey, eds., *Documenting Individual Identity: The Development of State Practices in the Modern World* (Princeton, NJ: Princeton University Press, 2001); Simon A. Cole, *Suspect Identities: A History of Fingerprinting and Criminal Identification* (Cambridge, MA: Harvard University Press, 2001). On normalization and surveillance, see Michel Foucault, *Discipline and Punish: The Birth of the Prison* (New York: Vintage, 1979).

4. Philip Corrigan and Derek Sayer, *The Great Arch: English State Formation as a Cultural Revolution* (London: Basil Blackwell, 1985), 4–5. For a somewhat similar discussion of the relation between the standardized "case" and the individualized "biography," see Carol A. Heimer, "Cases and Biographies: An Essay on Routinization and the Nature of Comparison," *Annual Review of Sociology* 27 (2001): 47–76.

5. In the next chapter, I return to the issue of the link between niche standardization and niche marketing, in my discussion of pharmaceutical marketing practices.

6. I. Young, "Polity and Group Difference." See also I. Young, *Justice and the Politics of Difference*; Kymlicka, *Multicultural Citizenship*. On the relation between affirmative action and the critique of the abstract individual citizen, see also John David Skrentny, *The Ironies of Affirmative Action: Politics, Culture, and Justice in America* (Chicago: University of Chicago Press, 1996), 19–23.

7. On the history of producing a "family" of dummies, see Margalit Fox, "Samuel Alderson, Crash-Test Dummy Inventor, Dies at 90," *New York Times*, February 18, 2005, A21.

8. Kate Zernike, "Sizing up America: Signs of Expansion from Head to Toe," *New York Times*, March 1, 2004, A1.

9. David John Frank and John W. Meyer, "The Profusion of Individual Roles and Identities in the Postwar Period," *Sociological Theory* 20, no. 1 (March 2002): 87, 95.

10. Alexis de Tocqueville, *Democracy in America* (1835 and 1840; New York: Harper & Row, 1966), 506-8.

11. Kim W. Williams, "Parties, Movements, and Constituencies in Categorizing Race," in *States, Parties, and Social Movements*, ed. Jack A. Goldstone, 197-225 (Cambridge: Cambridge University Press, 2003).

12. Indeed, group-based identities remain highly visible in much of the world, across a range of types of societies.

13. On evidence-based medicine, see Timmermans and Berg, *Gold Standard*. Clinical judgment and its role in the defense of professional autonomy is described in Eliot Freidson, *Profession of Medicine: A Study of the Sociology of Applied Knowledge* (Chicago: University of Chicago Press, 1988), 168-72. On the art/science divide, see Deborah R. Gordon, "Clinical Science and Clinical Expertise: Changing Boundaries between Art and Science in Medicine," in *Biomedicine Examined*, ed. Margaret Lock and Deborah R. Gordon, 257-95 (Dordrecht: Kluwer Academic Publishing, 1988).

14. Allan Roses, a key figure in the field, has proposed that pharmacogenomics will end the art/science divide in medicine by allowing for a scientific understanding of individual variation. Allen D. Roses, "Pharmacogenetics and the Practice of Medicine," *Nature* 405, no. 6788 (June 15, 2000): 857.

15. Michael J. Flower and Deborah Heath, "Micro-Anatomo Politics: Mapping the Human Genome Project," *Culture, Medicine and Psychiatry* 17 (1993): 33.

16. Reardon, *Race to the Finish*.

17. Linda Ann Sherman, Robert Temple, and Ruth B. Merkatz, "Women in Clinical Trials: An FDA Perspective," *Science* 269, no. 5225 (August 11, 1995): 793.

18. Jonathan Simon, "The Ideological Effects of Actuarial Practices," *Law and Society Review* 22, no. 4 (1988): 771-800.

19. Rabinow, *Essays on the Anthropology of Reason*, 91-111; Heath, Rapp, and Taussig, "Genetic Citizenship."

20. Lamont and Molnár, "Study of Boundaries in the Social Sciences," 187.

21. The question of whether categorical identities might usefully function as a *proxy* for behavioral risk practices is one that I take up in chapters 10 and 11.

22. "On the Pulse," *Washington Post*, December 20, 1994.

23. The anesthesiologist who conducted the research (using electric shocks) proposed a biological mechanism for redheads' sensitivity to pain: they produce more of a hormone that is related to skin and hair pigmentation but that also stimulates receptors in the brain linked to pain sensitivity. See Will Knight, "Red Heads Suffer More Pain," New Scientist.com News Service, October 15, 2002, www.newscientist.com/article.ns?id=dn2923. (My thanks to Wendy Espeland for bringing this example to my attention.)

24. Karen Weiss, "Gender Analysis in the Regulatory Setting," in *Science Meets Reality*, 66. On the sociological significance of APACHE scores, see Elizabeth Jennings, "Matters of Life and Death: Rationalizing Medical Decision-Making in a Managed Care Nation" (Ph.D. dissertation, University of California, San Diego, 2002).

25. Nancy Krieger, "Inequality, Diversity, and Health: Thoughts on 'Race/Ethnicity' and

'Gender,'" *Journal of the American Medical Women's Association* 51 (August–October 1996): 133–36. See also Hanson, *Social Assumptions, Medical Categories*.

26. Drawing on Michael Warner's discussion of the production of publics and public spheres, Charles Briggs has analyzed "the concept of 'public' that is embedded in notions of the 'public health'" in order to show how publics are produced via media representations of health and illness. See C. Briggs, "Why Nation-States and Journalists Can't Teach," 287; and Michael Warner, *Publics and Counterpublics* (New York: Zone Books, 2002).

27. See Hacking's discussion of "interactive kinds" in *Social Construction of What?* 104.

28. This construction of equivalences bears similarities to the "commensuration" practices described by Wendy Espeland and Mitchell Stevens, and it serves a similar function: It "offers standardized ways of constructing proxies for uncertain and elusive qualities [and] condenses and reduces the amount of information people have to process, [thereby] simplifying decision-making." Espeland and Stevens, "Commensuration as a Social Process," 316.

29. Shim, "Bio-Power and Racial, Class, and Gender Formation," 180. On the intersectional determinants of health, see also Schulz and Mullings, *Gender, Race, Class, and Health*.

30. Marcia Angell, interviewed by author.

31. Janet Wittes, interviewed by author.

32. Watanabe, "Amid Criticism, NCI Tries to Boost," 4–5.

33. Krieger and Fee, "Man-Made Medicine and Women's Health"; see also Hanson, *Social Assumptions, Medical Categories*. For a recent discussion of how to operationalize socioeconomic status in health research, see Paula A. Braveman et al., "Socioeconomic Status in Health Research: One Size Does Not Fit All," *Journal of the American Medical Association* 294, no. 22 (December 14, 2005): 2879–88.

34. On the construction of silences through classification, see Bowker and Star, *Sorting Things Out*.

35. Sheryl Gay Stolberg, "Concern among Jews Is Heightened as Scientists Deepen Gene Studies," *New York Times*, April 22, 1998, A24.

36. Abigail C. Saguy and Kevin W. Riley, "Weighing Both Sides: Morality, Mortality, and Framing Contests over Obesity," *Journal of Health Politics, Policy and Law* 30, no. 5 (October 2005): 869–923.

37. George Lundberg, interviewed by author.

38. Henrie M. Treadwell and Marguerite Ro, editorial, "Poverty, Race, and the Invisible Men," *American Journal of Public Health* 93, no. 5 (May 2003): 705–7; "Tailoring Care for Men," amednews.com, February 21, 2005, www.ama-assn.org/amednews/2005/02/21/edsa 0221.htm.

39. For creative thinking about men's health, see R. W. Connell, *The Men and the Boys* (Berkeley: University of California Press, 2000), chap. 10; Will H. Courtenay, "Constructions of Masculinity and Their Influence on Men's Well-Being: A Theory of Gender and Health," *Social Science and Medicine* 50 (2000): 1385–1401; Elianne Riska, *Masculinity and Men's Health: Coronary Heart Disease in Medical and Public Discourse* (Lanham, MD: Rowman & Littlefield, 2004).

40. Menstuff.org, "Latest NIH Report a Setback for Men's Health," 2001, www.menstuff. org/issues/byissue/healthgeneral.html; Menstuff.org, "The Myth: Medical Research Is Biased against Women," 2001, www.menstuff.org/issues/byissue/healthgeneral.html.

41. Cathy Young, "Ill-Considered: The Men's Rights Movement Takes on the NIH," *New Republic*, March 19, 2001, 18.

42. Office of Congressman Randy Cunningham, "Cunningham Delivers Father's Day Gift: Office of Men's Health," June 16, 2000, www.house.gov/cunningham/Press_Releases/cunningham_delivers_fathers_day_gift16jun00.htm. In 2005 Cunningham resigned his congressional seat and pled guilty to charges of accepting $2.4 million in bribes from military contractors; he was sentenced to eight years in prison. Randal C. Archibold, "Ex-Congressman Gets 8-Year Term in Bribery Case," *New York Times*, March 4, 2006, A1.

43. "Congressmen Move to Create Men's Health Office," *New York Times*, February 16, 2001.

44. On the "top-down" character of much men's health activism, see Dimock, "Demanding Disease Dollars."

45. Of course, it is not inconceivable that the racialization of biomedicine may eventually promote the emergence of white people's health as a recognized political project. Such a development would be consistent with the processes, in other social domains, by which the previously "unmarked" category of whiteness gradually emerges as the basis of a distinct social identity. There is a large literature in the area of "whiteness studies"; for its intersection with biomedicine, see Warwick Anderson, *The Cultivation of Whiteness: Science, Health, and Racial Destiny in Australia* (New York: Basic, 2003).

46. Bourdieu, *Practical Reason*, 45 (emphasis in the original).

47. Skrentny, *Minority Rights Revolution*, esp. 85-142.

48. Rueben C. Warren et al., editorial, "The Use of Race and Ethnicity in Public Health Surveillance," *Public Health Reports* 109, no. 1 (January-February 1994): 5.

49. Robert A. Hahn and Donna F. Stroup, "Race and Ethnicity in Public Health Surveillance: Criteria for the Scientific Use of Social Categories," *Public Health Reports* 109, no. 1 (1994): 7-8.

50. Robert A. Hahn, "The State of Federal Health Statistics on Racial and Ethnic Groups," *Journal of the American Medical Association* 267, no. 2 (1992): 269.

51. I return to these dilemmas of racial classification in chapter 10.

52. This importation process is also an example of what William Sewell has called the "transposition" of cultural schemas: "a concrete application of a rule to a new case, but in such a way that the rule will have subtly different forms in each of its applications." Sewell, "Theory of Structure," 17 n. 9. On policy legacies, see the references in chap. 1, n. 56.

53. NIH, "NIH Guidelines on the Inclusion of Women and Minorities," 14511.

54. Michael Omi, "Our Private Obsession, Our Public Sin: Racial Identity and the State: The Dilemmas of Classification," *Law and Inequality* (winter 1997).

55. Dvora Yanow, *Constructing "Race" and "Ethnicity" in America: Category-Making in Public Policy and Administration* (Armonk, NY: M. E. Sharpe, 2003), 116.

56. NIH, "NIH Guidelines on the Inclusion of Women and Minorities," 14511.

57. Lawrence Wright, "One Drop of Blood," *New Yorker*, July 25, 1994, 46-55; David Theo Goldberg, *Racial Subjects: Writing on Race in America* (New York: Routledge, 1997), 27-58.

58. Melissa Nobles, *Shades of Citizenship: Race and the Census in Modern Politics* (Stanford, CA: Stanford University Press, 2000), xi. On the census as a technology for organizing the U.S. state and society, see Desrosières, *Politics of Large Numbers*, 188. On censuses and racialization, see also Espiritu, *Asian American Panethnicity*, 112-33; D. Goldberg, *Racial*

Subjects, 27–58; Yanow, *Constructing "Race" and "Ethnicity"*; Telles, *Race in Another America*, 78–106.

59. Wright, "One Drop of Blood," 47.

60. The OMB revisions were posted in 1997. Executive Office of the President, Office of Management and Budget, "Revisions to the Standards for the Classification of Federal Data on Race and Ethnicity," *Federal Register* 62, no. 210 (October 30, 1997): 58782–83. On the politics behind these changes, see Wright, "One Drop of Blood," 46–55; David R. Harris and Jeremiah Joseph Sim, "Who Is Multiracial? Assessing the Complexity of Lived Race," *American Sociological Review* 67 (August 2002): 614–27; K. Williams, "Parties, Movements, and Constituencies." There has been little empirical study of the broader implications for people who identify as multiracial of the use of racial categories in the health domain. For one discussion, see Cathy J. Tashiro, "Mixed but Not Matched: Multiracial People and the Organization of Health Knowledge," in *The Sum of Our Parts: Mixed-Heritage Asian Americans*, ed. Teresa Williams-León and Cynthia L. Nakashima (Philadelphia: Temple University Press, 2001), 173–82.

61. NIH, "NIH Policy on Reporting Race and Ethnicity Data: Subjects in Clinical Research (Notice # NOT-OD-01-053)" (Washington, DC: U.S. Department of Health & Human Services, August 8, 2000).

62. Vivian Pinn, interviewed by author. See chapter 8 for a discussion of NIH efforts to track minority inclusion.

63. U.S. Census Bureau, "The Two or More Races Population: 2000" (Washington, DC: U.S. Department of Commerce, November 2001); Mireya Navarro, "Going beyond Black and White, Hispanics Choose 'Other,'" *New York Times*, November 9, 2003, A1. On the general implications for policy of the ability to select more than one racial category, see Joel Perlmann and Mary C. Waters, eds., *The New Race Question: How the Census Counts Multiracial Individuals* (New York: Russell Sage, 2002).

64. As opposed to rules, FDA guidances are nonbinding. See FDA, "Guidance for Industry: Collection of Race and Ethnicity Data in Clinical Trials," January 2003; FDA, "Guidance for Industry: Collection of Race and Ethnicity Data in Clinical Trials," September 2005.

65. The 2005 FDA guidance on racial categories takes a similar approach to this question; see FDA, "Guidance for Industry 2005," 5.

66. NIH, "NIH Policy on Reporting Race and Ethnicity Data." The instructions changed slightly in 2004.

67. Hayunga, interview.

68. Richard Levy, interviewed by author; Temple, interview.

69. Lionel D. Edwards, "Acceptability of Foreign Data: Genetic, Cultural and Environmental Differences—Do They Matter?" in *The Relevance of Ethnic Factors in the Clinical Evaluation of Medicines*, ed. Stuart Walker, Cyndy Lumley, and Neil McAuslane (Dordrecht: Kluwer Academic Publishers, 1994), 10.

70. On the ICH, see Daemmrich, *Pharmacopolitics*, 157–60, 219.

71. "International Conference on Harmonisation: Guidance on Ethnic Factors in the Acceptability of Foreign Clinical Data; Availability," *Federal Register* 63, no. 111 (1998): 31790–96.

72. Ibid., 31793–94.

73. Temple, interview.

74. On the transnational dimensions of pharmaceutical drug development, see also Lakoff, *Pharmaceutical Reason*; Petryna, Lakoff, and Kleinman, *Global Pharmaceuticals*. On the enduring significance of national differences in the politics of science, see Jasanoff, *Designs on Nature*.

CHAPTER EIGHT

1. One dimension of scientific work that is reshaped by the inclusion-and-difference paradigm—the practical work of finding research subjects for clinical studies—is such a weighty topic that it merits its own chapter. I reserve that discussion for the chapter following this one.

2. Hayunga and Pinn, "NIH Response to Researchers' Concerns," 59-64, quotation from 59.

3. Hayunga and Pinn, "Implementing the 1994 NIH Guidelines," 35-40, quotation from 36.

4. Vivian W. Pinn et al., "Monitoring Adherence to the NIH Policy on the Inclusion of Women and Minorities as Subjects in Clinical Research: Comprehensive Report (Fiscal Year 1999 & 2000 Tracking Data)" (Bethesda, MD: NIH, December 2002).

5. Duane Alexander, interviewed by author.

6. I am grateful to my research assistant, Devon Smith, for her work compiling these figures using the NIH Web site http://ClinicalTrials.gov.

7. Wendy Baldwin, interviewed by author.

8. Janet K. Shim, "Race, Class, and Gender across the Science-Lay Divide: Expertise, Experience, and 'Difference' in Cardiovascular Disease" (Ph.D. dissertation, University of California, San Francisco, 2002), 118.

9. Duane Alexander characterized the question of "whether we were going to require head counts" as "probably . . . the most significant debate that we had" in devising the children's inclusion policy. But clearly what weighed on Alexander and others within NIH was the risk of further alienating the scientific community, along with the perception that having to fill out forms documenting the numbers of those included was the part of the guidelines on women and minorities that investigators resented the most. Alexander, interview.

10. Eugene G. Hayunga, Margaret D. Costello, and Vivian W. Pinn, "Demographics of Study Populations," *Applied Clinical Trials* 6, no. 1 (1997): 41-45.

11. However, the greater representation of women overall substantially reflected the boom in women-only trials, including the enormous Women's Health Initiative. In 2000, there were 975 female-only trials and 360 male-only trials. Excluding the single-sex trials, women and men were at near parity (Pinn et al., "Monitoring Adherence—Fiscal Years 1999 & 2000," 16-21). By 2004, with the Women's Health Initiative completed, there were still many more women-only trials than men-only trials, but women's representation had dropped slightly to 57.6 percent of all participants in clinical studies and 55.5 percent of participants in Phase 3 trials. Vivian W. Pinn et al., "Monitoring Adherence to the NIH Policy on the Inclusion of Women and Minorities as Subjects in Clinical Research: Comprehensive Report: Tracking of Human Subjects Research as Reported in Fiscal Year 2003 and Fiscal Year 2004" (Bethesda, MD: NIH, 2005), 16, 18.

12. Pinn et al., "Monitoring Adherence—Fiscal Years 1999 & 2000," 19, 31-44.

13. Pinn et al., "Monitoring Adherence—Fiscal Years 2003 & 2004," 21–22.

14. Allen L. Gifford et al., "Participation in Research and Access to Experimental Treatments by HIV-Infected Patients," *New England Journal of Medicine* 346, no. 18 (May 2, 2002): 1373–82, esp. 1375.

15. Talmadge E. King, "Racial Disparities in Clinical Trials," *New England Journal of Medicine* 346, no. 18 (May 2, 2002): 1402.

16. David J. Harris and Pamela S. Douglas, "Enrollment of Women in Cardiovascular Clinical Trials Funded by the National, Heart, Lung, and Blood Institute," *New England Journal of Medicine* 343, no. 7 (August 17, 2000): 478. To be sure, as Julie Buring noted in an accompanying editorial, the question of the appropriate balance between two goals—including women in mixed-sex studies and conducting separate studies of women only—is a complex one. Buring, "Women in Clinical Trials," 505–506.

17. Baird, "New NIH and FDA Medical Research Policies." See also Karen L. Baird, *Gender Justice and the Health Care System* (New York: Garland, 1998).

18. Jill A. Fisher, "Pharmaceutical Paternalism and the Privatization of Clinical Trials" (Ph.D. dissertation, Rensselaer Polytechnic Institute, 2005); and on overall biomedical research spending (not just on clinical research), see Moses et al., "Financial Anatomy of Biomedical Research," 1333–42.

19. Gardiner Harris, "Congressional Investigators Are Critical of F.D.A.'s Efforts to Detect Drug Dangers," *New York Times*, April 24, 2006, A12.

20. Robert Temple, interviewed by author; Alexander, interview.

21. Robert Steinbrook, "Testing Medications in Children," *New England Journal of Medicine* 347, no. 18 (October 31, 2002): 1462.

22. Sheryl Gay Stolberg, "Children Test New Medicines Despite Doubts," *New York Times*, February 11, 2001, A1, A22.

23. FDA, "The Pediatric Exclusivity Provision: January 2001 Status Report to Congress," January 2001, ii, 33–35. See also Alan F. Holmer, "Progress against Diseases of Children Continues with 205 Medicines and Vaccines in Development" (Washington, DC: PhRMA, May 2001).

24. FDA, news release, "FDA Joins Children's Health Groups to Mark Historic Milestone for Pediatric Drugs," December 19, 2005, www.fda.gov/bbs/topics/NEWS/2005/NEW01280 .html. For a list of the one hundred drugs, see www.fda.gov/cder/pediatric/labelchange.htm. Recently, critics have complained that these studies resulting in labeling changes are not being reported in medical journals; see Daniel K. Benjamin et al., "Peer-Reviewed Publication of Clinical Trials Completed for Pediatric Exclusivity," *New England Journal of Medicine* 296, no 10 (September 13, 2006): 1266–73.

25. FDA, "Pediatric Exclusivity Provision," iii.

26. See the discussion in chapter 6.

27. Jerome Groopman, "The Pediatric Gap," *New Yorker*, January 10, 2005.

28. Patrick Y. Lee and Karen P. Alexander, "Representation of Elderly Persons and Women in Published Randomized Trials of Acute Coronary Syndromes," *Journal of the American Medical Association* 286, no. 6 (August 8, 2001): 710.

29. Robert N. Butler and James P. Nyberg, "Clinical Trials and Older Persons: The Need for Greater Representation" (New York: International Longevity Center—USA, November–December 2002), 4.

30. Kimberly A. Struble et al., "Enrollment of Women in HIV Clinical Trials (Abstract

Thb.4147)" (*Proceedings of the Conference on IX International AIDS Conference*, Vancouver, British Columbia, Canada, July 1996).

31. Cullen T. Vogelson, "Sex, Drugs, and Risk's Role," *Modern Drug Discovery*, October 2001, 27–28, 30.

32. B. Evelyn et al., Office of Special Health Issues, FDA, "Women's Participation in Clinical Trials and Gender-Related Labeling: A Review of New Molecular Entities Approved 1995–1999," June 2001. A similar study, funded by the FDA's Office of Women's Health, examined the "biologics" approved over the same time period and arrived at comparable results. FDA Scholarship in Women's Health Program, FDA, "Participation of Females in Clinical Trials and Gender Analysis of Data in Biologic Product Applications," April 3, 2001.

33. B. Evelyn et al., Office of Special Health Issues, FDA, "Participation of Racial/Ethnic Groups in Clinical Trials and Race-Related Labeling: A Review of New Molecular Entities Approved 1995–1999," October 16, 2001.

34. I am grateful to my research assistant, Nielan Barnes, for her work reviewing the labeling information. For the year 1998, ten labels were not legible on the FDA's Web site (www.fda.gov/cder/approval/index.htm) and are not included in the counts reported here. A different study of new drug approvals from 1995 through 1998 found fifteen cases where a racial or ethnic difference in the drug's effectiveness was described in the drug labeling information; see Sarah K. Tate and David B. Goldstein, "Will Tomorrow's Medicines Work for Everyone?" *Nature Genetics* 36, no. 11 (November 2004): S34.

35. A. Sonia Buist and Merwyn R. Greenlick, "Response to 'Inclusion of Women and Minorities in Clinical Trials and the NIH Revitalization Act of 1993—the Perspective of NIH Clinical Trialists,'" *Controlled Clinical Trials* 16, no. 5 (October 1995): 297.

36. Shim, "Race, Class, and Gender across the Science-Lay Divide," 195.

37. "Science Meets Reality" workshop (author's field notes); Brian Vastag, "Researchers Say Changes Needed in Recruitment Policies for NIH Trials," *Journal of the American Medical Association* 289, no. 5 (February 5, 2003).

38. "Science Meets Reality" workshop (author's field notes); Steven Piantadosi, "Why Sex Doesn't Matter," *Science Meets Reality*, 60.

39. Vastag, "Researchers Say Changes Needed."

40. Spero Manson, interviewed by author.

41. This individual offered his recollections on the condition that he not be identified by name.

42. NIH, "NIMH Policy for Recruitment of Participants in Clinical Research," Notice no. NOT-MH-05-013, July 29, 2005, http://grants.nih.gov/grants/guide/notice-files/NOT-MH-05-013.html.

43. Weiss, "Gender Analysis in the Regulatory Setting," 64.

44. Temple, interview.

45. Manson, interview.

46. Anna Nápoles-Springer, interviewed by author.

47. Manson, interview. Another issue raised by those disappointed by the pace of reform concerns how thoroughly the inclusionary mandate has trickled down to the IRBs that review the ethics of research protocols around the country. Certainly it is difficult to say how attentively the average IRB reviews responses to questions on inclusion—or even if there is such a thing as an "average IRB," as each one seems to develop its own culture.

48. Janet Heinrich, "Women's Health: Women Sufficiently Represented in New Drug

Testing, but FDA Oversight Needs Improvement," GAO-01-754 (Washington, DC: GAO, July 2001).

49. Janet Heinrich, "Drug Safety: Most Drugs Withdrawn in Recent Years Had Greater Health Risks for Women," GAO 01-286R (Washington, DC: GAO, January 19, 2001).

50. Victoria Stagg Elliott, "Early Testing of New Drugs Remains Mostly a Guy's Game," amednews.com, September 3, 2001.

51. Janet Heinrich, "Women's Health: NIH Has Increased Its Efforts to Include Women in Research," GAO/HEHS-00-96 (Washington, DC: GAO, May 2000), 2, 22; Laura Helmuth, "Reports See Progress, Problems, in Trials," *Science*, June 2, 2000, 1562.

52. "Society Recommendations Implemented by NIH," *Sexx Matters: Research News from the Society for Women's Health Research*, summer 2000, 1.

53. NIH, "NIH Guidelines on the Inclusion of Women and Minorities as Subjects in Clinical Research—Updated August 2, 2000," http://grants1.nih.gov/grants/guide/notice-files/NOT-OD-00-048.html.

54. Regina M. Vidaver et al., "Women Subjects in NIH-Funded Clinical Research Literature: Lack of Progress in Both Representation and Analysis by Sex," *Journal of Women's Health* 9, no. 5 (2000): 497. For corroborating findings, see also K. Ramasubbu, H. Curm, and D. Litaker, "Gender Bias in Clinical Trials: Do Double Standards Still Apply?" *Journal of Women's Health and Gender-Based Medicine* 10, no. 8 (2001): 757–64.

55. Heinrich, "Women's Health: NIH Has Increased Its Efforts," 9.

56. Vivian W. Pinn, "NIH Studies Include Women," *USA Today*, May 5, 2000, A16.

57. "Correction," *Journal of Women's Health and Gender-Based Medicine* 9, no. 9 (2000): 1043. The correction also presented a revised figure of the fraction of studies that failed to describe sex/gender analysis; this was now said to be between one-half and three-fifths.

58. Pinn, "NIH Studies Include Women," A16.

59. Vidaver et al., "Women Subjects," 499.

60. Helmuth, "Reports See Progress, Problems, in Trials," 1562.

61. Delores Parron, interviewed by author.

62. Marcia Angell, interviewed by author.

63. Agency for Healthcare Research and Quality, "Results of Systematic Review of Research on Diagnosis and Treatment of Coronary Heart Disease in Women," AHRQ Publication No. 03-E034 (Rockville, MD: Agency for Healthcare Research and Quality, May 2003).

64. On this point see Marianne N. Prout and Susan S. Fish, "Participation of Women in Clinical Trials of Drug Therapies: A Context for the Controversies," *Medscape Women's Health* 6, no. 5 (2001).

65. I return to this issue in the next chapter.

66. This phrasing is the reconstruction offered by an anonymous informant who is a university-based researcher, and it is not offered as an exact quotation of any NIH employee.

67. The classic discussion of the tension between formal and substantive rationality is in Max Weber, *Economy and Society* (Berkeley: University of California Press, 1978), 85–86. For a detailed analysis of another case involving this tension in the biomedical arena, see Evans, *Playing God?*

68. Lauren B. Edelman, "Legal Ambiguity and Symbolic Structures: Organizational Mediation of Civil Rights Law," *American Journal of Sociology* 97, no. 6 (May 1992): 1531–76. For an example of symbolic rituals of compliance in the domain of science, see Laurel

Smith-Doerr's analysis of how scientists comply with NIH requirements that they demon-
strate knowledge of research ethics. Laurel Smith-Doerr, "Learning to Reflect or Deflect?
U.S. Policies and Graduate Programs' Ethics Training for Life Scientists," in *New Political
Sociology of Science*, ed. Frickel and Moore, 405–31.

69. James Scott, *Seeing Like a State*, 310; Star, "Politics of Formal Representations," esp.
100–104.

70. Baldwin and Seto, interview; Hayunga, interview.

71. Claude Lenfant, interviewed by author.

72. James Jackson, interviewed by author.

73. Vivian Pinn, interviewed by author; Vivian W. Pinn, "The Role of the NIH's Office
of Research on Women's Health," *Academic Medicine* 69, no. 9 (September 1994): 698–
702; Jacquelyn Stone et al., "Evaluation of the First 10 Years of the Office of Research on
Women's Health at the National Institutes of Health: Selected Findings," *Journal of Women's
Health* 15, no. 3 (2006): 234–47.

74. Office of Research on Women's Health, NIH, "Comprehensive 1991–2003 Report
on Women's Health Research (by Institute/Center) Funded or Co-Funded by the Office of
Research on Women's Health," October 2003.

75. On NCMHD programs, see http://ncmhd.nih.gov/default.html.

76. On the Pediatric Pharmacology Research Unit program see www.nichd.nih.gov/
about/crmc/eng/ped/ped2.htm.

77. Lynn Rosenberg, Lucille Adams-Campbell, and Julie Palmer, "The Black Women's
Health Study: A Follow-up Study for Causes and Preventions of Illness," *Journal of the
American Medical Women's Association* 50, no. 2 (March–April 1995): 56–58.

78. Women's Health Initiative Study Group, "Design of the Women's Health Initiative
Clinical Trial and Observational Study," *Controlled Clinical Trials* 19, no. 1 (February 1998):
61–109.

79. Jacques E. Rossouw and Suzanne Hurd, "The Women's Health Initiative: Recruitment Complete—Looking Back and Looking Forward," *Journal of Women's Health* 8, no. 1
(1999): 3–5.

80. Pinn, "Role of the NIH's Office of Research on Women's Health," 700.

81. *Children's Health Act of 2000*, Public Law 106–310, 106th Congress, October 17, 2000;
National Institute of Child Health and Human Development, "The National Children's
Study," n.d. (accessed June 11, 2006), http://nationalchildrensstudy.gov/. As of this writing,
planning has been completed, but the study has not yet begun and its funding is not assured.

82. See, for example, the June 2003 special issue of *Academic Medicine*, which is devoted
to the theme of cultural competence, with particular attention to medical education.

83. Ciro V. Sumaya, Vivian W. Pinn, and Susan J. Blumenthal, "Women's Health in the
Medical School Curriculum: Report of a Survey and Recommendations," DHHS Publication no. HRSA-A-OEA-96-1 (Bethesda, MD: National Institutes of Health, 1996).

84. Sarah K. Keitt et al., "Positioning Women's Health Curricula in US Medical Schools,"
Medscape General Medicine 5, no. 2 (May 28, 2003).

85. Deborah Cotton, interviewed by author.

86. Peter Applebome, "A Lesson for Residents: They're Not Like Men," *New York Times*,
June 22, 1997.

87. "Uniform Requirements for Manuscripts Submitted to Biomedical Journals," *New
England Journal of Medicine* 336, no. 4 (January 23, 1997).

88. Nancy Krieger and Sally Zierler, "Accounting for Health of Women," *Current Issues in Public Health* 1 (1995): 251; Eckman, "Beyond 'the Yentl Syndrome,'" 133.

89. Catherine D. DeAngelis and Margaret A. Winker, "Women's Health—Filling the Gaps," *Journal of the American Medical Association* 285, no. 11 (March 21, 2000): 1508-9.

90. Catherine D. DeAngelis and Richard M. Glass, "Women's Health—Advances in Knowledge and Understanding," *Journal of the American Medical Association* 295, no. 12 (March 22, 2006): 1448-50. Later in 2006 *JAMA* also published a theme issue on the topic of men's health.

91. Policies of AMA House of Delegates, retrieved from PolicyFinder A-98 edition (downloadable from www.ama-assn.org/ad-com/polfind/announce.htm), current as of June 1998.

92. Council on Scientific Affairs, American Medical Association, "Featured CSA Report: Women's Health: Sex- and Gender-Based Differences in Health and Disease," CSA Report 4, I-00, 2000, www.ama-assn.org/ama/pub/print/article/2036-4946.html.

93. Damon Adams, "Minority Mistrust Still Haunts Medical Care," amednews.com, January 13, 2003, www.ama-assn.org/amednews/2003/01/13/prl20113.htm.

94. Kathleen Day, "In a Fever over Her Health Care," *Washington Post*, June 26, 1997, C1. On the history of the relation between marketing, consumption, and gender, see Victoria de Grazia, ed., *The Sex of Things: Gender and Consumption in Historical Perspective* (Berkeley: University of California Press, 1996).

95. David J. Morrow, "Women's Drugs: Big in Profits, Narrow in Scope," *New York Times*, June 13, 1999, 9.

96. Jonca Bull, interviewed by author.

97. Alan F. Holmer, "Women's Health Revolution Continues with 358 Medicines in the Pipeline for Diseases That Primarily Affect Women" (Washington, DC: PhRMA, October 2001), 1.

98. Michael Montoya, "Bioethnic Conscription: Genes, Race and Mexicana/o Ethnicity in Diabetes Research," *Cultural Anthropology* 22, no. 1 (February 2007). On the complex consequences of niche marketing in health, see also Roddey Reid, "Tensions within California Tobacco Control in the 1990s: Health Movements, State Initiatives, and Community Mobilization," *Science as Culture* 13, no. 4 (December 2004): 515-37.

99. Fourth Annual Multicultural Pharmaceutical Marketing and PR conference, sponsored by Strategic Research Institute, held March 18, 2003, in Princeton, NJ, www.srinstitute .com.

100. On post-Fordist economic restructuring. see Ash Amin, *Post-Fordism: A Reader* (Oxford: Blackwell, 1994).

101. Clarke et al., "Biomedicalization," 169. See also Adele E. Clarke and Virginia L. Olesen, "Revising, Diffracting, Acting," in *Revisioning Women, Health, and Healing*, ed. Clarke and Olesen, 18.

102. N. Klein, *No Logo*, 110-17.

103. Holmer, "Women's Health Revolution Continues."

104. Nathan Greenslit, "Pharmaceutical Branding: Identity, Individuality, and Illness," *Molecular Interventions* 2, no. 6 (October 2002): 342-45. On the repositioning of existing pharmaceutical products for sale to women, see also Courtney Kane, "The Two Faces of Athlete's Foot Cream: One Product Marketed Separately to Men and Women," *New York Times*, July 26, 2002, C7.

105. Robert Pear, "Congress Weighs Drug Comparisons," *New York Times*, August 24, 2003, 16.

106. Levy, *Ethnic and Racial Differences*, v.

107. Robert Temple, interviewed by author; Andrew Pollack, "Drug to Treat Bowel Illness Is Approved by the F.D.A.," *New York Times*, July 25, 2002, A12.

108. Andrew Pollack, "Drug Approved for Heart Failure in Black Patients," *New York Times*, July 20, 2004, C1.

109. This is the argument made in Raymond L. Woosley, Marietta Anthony, and Carl C. Peck, editorial, "Biological Sex Analysis in Clinical Research," *Journal of Women's Health and Gender-Based Medicine* 9, no. 9 (2000): 933–94.

110. On the racializing of BiDil, see, in particular, Jonathan Kahn, "How a Drug Becomes 'Ethnic.'"

CHAPTER NINE

1. Through the influence of actor-network theory in science and technology studies, it has become commonplace to assert that successful scientific work is crucially dependent on "enrollment": Scientists build facts and extend the reach of their claims by enlisting people and objects behind their banner and assigning to them distinct roles in the knowledge production process. But while *enrollment*, in this sense, is a term used by those who study scientists to describe practices that those actors perhaps more typically understand in other ways, sometimes enrollment is precisely what scientists themselves take as their mission. See Michel Callon, "Some Elements of a Sociology of Translation: Domestication of the Scallops and the Fishermen of St. Brieuc Bay," in *Power, Action, and Belief*, ed. John Law (London: Routledge & Kegan Paul, 1986), esp. 211–14; Latour, *Science in Action*.

2. In the language of technology studies, researchers testing pharmaceutical drugs need to "configure" the activities of the research subject as a first step toward eventually "configuring the user"—shaping the behavior of the downstream consumer of the product. See Nelly Oudshoorn, *The Male Pill: A Biography of a Technology in the Making* (Durham, NC: Duke University Press, 2003); and more generally on configuring the user, see Steve Woolgar, "Configuring the User: The Case of Usability Trials," in *A Sociology of Monsters: Essays on Power, Technology and Domination*, ed. John Law (London: Routledge, 1991), 57–99.

3. Daramola N. Cabral et al., "Population- and Community-Based Recruitment of African Americans and Latinos: The San Francisco Bay Area Lung Cancer Study," *American Journal of Epidemiology* 158, no. 3 (August 2003): 272.

4. NIH, Office of Research on Women's Health, "Recruitment and Retention of Women in Clinical Studies," NIH Publication no. 95-3756, 1995; NIH, "Outreach Notebook for the Inclusion, Recruitment and Retention of Women"; "Science Meets Reality: Recruitment and Retention of Women in Clinical Studies, and the Critical Role of Relevance," NIH Publication no. 03-5403 (Washington, DC: National Institutes of Health, January 6–9, 2003); *Science Meets Reality*, http://orwh.od.nih.gov/pubs/SMR_Final.pdf.

5. Epstein, *Impure Science*, 181–234.

6. Rebecca Dresser, "Surfing for Studies: Clinical Trials on the Internet," *Hastings Center Report*, November–December 1999, 26. In its current form, this database can be found at www.clinicaltrials.gov/.

7. Harry M. Collins, "The TEA Set: Tacit Knowledge and Scientific Networks," *Science Studies* 4 (1974); Clarke and Fujimura, *Right Tools for the Job*.

8. Epstein, "Activism, Drug Regulation," 691–92. See also Marcia Lynn Meldrum, "'Departing from the Design': The Randomized Clinical Trial in Historical Context, 1946–1970" (Ph.D. dissertation, State University of New York at Stony Brook, 1994), 384–86; Clarke, "Human Materials as Contested Objects"; Oudshoorn, *Male Pill*, 171–73.

9. Jennifer Fishman has described the manifold roles of clinical trial researchers in Jennifer R. Fishman, "Manufacturing Desire: The Commodification of Female Sexual Dysfunction," *Social Studies of Science* 34, no. 2 (April 2004): 187–218.

10. On the role of nurses serving as clinical trial coordinators in performing much of the backstage work of running clinical trials, see Mary-Rose Mueller, "Science versus Care: Physicians, Nurses, and the Dilemma of Clinical Research," in *Sociology of Medical Science and Technology*, ed. Elston, 57–78.

11. The estimate is from CenterWatch and applies to the year 2002. Diana L. Anderson, "The Patient Recruitment Market: An Overview of Today's Issues," *Applied Clinical Trials*, November 2003, 14.

12. Steven Folmar et al., "Recruitment of Participants for the Estrogen Replacement and Atherosclerosis (ERA) Trial: A Comparison of Costs, Yields, and Participant Characteristics from Community- and Hospital-Based Recruitment Strategies," *Controlled Clinical Trials* 22, no. 1 (February 2001): 23.

13. Patrick Jordan, "The Patient Recruitment Frontier: New Technologies for Forecasting and Measuring How Well They Work," Quintiles Transnational Corp., June 20, 2002, www.quintiles.com/Performance/Presentations.htm?year=2002. The statistic was attributed to the organization Centerwatch.

14. In the United States, the clock begins ticking on the twenty-year duration of a patent for a pharmaceutical product with the initial filing with the FDA, well before drug approval.

15. Fisher, "Pharmaceutical Paternalism"; Philip Mirowski and Robert Van Horn, "The Contract Research Organization and the Commercialization of Scientific Research," *Social Studies of Science* 35, no. 4 (August 2005): 503–48. Recruiting may be outsourced either to "contract research organizations" (CROs) that perform many tasks related to the conduct of clinical trials or to more specialized "central patient recruitment companies" that focus on recruitment and retention. All this is just part of what Fisher describes as the general increasing tendency toward outsourcing in private-sector clinical research.

16. Mirowski and Van Horn, "Contract Research Organization," 506.

17. Anderson, "Patient Recruitment Market," 16.

18. "Anaclim Established to Address Minority Clinical Trial Participation," *CW* [*CenterWatch*] *Weekly*, January 3, 2005, 1. I am grateful to Jill Fisher for forwarding me this information.

19. Quoted in Mark S. Lesney, "The Assent of Children," *Modern Drug Discovery*, October 2002, 19, 24.

20. Barbara Howard, interviewed by author.

21. Otis Brawley, interviewed by author.

22. Robert J. Levine, "Recruitment and Retention of Women in Clinical Studies: Ethical Considerations," in *Women and Health Research*, ed. Mastroianni, Faden, and Federman, 2:57; Fisher, "Pharmaceutical Paternalism."

23. Fisher, "Pharmaceutical Paternalism."

24. When the National Commission for the Protection of Human Subjects laid down its guidelines in the Belmont Report in 1979, it noted that voluntary consent to participate in research implied freedom not only from coercion but also from undue influence, which they defined as "an offer of an excessive, unwarranted, inappropriate or improper reward." National Commission for the Protection of Human Subjects of Biomedical and Behavioral Research, "Belmont Report," 6.

25. Catherine Waldby, *The Visible Human Project: Informatic Bodies and Posthuman Medicine* (London: Routledge, 2000), 19; Catherine Waldby, "Stem Cells, Tissue Cultures and the Production of Biovalue," *Health* 6, no. 3 (2002): 305–23. For a related analysis of "liquidity" in pharmaceutical research, see Lakoff, "Diagnostic Liquidity."

26. Neal Dickert and Christine Grady, "What's the Price of a Research Subject? Approaches to Payment for Research Participation," *New England Journal of Medicine* 341, no. 3 (July 15, 1999): 198–203.

27. Stacey Schultz, "Drug Trials Are Clamoring for Kids, but Scrutinize the Study before Signing Up," *U.S. News and World Report*, April 17, 2002, 62–63.

28. Lesney, "Assent of Children," 19, 24.

29. David D. Kirkpatrick, "E.P.A. Halts Florida Test on Pesticides," *New York Times*, April 9, 2005, A12.

30. Stolberg, "Children Test New Medicines," A1, A22.

31. Jeffrey Brainard, "2 Advisory Panels Suggest Improved Oversight of Research Involving Children," *Chronicle of Higher Education*, March 30, 2004.

32. For a critical discussion of informed consent and the notions of autonomy and choice on which it is based, see Oonagh Corrigan, "Empty Ethics: The Problem with Informed Consent," *Sociology of Health and Illness* 25, no. 7 (November 1, 2003): 768–92. I am grateful to Robert Levine for his discussion with me of the history of informed consent. Robert Levine, interviewed by author.

33. Robert Langer, interviewed by author.

34. Spero Manson, interviewed by author. On such mechanisms of group consent and their complexities in another domain of research in the biosciences, see the important discussion in Reardon, *Race to the Finish*, chap. 5. On the distinction in medical research between risks to the individual and collective risks to the group, see also Morris W. Foster and Richard R. Sharp, "Genetic Research and Culturally Specific Risks: One Size Does Not Fit All," *Genetics and Society* 16, no. 2 (February 2000): 93–95.

35. James Connor, interviewed by author.

36. Stanley Szefler, interviewed by author. Of course, gauging the desires and perceptions of children can be difficult. According to Diane Murphy, an FDA official familiar with pediatric issues: "The Academy of Pediatrics suggests that about the age of 7, children cognitively begin to understand risk. Somewhere around 7, the kid can begin to understand what you tell them. But that process is very time-consuming and very difficult and has to be done by people who know how to put it in language that kids can understand." Alexis Jetter, "A Conversation with Diane Murphy: Trying to End Guesswork in Dosing Children," *New York Times*, September 12, 2000, F7.

37. Marcel Mauss, *The Gift: Forms and Functions of Exchange in Archaic Societies* (Glencoe, IL: Free Press, 1954). I am grateful to Martha Poon for suggestions about the relevance of the gift relationship in the context of biomedical research.

38. Richard M. Titmuss, *The Gift Relationship: From Human Blood to Social Policy* (New York: Pantheon, 1971).

39. Organ donation is another prominent biomedical example where individuals often are called upon to make gifts for the benefit of their racial or ethnic group.

40. Such efforts to impute responsibilities to the group may invoke and reinforce very particular ideas about what groups are "really like." For example, in her dissertation on breast cancer chemoprevention, Jennifer Fosket found that investigators constructed highly gendered images of the ideal participant—images that "draw on cultural ideologies that equate womanhood and femininity with self-sacrifice and nurturing as well as more modernist images of the active, involved, and decisive woman." Jennifer Ruth Fosket, "Breast Cancer Risk and the Politics of Prevention: Analysis of a Clinical Trial" (Ph.D. dissertation, University of California, San Francisco, 2002), 251. And in her ethnographic work with members of the clinical trial industry in the U.S. Southwest, Jill Fisher found that many professionals working in the trenches operate with a series of working stereotypes according to race: Asians lack altruism, and blacks are suspicious, but Hispanics are compliant. Fisher, "Pharmaceutical Paternalism."

41. As Jill Fisher has observed, the increasingly pervasive public advertising for clinical trial participants mirrors the direct-to-consumer advertising of pharmaceutical products that is now ubiquitous in the United States. See Fisher, "Pharmaceutical Paternalism."

42. Philip Gorelick, interviewed by author.

43. Norman Lasser, interviewed by author.

44. Gina P. Vozenilek, "Meeting the Challenges of Recruiting and Retaining Participants in Clinical Trials," *Journal of the American Dietetic Association* 99, no. 10 (October 1999): 1190–91.

45. Rossouw and Hurd, "Women's Health Initiative," 3–5; Mona N. Fouad et al., "Special Populations Recruitment for the Women's Health Initiative: Successes and Limitations," *Controlled Clinical Trials* 25, no. 4 (August 2004): 335–52.

46. Virginia Nacif de Brey and Virginia M. Gonzalez, "Recruiting for Arthritis Studies in Hard-to-Reach Populations: A Comparison of Methods Used in an Urban Spanish-Speaking Community," *Arthritis Care and Research* 10, no. 1 (February 1997): 64.

47. For an example of the former, see Folmar et al., "Recruitment of Participants," 13–25; and of the latter, see Paul K. Whelton et al., "Recruitment Experience in the African American Study of Kidney Disease and Hypertension (AASK) Pilot Study," *Controlled Clinical Trials* 17, no. 4, suppl. 1 (August 1996): S17–S33.

48. Foucault, *Discipline and Punish*.

49. Science studies has long been interested in understanding the link between the construction of natural order and social order. See Shapin and Schaffer, *Leviathan and the Air-Pump*. Recently this issue has been investigated under the rubric of "co-production." According to Sheila Jasanoff: "co-production is shorthand for the proposition that the ways in which we know and represent the world (both nature and society) are inseparable from the ways in which we choose to live in it." Jasanoff, "Idiom of Co-Production," 2–3. My reference to "mapping" is also meant to invoke Thomas Gieryn's analysis of how varied social groups make sense of science through "cultural cartography." Gieryn, *Cultural Boundaries of Science*.

50. For example, at a conference on health research in communities of color, Anna Nápoles-Springer at the Center for Aging in Diverse Communities of the University of

California, San Francisco, reported on focus groups conducted with older Latinos and African Americans, as well as results from a questionnaire mailed to key informants at 117 community-based organizations serving those groups. The themes that surfaced repeatedly were a distrust of researchers, a lack of information about medical research, a fear of experimentation, and a perceived lack of benefits. "Health Research in Communities of Color: Are We Making a Difference?" forum sponsored by Center for Aging in Diverse Communities at the University of California, San Francisco, March 23, 1999 (author's field notes).

51. Kathryn Whetten-Goldstein, "Rural Populations: Challenges in Recruitment, Retention, and Relevance," in *Science Meets Reality*, 121–23.

52. "Science Meets Reality" workshop (author's field notes). The term was used by Kwame Osei.

53. For examples, see A. C. King, R. B. Harris, and W. L. Haskell, "Effect of Recruitment Strategy on Types of Subjects Entered into a Primary Prevention Clinical Trial," *Annals of Epidemiology* 4, no. 4 (July 1994): 312–20; DPP Research Group, "The Diabetes Prevention Program: Recruitment Methods and Results," *Controlled Clinical Trials* 23 (2002): 157–71, esp. 166–67; Cabral et al., "Population- and Community-Based Recruitment," 272–79.

54. Kusek, interview. See also Stephen B. Thomas and Sandra Crouse Quinn, "The Tuskegee Syphilis Study, 1932 to 1972: Implications for HIV Education and AIDS Risk Education Programs in the Black Community," *American Journal of Public Health* 81, no. 11 (November 1991): 1498–1505.

55. See, for example, Giselle Corbie-Smith, "The Continuing Legacy of the Tuskegee Syphilis Study: Considerations for Clinical Investigation," *American Journal of the Medical Sciences* 317, no. 1 (January 1999): 5–8; Vickie L. Shavers, Charles F. Lynch, and Leon F. Burmeister, "Knowledge of the Tuskegee Study and Its Impact on the Willingness to Participate in Medical Research Studies," *Journal of the National Medical Association* 92 (2000): 563–72; Giselle Corbie-Smith, Stephen B. Thomas, and Diane Marie M. St. George, "Distrust, Race, and Research," *Archives of Internal Medicine* 162 (November 25, 2002): 2458–63; Vickie L. Shavers, Charles F. Lynch, and Leon F. Burmeister, "Racial Differences in Factors That Influence the Willingness to Participate in Medical Research Studies," *Annals of Epidemiology* 12, no. 4 (May 2002): 248–56.

56. Shavers, Lynch, and Burmeister, "Racial Differences in Factors," 252.

57. Gamble, "Under the Shadow of Tuskegee," 1773. See also D. T. Brandon, L. A. Isaac, and T. A. LaVeist, "The Legacy of Tuskegee and Trust in Medical Care: Is Tuskegee Responsible for Race Differences in Mistrust of Medical Care?" *Journal of the National Medical Association* 97, no. 7 (July 2005): 951–56.

58. Corbie-Smith, Thomas, and St. George, "Distrust, Race, and Research," 2458.

59. Health Research in Communities of Color forum (author's field notes).

60. Giselle Corbie-Smith, interviewed by author.

61. Julia Scott, interviewed by author.

62. Gina Moreno-John et al., "Ethnic Minority Older Adults Participating in Clinical Research: Developing Trust," *Journal of Aging and Health* 16, no. 5 suppl. (November 2004): 98S. See also Barbara W. Lex and Janice Racine Norris, "Health Status of American Indian and Alaska Native Women," in *Women and Health Research*, ed. Mastroianni, Faden, and Federman, 2:192–215.

63. Moreno-John et al., "Ethnic Minority Older Adults," 101S.

64. Mary-Rose Mueller, "Involvement and (Potential) Influence of Care Providers in the Enlistment Phase of the Informed Consent Process: The Case of AIDS Clinical Trials," *Nursing Ethics* 11, no. 1 (2004): 42–52.

65. Ibid., 47.

66. The phrase "technology of trust" is from Oudshoorn, *Male Pill*, 225–41. More generally, on the centrality of trust relationships to the maintenance of moral order in modern science, see Steven Shapin, *A Social History of Truth: Civility and Science in Seventeenth-Century England* (Chicago: University of Chicago Press, 1994).

67. Deborah J. Cotton et al., "Determinants of Accrual of Women to a Large, Multicenter Clinical Trials Program of Human Immunodeficiency Virus Infection," *Journal of Acquired Immune Deficiency Syndromes* 6, no. 12 (1993): 1327; Estina E. Thompson et al., "Recruitment and Retention of African American Patients for Clinical Research: An Exploration of Response Rates in an Urban Psychiatric Hospital," *Journal of Consulting and Clinical Psychology* 64, no. 5 (1996): 864; Nancy Stark et al., "Increasing Participation of Minorities in Cancer Clinical Trials: Summary of the 'Moving beyond the Barriers' Conference in North Carolina," *Journal of the National Medical Association* 94, no. 1 (January 2002): 34.

68. Claude Lenfant, interviewed by author; Kusek, interview.

69. Victoria Cargill, "Recruitment and Retention in the Real World," in *Science Meets Reality*, 112.

70. Personal communication, 1999.

71. Gay Men's Health Summit II, Boulder, CO, July 19–23, 2000 (author's field notes).

72. Moreno-John et al., "Ethnic Minority Older Adults," 104S.

73. Ibid., 114S, 117S.

74. Barbara L. Dancy et al., "Community-Based Research: Barriers to Recruitment of African Americans," *Nursing Outlook* 52, no. 5 (2004): 234–40; see also Giselle Corbie-Smith, Sandra Moody-Ayers, and Angela D. Thrasher, "Closing the Circle between Minority Inclusion in Research and Health Disparities," *Archives of Internal Medicine* 164 (July 12, 2004): 1362–64. More generally, on the use of participatory action research in the domain of health, see N. Khanlou and E. Peter, "Participatory Action Research: Considerations for Ethical Review," *Social Science and Medicine* 60, no. 10 (2005): 2333–40.

75. Neal Dickert and Jeremy Sugarman, "Ethical Goals of Community Consultation in Research," *American Journal of Public Health* 95, no. 7 (July 2005); Reardon, *Race to the Finish*.

76. Barbara V. Howard, "Recruitment and Retention in American Indian/Alaska Native Communities," in *Science Meets Reality*, 49.

77. Ilena M. Norton and Spero M. Manson, "Research in American Indian and Alaska Native Communities: Navigating the Cultural Universe of Values and Processes," *Journal of Consulting and Clinical Psychology* 64, no. 5 (1996): 858.

78. J. Goodman, Anthony McElligott, and Lara Marks, "Making Human Bodies Useful: Historicizing Medical Experiments in the Twentieth Century," in *Useful Bodies*, ed. Goodman, McElligott, and Marks, 13.

79. "Human Subject Protection; Foreign Clinical Studies Not Conducted under an Investigational New Drug Application," *Federal Register* 69, no. 112 (June 10, 2004): 32471.

80. Adriana Petryna, "Globalizing Human Subjects Research," in *Global Pharmaceuticals: Ethics, Markets, Practices*, ed. Adriana Petryna, Andrew Lakoff, and Arthur Kleinman (Durham, NC: Duke University Press, 2006), 37.

81. David J. Rothman, "The Shame of Medical Research," *New York Review of Books*, November 30, 2000, 63. See also Samiran Nundy and Chandra M. Gulhati, "A New Colonialism? Conducting Clinical Trials in India," *New England Journal of Medicine* 352, no. 16 (April 21, 2005): 1634.

82. LatinTrials, "Why Latin America?" n.d. (accessed July 10, 2005), www.latintrials .com/why.htm.

83. Ray Marcelo, "India Beckons as a Test-Bed for Western Drug Companies," *Financial Times*, 14 October 2003, 24.

84. Nundy and Gulhati, "New Colonialism?" 1634.

85. Ibid., 1635.

86. Certain implications of globalized research are discussed in other chapters, including the complexities of the NIH reporting requirements on the racial and ethnic compositions of foreign study populations (chapter 7) and the potential spread of inclusionary requirements to other countries (chapter 12).

87. "FDA Panel Debates Issues Involved in HIV Perinatal Transmission Trials," *Reuters Medical News*, October 10, 1999.

88. Peter Lurie and Sidney M. Wolfe, "Unethical Trials of Interventions to Reduce Perinatal Transmission of the Human Immunodeficiency Virus in Developing Countries," *New England Journal of Medicine* 337, no. 12 (September 18, 1997): 853-56.

89. Marcia Angell, "The Ethics of Clinical Research in the Third World," *New England Journal of Medicine* 337, no. 12 (September 18, 1997): 847-49. Angell became editor-in-chief in 1999.

90. Sheryl Gay Stolberg, "Defense for Third-World H.I.V. Experiments," *New York Times*, October 2, 1997, A10. On the use of the Tuskegee metaphor, see also Amy L. Fairchild and Ronald Bayer, "Uses and Abuses of Tuskegee," *Science* 284 (May 7, 1999): 919-21.

91. George J. Annas and Michael A. Grodin, "Human Rights and Maternal-Fetal HIV Transmission Prevention Trials in Africa," *American Journal of Public Health* 88, no. 4 (April 1998): 560-63; Robert J. Levine, "The Need to Revise the Declaration of Helsinki," *New England Journal of Medicine* 341, no. 7 (August 12, 1999): 531-34; Rothman, "Shame of Medical Research," 60-64.

92. On the transnational diffusion of the inclusion-and-difference paradigm, see chapter 12.

CHAPTER TEN

1. See the references in the introduction, n. 21.

2. One exception to the pattern of separating consideration of racial profiling from that of sex profiling is the work of Anne Fausto-Sterling, who is following up on a critical examination of the use of sex and gender categories in one domain of medical research (bone diseases) with a forthcoming article on racial categories in the same domain. See Anne Fausto-Sterling, "The Bare Bones of Sex: Part 1—Sex and Gender," *Signs* 30, no. 2 (2005): 1491-1527.

3. Hahn, "State of Federal Health Statistics," 269.

4. Williams, "Race and Health," 324.

5. Hahn and Stroup, "Race and Ethnicity in Public Health Surveillance," 7-8.

6. Newton G. Osborne and Marvin Feit, "The Use of Race in Medical Research," *Journal of the American Medical Association* 267, no. 2 (January 8, 1992): 275.

7. Leon D. Hankoff, letter to the editor, *Journal of the American Medical Association* 267, no. 23 (17 June 1992): 3150.

8. Newton G. Osborne, "Reply to Letters to the Editor," *Journal of the American Medical Association* 267, no. 23 (June 17, 1992): 3151.

9. Fullilove, "Abandoning 'Race' as a Variable," 1297–98.

10. Harold P. Freeman, "The Meaning of Race in Science—Considerations for Cancer Research: Concerns of Special Populations in the National Cancer Program," *Cancer* 82, no. 1 (1998): 220.

11. "Uniform Requirements for Manuscripts," *New England Journal of Medicine*.

12. George Lundberg, interviewed by author. By contrast, certain journals, such as the *BMJ* (*British Medical Journal*), have published more specific guidelines calling for complete descriptions of populations and the criteria used for classification. For example, contributors are advised to use descriptors such as "self-assigned as black Caribbean" in place of "black," and "UK-born individuals of Vietnamese ancestry" in place of "Asian." Trude Bennett and Raj Bhopal, "US Health Journal Editors' Opinions and Policies on Research in Race, Ethnicity and Health," *Journal of the National Medical Association* 90, no. 7 (1998): 402.

13. Frederick P. Rivara and Laurence Finberg, "Use of the Terms Race and Ethnicity," *Archives of Pediatrics and Adolescent Medicine* 155, no. 2 (February 2001): 119.

14. S. Nelson, "Reply to 'MEDLINE Definitions of Race and Ethnicity,'" 120.

15. Thomas H. Maugh II, "Scientists Offer Explanation of HIV Resistance," *Los Angeles Times*, August 9, 1996, A1.

16. Jeremy J. Martinson et al., "Global Distribution of the *CCR5* Gene 32-Basepair Deletion," *Nature Genetics* 16 (May 1997): 100.

17. Priscilla Wald cites examples and discusses this incident in Priscilla Wald, "Future Perfect: Grammar, Genes, and Geography," *New Literary History* 31, no. 4 (fall 2000): 689.

18. Edward M. Sellers, "Pharmacogenetics and Ethnoracial Differences in Smoking," *Journal of the American Medical Association* 280, no. 2 (July 8, 1998): 179.

19. Ibid. Results from studies of CYP2A6 and smoking have been inconsistent, and the data on distribution of the allele do not necessarily correspond in a predictable way with the data on the epidemiology of smoking-related illnesses. For critical analyses of the literature on the genetics of smoking, see Shields et al., "Use of Race Variables in Genetic Studies"; and S. Lee, Mountain, and Koenig, "Meanings of 'Race' in the New Genomics," 55.

20. Matthew W. Weir et al., "Differing Mechanisms of Action of Angiotensin-Converting Enzyme Inhibition in Black and White Hypertensive Patients," *Hypertension* 26, no. 1 (July 1995): 124–30; A. D. Richardson and R. W. Piepho, "Effect of Race on Hypertension and Antihypertensive Therapy," *International Journal of Clinical Pharmacology and Therapeutics* 38, no. 2 (2000): 75–79; Antihypertensive and Lipid-Lowering Treatment to Prevent Heart Attack Trial, "Frequently Asked Questions for Clinicians," May 1, 2003, http://allhat.sph.uth.tmc.edu/results/faqsclinicians.cfm.

21. National Heart Lung and Blood Institute, NIH, "The Seventh Report of the Joint National Committee on Prevention, Detection, Evaluation, and Treatment of High Blood Pressure," NIH Publication no. 03–5233, May 2003. See also the somewhat differing guidelines of the International Society on Hypertension in Blacks, which likewise recommends combination therapy for African Americans. Janice G. Douglas et al., "Management of High Blood Pressure in African Americans: Consensus Statement of the Hypertension in

African Americans Working Group of the International Society on Hypertension in Blacks," *Archives of Internal Medicine* 163, no. 5 (March 10, 2003): 525–41.

22. For a discussion see Tate and Goldstein, "Will Tomorrow's Medicines Work for Everyone?" S35. Some also have hypothesized that African American hypertension differences reflect genetic selection effects related to the hardships of slavery and the Middle Passage; for a critical debunking, see Richard S. Cooper, Charles N. Rotimi, and Ryk Ward, "The Puzzle of Hypertension in African-Americans," *Scientific American*, February 1999, 63; Kaufman and Hall, "Slavery Hypertension Hypothesis," 111–26.

23. Kenneth A. Jamerson, "Prevalence of Complications and Response to Different Treatments of Hypertension in African Americans and White Americans in the U.S.," *Clinical and Experimental Hypertension* 15, no. 6 (November 1993): 979–95.

24. Tate and Goldstein, "Will Tomorrow's Medicines Work for Everyone?" S34.

25. See table 1 in ibid., S36–S37.

26. Jonathan Kahn, "From Disparity to Difference: How Race-Specific Medicines May Undermine Policies to Address Inequalities in Health Care," *Southern California Interdisciplinary Law Journal* 15 (2005): 105–29.

27. Carolyn Abraham, "The New Science of Race," *Globe and Mail*, June 18, 2005. See also S. Lee, Mountain, and Koenig, "Meanings of 'Race' in the New Genomics," 36–37.

28. Vence L. Bonham, Esther Warshauer-Baker, and Francis S. Collins, "Race and Ethnicity in the Genome Era: The Complexity of the Constructs," *American Psychologist* 60, no. 1 (January 2005): 11–12.

29. Templeton, "Human Races in the Context of Recent Human Evolution," 252; A. Goodman, "Two Questions about Race"; Audrey Smedley and Brian D. Smedley, "Race as Biology Is Fiction, Racism as Social Problem Is Real: Anthropological and Historical Perspectives on the Social Construction of Race," *American Psychologist* 60, no. 1 (January 2005): 16–26.

30. "Remarks Made by the President, Prime Minister Tony Blair of England (via Satellite), Dr. Francis Collins, Director of the National Human Genome Research Institute, and Dr. Craig Venter, President and Chief Scientific Officer, Celera Genomics Corporation, on the Completion of the First Survey of the Entire Human Genome Project," press release (Office of the Press Secretary, White House, June 26, 2000, www.genome.gov/10001356.

31. Susanne B. Haga and J. Craig Venter, "FDA Races in Wrong Direction," *Science* 301, no. 5632 (July 25, 2003): 466.

32. A single nucleotide polymorphism is a common variation of a nucleotide (one of the structural components of DNA) at a given point in the genetic sequence.

33. Alleles are alternative forms of a single gene, and *frequency* refers to their prevalence within a defined population.

34. Rick A. Kittles and Kenneth M. Weiss, "Race, Ancestry, and Genes: Implications for Defining Disease Risk," *Annual Review of Genomics and Human Genetics* 4, no. 1 (2003): 37–38.

35. J. Marks, *Human Biodiversity*, 112, 162.

36. Lynn B. Jorde and Stephen P. Wooding, "Genetic Variation, Classification and 'Race,'" *Nature Genetics* 36, no. 11 (November 2004): S32.

37. Wailoo, *Drawing Blood*, 134–61; Tapper, *In the Blood*; Wailoo, "Inventing the Heterozygote." As Charles Rotimi at Howard University's National Human Genome Center has noted, "The label 'black disease' . . . rendered the distribution of sickle cell anemia invisible

in other populations, leading to erroneous understanding of the geographical distribution of the underlying genetic variants. This is one reason why many people, including physicians, are unaware that the town of Orchomenos in central Greece has a rate of sickle cell anemia that is twice that of African Americans and that black South Africans do not carry the sickle-cell trait." Charles N. Rotimi, "Are Medical and Nonmedical Uses of Large-Scale Genomic Markers Conflating Genetics and 'Race'?" *Nature Genetics* 36, no. 11 (November 2004): S45.

38. Graves, *Emperor's New Clothes*, chap. 11.

39. Neil Risch et al., "Categorization of Humans in Biomedical Research: Genes, Race and Disease," *Genome Biology* 3, no. 7 (2002): 2007.6 See also Esteban González Burchard et al., "The Importance of Race and Ethnic Background in Biomedical Research and Clinical Practice," *New England Journal of Medicine* 348, no. 12 (March 20, 2003): 1170–75; Joanna L. Mountain and Neil Risch, "Assessing Genetic Contributions to Phenotypic Differences among 'Racial' and 'Ethnic' Groups," *Nature Genetics* 36, no. 11S (November 2004): S48–S53.

40. James F. Wilson et al., "Population Genetic Structure of Variable Drug Response," *Nature Genetics* 29, no. 3 (October 29, 2001): 266.

41. Lundy Braun, "Genetic Explanations for Health Disparities: What Is at Stake?" in *Proceedings of the Conference on Genetics and Health Disparities* (Ann Arbor: University of Michigan, Survey Research Center, Institute for Social Research, March 20–21, 2004), 127. On the appeal of Risch's claims and rhetoric, see also Fausto-Sterling, "Refashioning Race," 9–10; and for an evaluation of the debate, see Sankar and Cho, "Toward a New Vocabulary of Human Genetic Variation," 1337–38.

42. On the cultural appeal of genetic explanations and on genetics in the mass media, see Nelkin and Lindee, *DNA Mystique*; Peter Conrad, "Public Eyes and Private Genes: Historical Frames, News Constructions, and Social Problems," *Social Problems* 44, no. 2 (May 2001): 139–54; Peter Conrad and Susan Markens, "Constructing the 'Gay Gene' in the News: Optimism and Skepticism in the US and British Press," *Health* 5, no. 3 (July 2001): 373–400. On the complexities of lay understandings of genetics and race, see Celeste M. Condit et al., "The Role of 'Genetics' in Popular Understandings of Race in the United States," *Public Understanding of Science* 13, no. 3 (July 2004): 249–72.

43. Robert S. Schwartz, editorial, "Racial Profiling in Medical Research," *New England Journal of Medicine* 344, no. 18 (3 May 2001): 1392.

44. Ibid., 1393.

45. Lila Guterman, "Shades of Doubt and Fears of Bias in the Doctor's Office," *Chronicle of Higher Education*, May 25, 2001.

46. Sheryl Gay Stolberg, "Skin Deep: Shouldn't a Pill Be Colorblind?" *New York Times*, May 13, 2001, 4–1. On the role of professional groups such as the Association of Black Cardiologists in "the aggressive pursuit of trial diversity," see also Susanna Space, "Advocacy Groups Lead in Diversity," *Center Watch Monthly* 12, no. 11 (November 2005): 13.

47. Jamerson had argued that "African American race is not a clinically significant predictor of poor response to any class of antihypertensive therapy and there is little justification to use racial profiling as a criterion for choice of medication." Jamerson, "Prevalence of Complications," 979.

48. John Kifner and David M. Herszenhorn, "Racial 'Profiling' at Crux of Inquiry into Shooting by Troopers," *New York Times*, May 8, 1998, B1.

49. Helen Peterson, "Gore Promises NAACP: I'll End Racial Profiling," *New York Daily News*, July 16, 1999, 82.

50. On racial profiling in general, see Frederick Schauer, *Profiles, Probabilities, and Stereotypes* (Cambridge, MA: Harvard University Press, 2003); Rodney D. Coates, "Introduction: Critical Racial and Ethnic Studies—Profiling and Reparations," *American Behavioral Scientist* 47, no. 7 (March 2004): 873-78.

51. Sally Satel, "I Am a Racially Profiling Doctor," *New York Times Magazine*, May 5, 2002, 56. See also Sally Satel, "Medicine's Race Problem," *Policy Review*, December 2001.

52. Satel, "Science by Quota," 14-15.

53. Satel, *P.C., M.D.*

54. See, for example, the debate in the *New England Journal* in 2003: Burchard et al., "Importance of Race and Ethnic Background," 1170-75; Cooper, Kaufman, and Ward, "Race and Genomics," 1166-70; Elizabeth G. Phimister, "Medicine and the Racial Divide," *New England Journal of Medicine* 348, no. 12 (March 20, 2003): 1081-82.

55. Okay Odocha, "Race and Racialism in Scientific Research and Publication in the Journal of the National Medical Association," *Journal of the National Medical Association* 92, no. 2 (2000): 96.

56. Ian Hacking, "Why Race Still Matters," *Daedalus*, winter 2005, 107 (emphasis in the original).

57. Naomi Zack, *Philosophy of Science and Race* (London: Routledge, 2002), 100-101.

58. Root, "Problem of Race in Medicine"; Michael Root, "The Use of Race in Medicine as a Proxy for Genetic Differences," *Philosophy of Science* 70 (December 2003): 1173-83.

59. Rose, "Politics of Life Itself," 8. On the rise of the "risk factor" in modern medicine, see also chap. 2, n. 68. On the notion of the "risk group," see Alex Preda, *AIDS, Rhetoric, and Scientific Knowledge* (New York: Cambridge University Press, 2004).

60. Although donated blood is tested for the presence of antibodies to HIV, such antibodies do not form until two weeks to six months after infection, leaving a "window period" during which infected blood could enter the blood supply undetected.

61. Duster, "Buried Alive," 265 (emphasis in the original). On this point see also Paul Rabinow, "Galton's Regret and DNA Typing," *Culture, Medicine and Psychiatry* 17, no. 1 (March 1993): 63.

62. James Jackson, interviewed by author.

63. Keh-Ming Lin, "Ethical Aspects of Psychopharmacological Studies in Different Ethnic Groups," *Clinical Neuropharmacology* 15, suppl., pt. A (1992): 484A. See also Keh-Ming Lin, "Biological Differences in Depression and Anxiety across Races and Ethnic Groups," *Journal of Clinical Psychiatry* 62, suppl. 13 (2001): 17.

64. Ashwini R. Sehgal, "Overlap between Whites and Blacks in Response to Antihypertensive Drugs," *Hypertension* 43 (March 2004): 569-70.

65. Celeste Condit, Joseph Graves, and Michael Root all have made similar arguments. See Abraham, "New Science of Race"; Graves, *Emperor's New Clothes*; Linda Villarosa, "A Conversation with Joseph Graves: Beyond Black and White in Biology and Medicine," *New York Times*, January 1, 2002, D5; Root, "Use of Race in Medicine," 1178.

66. Yusuf et al., "Analysis and Interpretation of Treatment Effects," 94. See also Silverman, *Human Experimentation*, 134. In this regard, opponents of the NIH Revitalization Act (see chapter 5) were making an important point.

67. ISIS-2 Collaborative Group, "Randomised Trial of Intravenous Streptokinase," 356.

68. Barnett Kramer, editor of the *Journal of the National Cancer Institute*, quoted in Gina Kolata, "Science Needs a Healthy Negative Outlook," *New York Times*, July 7, 2002, 4–10. According to Salim Yusuf and coauthors, engaging in post hoc subgroup analysis "smacks of betting on a horse after the race is over." Yusuf et al., "Analysis and Interpretation of Treatment Effects," 95.

69. L. A. Weisberg, "The Efficacy and Safety of Ticlopidine and Aspirin in Non-Whites: Analysis of a Patient Subgroup from the Ticlopidine Aspirin Stroke Study," *Neurology* 43, no. 1 (January 1993): 27.

70. Philip B. Gorelick et al., "Aspirin and Ticlopidine for Prevention of Recurrent Stroke in Black Patients: A Randomized Trial," *Journal of the American Medical Association* 289, no. 22 (June 11, 2003): 2953–55. See also Saif S. Rathore and Harlan M. Krumholz, "Race, Ethnic Group, and Clinical Research," *BMJ* 327, no. 7418 (October 4, 2003): 763–64.

71. Vastag, "Researchers Say Changes Needed," 537. While perhaps the most immediate danger from "data-trolling" is harm to patients, there is also the more diffuse risk of damaging trust relationships between researchers and communities of color. A 1991 study (later disconfirmed) that suggested that the drug AZT was less effective in "minorities" left behind a lingering cloud of suspicion. Epstein, *Impure Science*, 261–62. Seven years later, Wafaa El-Sadr, a clinician and researcher at Harlem Hospital, observed that the study had "perpetuated a sense of mistrust against the biomedical environment in general." Wafaa El-Sadr, interviewed by author.

72. Keh-Ming Lin, interviewed by author.

73. Elijah Saunders, interviewed by author.

74. Levy, *Ethnic and Racial Differences*, iii–v, 3.

75. Valentine J. Burroughs, Randall W. Maxey, and Richard A. Levy, "Racial and Ethnic Differences in Response to Medicines: Toward Individualized Pharmaceutical Treatment," *Journal of the National Medical Association* 94, no. 10 (suppl.) (October 2002): 2.

76. Angell, *Truth about the Drug Companies*.

77. Pear, "Congress Weighs Drug Comparisons," 16.

78. Jonathan Kahn, "How a Drug Becomes 'Ethnic.'" See also M. Gregg Bloche, "Race-Based Therapeutics," *New England Journal of Medicine* 351, no. 20 (November 8, 2004): 2035–37.

79. Robin Marantz Henig, "The Genome in Black and White (and Gray)," *New York Times Sunday Magazine*, October 10, 2004.

80. A. Taylor et al., "Combination of Isosorbide Dinitrate and Hydralazine"; Stephanie Saul, "F.D.A. Approves a Heart Drug for African-Americans," *New York Times*, June 24, 2005, C2.

81. Bloche, "Race-Based Therapeutics," 2036.

82. Ibid.

83. Stephanie Saul, "U.S. to Review Drug Intended for One Race," *New York Times*, June 13, 2005, A12.

84. Jonathan Kahn, "From Disparity to Difference."

85. Saul, "F.D.A. Approves a Heart Drug for African-Americans," C2.

86. Kevin Moseby and Steven Epstein, "Racial Niche Marketing and the Particularities of Racialization in Biomedicine: A Comparison of AIDSVAX and BiDil" (paper presented at the Annual Meeting of the Society for Social Studies of Science, Pasadena, October 21, 2005).

87. Andrew Pollack and Lawrence K. Altman, "Large Trial Finds AIDS Vaccine Fails to Stop Infection," *New York Times*, February 24, 2003, A1.

88. Carol Ezzell, "The Race Card," *Scientific American*, May 2003, 26.

89. Lawrence K. Altman, "Official Hopes to Explain AIDS Vaccine Disparities," *New York Times*, February 25, 2003, A23.

90. "The Diabolic Science: VaxGen's Claims of Vaccine Efficacy Evanesce in Autumn's Light," *TAGLine*, October 2003, 3.

91. Victoria Stagg Elliott, "Color-Blind? The Value of Racial Data in Medical Research," amednews.com, January 5, 2004.

92. Community HIV/AIDS Mobilization Project et al., letter to Dr. Debra B. Birnkrant, Director, FDA Division of Antiviral Products, April 20, 2006.

93. Kellee Terrell, "No Blacks Allowed? A Drug Trial Comes under Fire," POZ, April 5, 2006, www.poz.com/articles/401_2977.shtml.

94. "Activists: Hepatitis C Clinical Trial Unfairly Excludes Blacks," Advocate.com, April 4, 2006, www.advocate.com/news_detail.asp?id=28829.

95. Tate and Goldstein, "Will Tomorrow's Medicines Work for Everyone?" S39.

96. On pharmacogenomics generally, see Hedgecoe, *Politics of Personalized Medicine*; Mark A. Rothstein, ed., *Pharmacogenomics: Social, Ethical, and Clinical Dimensions* (Hoboken, NJ: Wiley, 2003).

97. Christine Gorman, "Drugs by Design," *Time*, January 11, 1999, 78. See also Gina Kolata, "Using Gene Testing to Decide a Patient's Treatment," *New York Times*, December 20, 1999, A1; Rick Weiss, "The Promise of Precision Prescriptions; 'Pharmacogenomics' Also Raises Issues of Race, Privacy," *Washington Post*, June 24, 2000.

98. For example, Valentine Burroughs and coauthors advise that "attention should be paid to the need to individualize drug therapy for specific population groups." Burroughs, Maxey, and Levy, "Racial and Ethnic Differences in Response to Medicines," 4. In chapter 7 I noted other examples of this tendency to refer to group-specific approaches as "individualization," and I suggested that an appeal to individualism provides legitimacy in a country where it serves as a cherished value.

99. Robert F. Service, "Pharmacogenomics: Going from Genome to Pill," *Science* 308, no. 5730 (June 24, 2005): 1858.

100. Howard L. McLeod, "Pharmacogenetics: More Than Skin Deep," *Nature Genetics* 29 (November 2001): 248-48.

101. Peter E. Cadman and Daniel T. O'Connor, "Pharmacogenomics of Hypertension," *Current Opinion in Nephrology and Hypertension* 12 (2003): 62.

102. Haga and Venter, "FDA Races in Wrong Direction," 466.

103. Satel, "I Am a Racially Profiling Doctor," 58.

104. Robert Temple, interviewed by author.

105. FDA, press release, "FDA Works to Speed the Advent of New, More Effective Personalized Medicines," March 22, 2005 www.fda.gov/bbs/topics/news/2005/NEW01167.html. See also the FDA Web page www.fda.gov/cder/genomics/default.htm.

106. See http://grants1.nih.gov/grants/guide/rfa-files/RFA-GM-99-004.html. The terms *pharmacogenetics* and *pharmacogenomics* are often used interchangeably, though the former has a longer history; on the differences, see Adam H. Hedgecoe, "Technology and the Construction of Scientific Disciplines: The Case of Pharmacogenomics," *Science, Technology, and Human Values* 28, no. 4 (fall 2003): 514.

107. Hedgecoe, "Technology and the Construction of Scientific Disciplines," 513–37; Hedgecoe, *Politics of Personalized Medicine*.

108. The Royal Society, "Medicines Personalised for Patients Still Decades Away," September 21, 2005, www.royalsoc.ac.uk/news.asp?year=&id=3781.

109. Morris W. Foster, Richard R. Sharp, and John J. Mulvihill, "Pharmacogenetics, Race, and Ethnicity: Social Identities and Individualized Medical Care," *Therapeutic Drug Monitoring* 23, no. 3 (2001): 233. See also Sandra Soo-Jin Lee, "Racializing Drug Design: Implications of Pharmacogenomics for Health Disparities," *American Journal of Public Health* 95, no. 12 (December 2005): 2134.

110. Mark A. Rothstein and Phyllis Griffin Epps, "Ethical and Legal Implications of Pharmacogenomics," *Nature Reviews: Genetics* 2 (March 2001): 229.

111. Temple, interview.

112. Henig, "Genome in Black and White (and Gray)."

113. Duster, "Race and Reification in Science," 1050.

114. Ariana Eunjung Cha, "Race Plays Role in New Drug Trials," *Washington Post*, July 28, 2003, A1.

115. Root, "Use of Race in Medicine," 1176.

116. S. Lee, Mountain, and Koenig, "Meanings of 'Race' in the New Genomics," 57. See also Jonathan Kahn, "From Disparity to Difference." For a parallel case involving the construal of environmental racism as a genetic issue, see Sara Shostak, "Environmental Justice and Genomics: Acting on the Futures of Environmental Health," *Science as Culture* 13, no. 4 (December 2004): 539–62.

117. Nancy Krieger, "Embodying Inequality: A Review of Concepts, Measures, and Methods for Studying Health Consequences of Discrimination," *International Journal of Health Services* 29, no. 2 (1999): 296.

118. Pilar Ossorio and Troy Duster, "Race and Genetics: Controversies in Biomedical, Behavioral, and Forensic Sciences," *American Psychologist* 60, no. 1 (January 2005): 116.

119. Fausto-Sterling, "Bare Bones of Sex: Part 1," 1510. See also Fausto-Sterling, "Refashioning Race," 13.

120. See n. 42 above.

121. O. E. Streeter and M. Roach, "Racial Differences in the Incidence, Behavior, and Management of Tumors of the Genitourinary Tract," in *Carcinoma of the Kidney and Testis, and Rare Urologic Malignancies: Innovations in Management*, ed. Z. Petrovich, L. Baert, and L. W. Brady (Berlin: Springer-Verlag, 1999), 433.

122. Peter B. Bach et al., "Survival of Blacks and Whites after a Cancer Diagnosis," *Journal of the American Medical Association* 287, no. 16 (April 24, 2002): 211–12.

123. Richard S. Cooper, "Hypertension in the African Diaspora: Genes and the Environment," in *Plain Talk about the Human Genome Project: A Tuskegee University Conference on Its Promise and Perils . . . And Matters of Race*, ed. Edward Smith and Walter Sapp (Tuskegee, AL: Tuskegee University Publications Office, 1997), 36. See also Cooper, Rotimi, and Ward, "Puzzle of Hypertension," 56–63.

124. Norman B. Anderson et al., "Hypertension in Blacks: Psychosocial and Biological Perspectives (Editorial Review)," *Journal of Hypertension* 7, no. 3 (1989): 161–72; Nancy Krieger, Stephen Sidney, and Eugenie Croakley, "Racial Discrimination and Skin Color in the Cardia Study: Implications for Public Health Research," *American Journal of Public Health* 88 (September 1998): 1308–13; Rebecca Din-Dzietham et al., "Perceived Stress

Following Race-Based Discrimination at Work Is Associated with Hypertension in African-Americans: The Metro Atlanta Heart Disease Study, 1999–2001," *Social Science and Medicine* 58, no. 3 (February 2004): 449–61.

125. Jing Fang, Shantha Madhavan, and Michael H. Alderman, "Influence of Nativity on Cancer Mortality among Black New Yorkers," *Cancer* 80, no. 1 (July 1997): 129–35.

126. Charlene Laino, "Racial Gap in Achievement of Hypertension Goals Grows," Medscape Medical News, November 14, 2003, www.medscape.com/viewarticle/464459.

127. Tate and Goldstein, "Will Tomorrow's Medicines Work for Everyone?" S35.

128. Bloche, "Race-Based Therapeutics," 2037.

129. Braun, "Race, Ethnicity, and Health," 159.

130. Ossorio and Duster, "Race and Genetics," 115–28.

131. I am grateful to Jenny Reardon for discussion of these issues.

132. See Fatimah Jackson, "African-American Responses to the Human Genome Project," *Public Understanding of Science* 8 (1999): 181–91, including her discussion (p. 185) of the "Manifesto on Genomic Studies among African-Americans."

133. King, "Dangers of Difference," 37; Patricia King, interviewed by author. For a somewhat similar perspective on the potential benefits of racial universalism in medicine, see Jacqueline Stevens, "Racial Meanings and Scientific Methods: Changing Policies for NIH-Sponsored Publications Reporting Human Variation," *Journal of Health Politics, Policy and Law* 28, no. 6 (December 2003): 1033–87, esp. 1077.

CHAPTER ELEVEN

1. Raymond Woosley, interviewed by author. Woosley maintains a list of pharmaceutical drugs linked to *torsades de pointes* at www.torsades.org. Many of them are associated with sex differences in risk. My account of the Seldane story also draws on Karen Young Kreeger, "The Inequality of Drug Metabolism," *Scientist* 16, no. 6 (March 18, 2002): 29. See also Woosley, Anthony, and Peck, "Biological Sex Analysis in Clinical Research," 933–34; Marietta Anthony, "Male/Female Differences in Pharmacology: Safety Issues with QT-Prolonging Drugs," *Journal of Women's Health* 14, no. 1 (2005): 47–52.

2. Jocelyn Kaiser, "Gender in the Pharmacy: Does It Matter?" *Science* 308, no. 5728 (June 10, 2005): 1572–74.

3. Viviana Simon, "Wanted: Women in Clinical Trials," *Science* 308, no. 5728 (10 June 2005): 1517.

4. Leslie Benet, interviewed by author. See also Benet's comments as quoted in Kaiser, "Gender in the Pharmacy," 1573.

5. Satel, *P.C., M.D.*, 125.

6. My searches for "sex profiling" and "gender profiling" in the National Library of Medicine's "PubMed" database retrieved null results. However, while this book was in production, I learned that Rebecca Young has used the phrase *sex profiling* from a critical perspective that is similar to my own. Rebecca Young, "Sexual Profiling: Contrasting Scientific Perspectives on Women's Health and the Embodiment of Marginality" (talk presented to the Barnard Center for Research on Women, New York City, April 2004).

7. However, Anne Fausto-Sterling is following up on a critical examination of the use of sex and gender categories in one domain of medical research (bone diseases) with a forthcoming article on the use of racial categories in the same domain. See Fausto-Sterling, "Bare Bones of Sex: Part 1."

8. Hacking, "Why Race Still Matters," 106.

9. Root, "Use of Race in Medicine," 1181.

10. For another example of the drawing of a clear distinction between sex and race in order to counter racial profiling in medicine, see Shields et al., "Use of Race Variables in Genetic Studies," 8. On boundary work in science, see the references in the introduction, n. 43.

11. Fausto-Sterling, "Five Sexes"; Anne Fausto-Sterling, "The Five Sexes, Revisited," *Sciences* (July/August 2000): 19–23. I expand on this point later in this chapter.

12. For a characteristic example, see Hara Estroff Marano, "The New Sex Scorecard," *Psychology Today*, July–August 2003, 38–46. On the debate over differences in brain function, see Angier and Chang, "Gray Matter and the Sexes." For critiques of biological reductionism in the understanding of male-female differences, see Roger N. Lancaster, *The Trouble with Nature: Sex in Science and Popular Culture* (Berkeley: University of California Press, 2003); Harding and O'Barr, *Sex and Scientific Inquiry*; Anne Fausto-Sterling, *Myths of Gender: Biological Theories about Women and Men* (New York: Basic, 1992); Tavris, *Mismeasure of Woman*; Fausto-Sterling, "Five Sexes," 20–26; Wijngaard, *Reinventing the Sexes*; Fausto-Sterling, "Five Sexes, Revisited," 19–23; Anne Fausto-Sterling, *Sexing the Body: Gender Politics and the Construction of Sexuality* (New York: Basic, 2000); Fausto-Sterling, "Bare Bones of Sex."

13. Bob Beale, "The Sexes: New Insights into the X and Y Chromosomes," *Scientist* 23 (July 2001): 18.

14. Mary J. Berg, "Pharmacological Differences between Men and Women," in *Principles of Clinical Pharmacology*, ed. Arthur J. Atkinson et al. (San Diego: Academic Press, 2001), 265–75.

15. Monica Gandhi et al., "Sex Differences in Pharmacokinetics and Pharmacodynamics," *Annual Review of Pharmacology and Toxicology* 44, no. 1 (2004): 499–523.

16. Ibid., 511–12.

17. Ibid., 512–13.

18. "FDA Commissioner & SWHR Outline Critical Steps to Improve Women's Health," *Sexx Matters*, fall 2003, 1.

19. See, for example, NIH, Office of Research on Women's Health, "Conference on Biologic and Molecular Mechanisms for Sex Differences in Pharmacokinetics, Pharmacodynamics, and Pharmacogenetics," May 5, 1999, www4.od.nih.gov/orwh/pharmacology.html.

20. Gail D. Anderson, "Sex and Racial Differences in Pharmacological Response: Where Is the Evidence? Pharmacogenetics, Pharmacokinetics, and Pharmacodynamics," *Journal of Women's Health* 14, no. 1 (2005): 25.

21. Rosaly Correa-de-Araujo, "Improving the Use and Safety of Medications in Women through Sex/Gender and Race/Ethnicity Analysis: Introduction," *Journal of Women's Health* 14, no. 1 (2005): 12.

22. "Medscape Women's Health eJournal: Instructions for Authors," www.medscape.com/viewpublication/128_guideline.

23. Doug Bowles, "A Radical Idea: Men and Women Are Different," *Cardiovascular Research* 61, no. 1 (January 2004): 5. See also Robert Preidt, "Nailing Down Differences in Heart Disease," HealthDayNews, December 16, 2003, www.healthscout.com/printer/1/516486/main.html.

24. Amanda Gardner, "The Gender Differences of Heart Disease," HealthScout News Service, February 21, 2004, www.healthday.com/printer.cfm?id=516951.

25. Denise Grady, "Many Women Face Hidden Risk of Heart Disease," *New York Times*, February 1, 2006.

26. Medscape, "Arrhythmias More Common in Men Than Women with Implanted Defibrillators," June 18, 2004, www.medscape.com/viewarticle/481325.

27. Michael E. Mendelsohn and Richard H. Karas, "Molecular and Cellular Basis of Cardiovascular Gender Differences," *Science* 308, no. 5728 (June 10, 2005): 1583–87.

28. Ridker et al., "Randomized Trial of Low-Dose Aspirin"; Mary Duenwald, "Aspirin Is Found to Protect Women from Strokes, Not Heart Attacks," *New York Times*, March 8, 2005, F5.

29. Richard I. Levin, "The Puzzle of Aspirin and Sex," *New England Journal of Medicine* 352, no. 13 (March 31, 2005): 1366. Levin did also observe that the Women's Health Study and the Physicians' Health Study were "not directly comparable," due to the time lag between them and the overall changes in mortality from cardiovascular causes in the interim (1367).

30. Marilynn Marchione, "Study: Aspirin Affects Sexes Differently," *San Diego Union-Tribune*, March 8, 2005, A1; Rob Stein, "Aspirin's Benefits Differ for Women," *Washington Post*, March 8, 2005, A1.

31. Theresa M. Wizemann and Mary-Lou Pardue, *Exploring the Biological Contributions to Human Health: Does Sex Matter?* (Washington, DC: National Academy Press, 2001), x.

32. Ibid., 178–79.

33. See the discussion in the preceding chapter.

34. "Sex Matters," *The NewsHour with Jim Lehrer*, PBS, April 25, 2001.

35. Robert Pear, "Sex Differences Called Key in Medical Studies," *New York Times*, April 25, 2001, A14.

36. Comments at "Science Meets Reality" workshop (author's field notes).

37. Five years later, the organization's president, Phyllis Greenberger, was named one of the one hundred "Most Powerful Women" in Washington, DC, by *Washingtonian* magazine. Society for Women's Health Research, "Society President Named One of 100 Most Powerful Women in Washington," June 6, 2006 www.womenshealthresearch.org/site/News2?page= NewsArticle&id=5808&JServSessionIdr002=6pgqjyjp23.app6b.

38. Florence B. Haseltine, conclusion to *Women's Health Research: A Medical and Policy Primer*, ed. Florence B. Haseltine and Beverly Greenberg Jacobson (Washington, DC: Health Press International, 1997), 331–36.

39. Florence Haseltine, interviewed by author.

40. Marianne J. Legato and Carol Colman, *The Female Heart: The Truth about Women and Coronary Artery Disease* (New York: Simon & Schuster, 1991); Marianne J. Legato, "Men, Women, and Brains: What's Hardwired, What's Learned, and What's Controversial," *Gender Medicine* 2, no. 2 (2005): 59–61.

41. Society for Women's Health Research, "What Is Sex-Based Biology?" www.womens healthresearch.org/site/PageServer?pagename=hs_sbb.

42. Society for the Advancement of Women's Health Research, "Annual Update on Women's Health Research: Discoveries and Implications" (Eighth Annual Scientific Advisory Meeting of the Society for the Advancement of Women's Health Research, Washington, DC, November 2, 1998).

43. For a few years, the title was changed to the *Journal of Women's Health and Gender-Specific Medicine*.

44. Sherry Marts, interviewed by author.

45. Karen Young Kreeger, "X and Y Chromosomes Concern More Than Reproduction," *Scientist* 16, no. 3 (February 4, 2002).

46. Susan Brenna, "Women's Health: Sex Matters," *New York Magazine*, February 8, 1999.

47. See the Partnership's Web site at www.cumc.columbia.edu/dept/partnership/.

48. Marianne J. Legato, "Why Do We Need an *Association for Gender-Specific Medicine?*" *Journal of Gender-Specific Medicine* 6, no. 1 (2003).

49. See www.gendermedicine.com/default.asp.

50. See womenshealth.stanford.edu/research/.

51. Karen Birmingham, "NIH Funds Gender Biology Research," *Nature Medicine* 6, no. 9 (September 2000): 950.

52. NIH, "Specialized Centers of Research on Sex and Gender Factors Affecting Women's Health (RFA-OD-02-002)" (Washington, DC: U.S. Department of Health & Human Services, December 18, 2001).

53. Viviana Simon et al., "National Institutes of Health: Intramural and Extramural Support for Research on Sex Differences, 2000–2003" (Washington, DC: Society for Women's Health Research, May 2005), www.womenshealthresearch.org/site/DocServer/CRISP report.pdf. The authors found that the percentage of funding devoted to the study of sex differences varied significantly from one institute to another, with the highest percentage, nearly 8 percent, at the National Institute on Alcohol Abuse and Alcoholism.

54. Society for Women's Health Research, press release, "Senate Appropriations Committee Instructs the National Institutes of Health to Make 'Sex-Based Biology an Integral Part' of Research," September 20, 2004, www.womenshealthresearch.org/site/News2? page=NewsArticle&id=5477; Correa-de-Araujo, "Improving the Use and Safety of Medications," 13. Recommendations contained in "report language" from Congress are not legally binding, but government agencies tend to take them seriously as indications of strong congressional concern about a topic.

55. Keating and Cambrosio, *Biomedical Platforms*, 19. See also Rae Bucher, "On the Natural History of Health Care Occupations," *Work and Occupations* 15, no. 2 (May 1988): 131–47.

56. Council on Scientific Affairs, American Medical Association, "Featured CSA Report: Women's Health: Sex- and Gender-Based Differences in Health and Disease" (CSA Report 4, I-00, 2000, www.ama-assn.org/ama/pub/print/article/2036-4946.html. Another indicator was the announcement in 2006 of funding from the Fannie E. Rippel Foundation to support investigators performing "sex-difference biomedical research and gender-specific medicine." Fannie E. Rippel Foundation, "Rippel Scholars Program—2006 Competition," April 25, 2006, http://foundationcenter.org/grantmaker/rippel/scholars.pdf.

57. Society for the Advancement of Women's Health Research, *Vive La Différence! [sic] A Comprehensive Introduction to Gender-Based Biology*, videotape (Washington, DC: Society for the Advancement of Women's Health Research, 1998).

58. See http://womenshealth.stanford.edu/research/.

59. Elizabeth Shaw, "What Your Doctor Didn't Learn in Med School," *American Health for Women* 17, no. 6 (July/August 1998): 42.

60. Rubin, "Traffic in Women," 179.

61. Nancy Chodorow, *The Reproduction of Mothering: Psychoanalysis and the Sociology of Gender* (Berkeley: University of California Press, 1978).

62. See Echols, *Daring to Be Bad.*

63. Vogel, *Woman Questions*, 111. See also Vogel, *Mothers on the Job*.

64. On symmetric versus asymmetric approaches, see Vogel, *Woman Questions*, 113–18; V. Taylor, *Rock-a-by Baby*, 166–68. I return to the issue of the "equality versus difference" debate in the conclusion.

65. Katha Pollitt, *Reasonable Creatures: Essays on Women and Feminism* (New York: Knopf, 1994), 58.

66. Healy, "Challenging Sameness," 18.

67. Marano, "New Sex Scorecard."

68. Marianne J. Legato, "Gender-Specific Physiology: How Real Is It? How Important Is It?" *International Journal of Fertility and Women's Medicine* 42, no. 1 (1997): 26.

69. Marts, interview.

70. Angier and Chang, "Gray Matter and the Sexes."

71. Legato, "Men, Women, and Brains," 59. Legato did not entirely endorse Summers's remarks; she commented that "what Dr. Summers might have more accurately expressed is that when vast numbers of people are tested, there are well-documented differences in some abilities between the sexes" (60).

72. Ibid., 61. For a critique of claims of sex differences in brain anatomy, see Fausto-Sterling, *Sexing the Body*, 115–45.

73. On the U.S. women's health movement generally, see the references in chap. 3, n. 9.

74. Sheryl Burt Ruzek and Julie Becker, "The Women's Health Movement in the United States: From Grass-Roots Activism to Professional Agendas," *Journal of the American Medical Women's Association* 54, no. 1 (winter 1999): 7; Judy Norsigian, interviewed by author; Julia Scott, interviewed by author; Cynthia Pearson, interviewed by author. Another interesting difference is the increasingly gender-neutral framing of the political project mounted by the medically minded professionals: although clearly the new advocacy groups remain recognizably focused on health as a women's issue, the goal of sex-based biology is promoted in terms of its benefits to both sexes. Marianne J. Legato, "Research on the Biology of Women Will Improve Health Care for Men, Too," *Chronicle of Higher Education*, May 15, 1998, B5. It is worth noting the emergence of a men's sex-based biology movement, as reflected by the launch, in 2004, of the *Journal of Men's Health and Gender*.

75. On SWHR, see www.womenshealthresearch.org/about/corppart.htm; on Legato's Partnership, see Gigi Verna, "Partners to Study Gender Medicine," *American City Business Journal*, March 24, 1997.

76. Vivian Pinn, interviewed by author.

77. Treichler, Cartwright, and Penley, "Paradoxes of Visibility," 5.

78. Eckman, "Beyond 'the Yentl Syndrome,'" 145.

79. Ibid., 149.

80. Haseltine, conclusion to *Women's Health Research*, 333; Legato and Colman, *Female Heart*.

81. "Men and Women Are Different," *USA Today (Magazine)*, April 2003, 8.

82. Hirschauer and Mol, "Shifting Sexes, Moving Stories," 377.

83. Woosley, interview.

84. Judith Lorber, "Believing Is Seeing: Biology as Ideology," *Gender and Society* 7, no. 4 (December 1993): 571. See also Jeanne Mager Stellman and Joan E. Bertin, editorial, "Science's Anti-Female Bias," *New York Times*, June 4, 1990, A23; Joan E. Bertin and Laurie R. Beck, "Of Headlines and Hypotheses: The Role of Gender in Popular Press Coverage of

Women's Health and Biology," in *Man-Made Medicine*, ed. Moss, 37–56. Such work draws on an earlier history of critique of scientific studies of sex differences; see, for example, Susan Leigh Star, "Sex Differences and the Dichotomization of the Brain: Methods, Limits and Problems in Research on Consciousness," in *Genes and Gender II*, ed. Hubbard and Lowe, 113–30; Harding and O'Barr, *Sex and Scientific Inquiry*.

85. On this point see Hanson, *Social Assumptions, Medical Categories*.

86. Barbara Hanson, "Gender Blind, Sex Bind: Sex Categories as Problematic to Cancer Research and Intervention" (Annual Meeting of the American Sociological Association, Chicago, August 1999).

87. Sheryl Burt Ruzek, Adele K. Clarke, and Virginia L. Olesen, "What Are the Dynamics of Differences?" in *Women's Health: Complexities and Differences*, ed. Ruzek, Olesen, and Clarke, 52.

88. Nieca Goldberg, *Women Are Not Small Men: Life-Saving Strategies for Preventing and Healing Heart Disease in Women* (New York: Ballantine, 2002). Missing from most of this literature is an understanding of the "intersectionality" of identities. See Crenshaw, "Mapping the Margins." Ironically, in her ethnographic work with sufferers of cardiovascular disease, Janet Shim discovered that understandings of intersectionality are alive and well among laypeople of color. Shim, "Race, Class, and Gender across the Science-Lay Divide." On the implications of intersectionality for health, see also Schulz and Mullings, *Gender, Race, Class, and Health*. On health activism on behalf of women of color, see Avery, "Breathing Life into Ourselves"; Grayson, "Necessity Was the Midwife of Our Politics."

89. Yusuf et al., "Analysis and Interpretation of Treatment Effects," 94.

90. Star, "Sex Differences and the Dichotomization of the Brain," 114–15.

91. Robert Temple, interviewed by author; Pollack, "Drug to Treat Bowel Illness Is Approved by the F.D.A.," A12.

92. Marts, interview.

93. Simon, "Wanted: Women in Clinical Trials," 1517.

94. Fausto-Sterling, *Myths of Gender*, 269.

95. Fausto-Sterling, "Five Sexes."

96. Fausto-Sterling, "Five Sexes, Revisited," 22.

97. Alice Domurat Dreger, *Hermaphrodites and the Medical Invention of Sex* (Cambridge, MA: Harvard University Press, 1998)

98. Hirschauer, "Performing Sexes and Genders in Medical Practices"; Meyerowitz, *How Sex Changed*.

99. J. Butler, *Gender Trouble*; Haraway, *Simians, Cyborgs, and Women*, 127–48; Oudshoorn, *Beyond the Natural Body*; Clarke, *Disciplining Reproduction*; Fausto-Sterling, "Bare Bones of Sex: Part 1," 1493–95.

100. Oudshoorn, *Beyond the Natural Body*; Nelly Oudshoorn, "The Birth of Sex Hormones," in *Feminism and the Body*, ed. Londa Schiebinger, 87–117 (Oxford: Oxford University Press, 2000).

101. Judith Lorber, "Beyond the Binaries: Depolarizing the Categories of Sex, Sexuality, and Gender," *Sociological Inquiry* 66, no. 2 (1996): 143–59; Hirschauer, "Performing Sexes and Genders in Medical Practices"; Kessler, *Lessons from the Intersexed*; Katrina Alicia Karkazis, "Beyond Treatment: Mapping the Connections among Gender, Genitals, and Sexuality in Recent Controversies over Intersexuality" (Ph.D. dissertation, Columbia University, 2002); Meyerowitz, *How Sex Changed*.

102. Krieger, "Embodying Inequality," 296; Fausto-Sterling, "Bare Bones of Sex: Part 1." For an integrated model for the study of biological and social aspects of men's and women's health, see Chloe E. Bird and Patricia P. Rieker, "Gender Matters: An Integrated Model for Understanding Men's and Women's Health," *Social Science and Medicine* 48, no. 6 (March 1999): 745–55.

103. NIH, "Women's Mental Health and Sex/Gender Differences Research (PA-03-143)," June 20, 2003, http://grants1.nih.gov/grants/guide/pa-files/PA-03-143.html. This program announcement replaced a prior one that used the term *gender*, rather than *sex/gender*.

104. Karen Young Kreeger, "Sex-Based Longevity," *Scientist* 16, no. 10 (May 13, 2002): 34.

105. Sergey V. Nikiforov and Valery B. Mamaev, "The Development of Sex Differences in Cardiovascular Disease Mortality: A Historical Perspective," *American Journal of Public Health* 88, no. 9 (September 1998): 1348–53.

106. H. M. Richards, M. E. Ried, and G. C Watt, "Why Do Men and Women Respond Differently to Chest Pain? A Qualitative Study," *Journal of the American Medical Women's Association* 57, no. 2 (spring 2002): 79–81.

107. Reynolds Farley, "Racial Identities in 2000: The Response to the Multiple-Race Response Option," in *The New Race Question*, ed. Perlmann and Waters, 33–61; Harris and Sim, "Who Is Multiracial?"

CHAPTER TWELVE

1. Valerie Jenness, "Social Movement Growth." See also Jenness, "Managing Differences and Making Legislation"; Jenness and Grattet, *Making Hate a Crime*.

2. Skrentny, *Minority Rights Revolution*; Katzenstein and Reppy, "Rethinking Military Culture."

3. On the diffusion of repertoires and frames from one social movement to another, see chap. 1, n. 47. On the effects of policy legacies and path dependence on organizations, see chap. 1, n. 56. On the diffusion of organizational solutions, see chap. 6, n. 3.

4. Of course, possibilities for domain expansion vary depending on the institutional setting, so it can be dangerous to generalize about these processes. For example, U.S. courts may be particularly resistant to expanding the list of groups that count as "protected classes." Kenji Yoshino, *Covering: The Hidden Assault on Our Civil Rights* (New York: Random House, 2006).

5. Health politics in the city of San Francisco provides an interesting example of how the expansion of claims for medical attention can proceed through the subdividing of groups into smaller and smaller subunits. A document from 2001 from the city's HIV Prevention Planning Council that establishes "resource allocation guidelines" breaks down the "behavioral risk population" into eight clusters that are further subdivided to yield thirty-six categories. These include, for example, "MSM" (men who have sex with men), "MSM/F" (men who have sex with both men and women), "TSM" (transgender who have sex with men), "TSM/F" (transgenders who have sex with both men and women), "TSF" (transgenders who have sex with women), "TST" (transgenders who have sex with transgenders"), etc. The list is impressive from the standpoint of logical completeness. See San Francisco HIV Prevention Planning Council, "Behavioral Risk Populations, Estimated New Infections, and Resource Allocation Guidelines," 2001.

6. Kate Barnhart, "Adolescent Underrepresention in Clinical AIDS Research," in *Gender Politics of HIV/AIDS in Women: Perspectives on the Pandemic in the United States*, ed. Nancy Goldstein and Jennifer J. Manlowe (New York: New York University Press, 1997), 74–85, esp. 75.

7. Jenness and Grattet, *Making Hate a Crime*, 14.

8. Skrentny, *Minority Rights Revolution*.

9. Ibid. See also Kingdon, *Agendas, Alternatives, and Public Policies*, 202–3; D. Richards, *Identity and the Case for Gay Rights*.

10. Skrentny, *Minority Rights Revolution*, 12.

11. Jenness, "Managing Differences and Making Legislation," 560–61.

12. Skrentny, *Minority Rights Revolution*, 12, 315.

13. Anne Schneider and Helen Ingram, "Social Construction of Target Populations: Implications for Politics and Policy," *American Political Science Review* 87, no. 2 (June 1993): 334. See also James A. Morone, *Hellfire Nation: The Politics of Sin in American History* (New Haven, CT: Yale University Press, 2003).

14. Suzanne Haynes, interviewed by author.

15. Jonathan Margulies, "Embryos Get 'Human Subjects' Status in Charter of New Federal Panel on Research Protection," *Chronicle of Higher Education*, October 31, 2002.

16. Merton, "Exclusion of Pregnant, Pregnable, and Once-Pregnable People."

17. Linda A. Goodrum et al., "Conference Report: Complex Clinical, Legal, and Ethical Issues of Pregnant and Postpartum Women as Subjects in Clinical Trials," *Journal of Women's Health* 12, no. 9 (2003): 860; Sumner Yaffe, interviewed by author.

18. Catherine S. Stika and Marilynn C. Frederiksen, "Drug Therapy in Pregnant and Nursing Women," in *Principles of Clinical Pharmacology*, ed. Arthur J. Atkinson et al. (San Diego: Academic Press, 2001), 277.

19. NIH, Office of Research on Women's Health, "Conference on Biologic and Molecular Mechanisms for Sex Differences in Pharmacokinetics, Pharmacodynamics, and Pharmacogenetics," May 5, 1999, www4.od.nih.gov/orwh/pharmacology.html.

20. Duane Alexander, interviewed by author; Yaffe, interview.

21. FDA, "Draft Guidance for Industry on Establishing Pregnancy Registries," *Federal Register* 64 (June 4, 1999).

22. U.S. House of Representatives, 107th Congress, 2nd Session, S. 2328 and H.R. 4602.

23. Dorothy Roberts, *Killing the Black Body: Race, Reproduction, and the Meaning of Liberty* (New York: Pantheon, 1997); Monica J. Casper, *The Making of the Unborn Patient: A Social Anatomy of Fetal Surgery* (New Brunswick, NJ: Rutgers University Press, 1998); Katha Pollitt, "'Fetal Rights': A New Assault on Feminism," in *The Politics of Women's Bodies: Sexuality, Appearance, and Behavior*, ed. Rose Weitz, 2nd ed., 290–99 (New York: Oxford University Press, 2003).

24. Steven Epstein, "Sexualizing Governance and Medicalizing Identities: The Emergence of 'State-Centered' LGBT Health Politics in the United States," *Sexualities* 6, no. 2 (May 2003): 131–71.

25. Ronald Bayer, "AIDS and the Gay Movement: Between the Specter and the Promise of Medicine," *Social Research* 52, no. 3 (1985): 581–606.

26. Ronald Bayer, *Homosexuality and American Psychiatry: The Politics of Diagnosis* (New York: Basic, 1981).

27. Epstein, *Impure Science*, 62–66.

28. Jennifer Terry, "Agendas for Lesbian Health: Countering the Ills of Homophobia,"

in *Revisioning Women, Health, and Healing*, ed. Clarke and Olesen, 324. See also Terry, *American Obsession*.

29. Bopper Deyton and Walter Lear, "A Brief History of the Gay/Lesbian Health Movement in the U.S.A," in *The Sourcebook on Lesbian/Gay Health Care*, ed. Michael Shernoff and William A. Scott (Washington, DC: National Lesbian and Gay Health Foundation, 1988), 15.

30. Anthony J. Silvestre, "Gay Male, Lesbian and Bisexual Health-Related Research Funded by the National Institutes of Health between 1974 and 1992," *Journal of Homosexuality* 37, no. 1 (1999): 81–94. See also Ulrike Boehmer, "Twenty Years of Public Health Research: Inclusion of Lesbian, Gay, Bisexual, and Transgender Populations," *American Journal of Public Health* 92, no. 7 (July 2002): 1125–30.

31. Obviously this is a highly truncated account of the histories of LGBT health advocacy. See Epstein, "Sexualizing Governance"; as well as Deyton and Lear, "Brief History of the Gay/Lesbian Health Movement," 15–19; Patricia E. Stevens, "Lesbian Health Care Research: A Review of the Literature from 1970 to 1990," *Health Care for Women International* 13 (1992): 91–120; Epstein, *Impure Science*; Risa Denenberg, "A History of the Lesbian Health Movement," in *The Lesbian Health Book: Caring for Ourselves*, ed. Jocelyn White and Marissa C. Martínez, 3–22 (Seattle: Seal Press, 1997); Marj Plumb, "Blueprint for the Future: The Lesbian Health Advocacy Movement," in *The Lesbian Health Book: Caring for Ourselves*, ed. Jocelyn White and Marissa C. Martínez (Seattle: Seal Press, 1997), 362–77; Michael Scarce, *Smearing the Queer: Medical Bias in the Health Care of Gay Men* (New York: Harrington Park, 1999); Eric Rofes, foreword to *Smearing the Queer*, by Scarce, xi–xiv; Terry, "Agendas for Lesbian Health," 324–42; Viviane K. Namaste, *Invisible Lives: The Erasure of Transsexual and Transgendered People* (Chicago: University of Chicago Press, 2000), chap. 7; Eric Rofes, "Resuscitating the Body Politic: Creating a Gay Men's Health Movement," *Baltimore Alternative*, August 8, 2000, 21; Michael Scarce, editorial, "The Second Wave of the Gay Men's Health Movement: Medicalization and Cooptation as Pitfalls of Progress," *Journal of the Gay and Lesbian Medical Association* 4, no. 1 (2000): 3–4; Sarah Wilcox, "Framing AIDS and Breast Cancer as Lesbian Health Issues: Social Movements and the Alternative Press" (unpublished manuscript, Department of Sociology, University of Pennsylvania, February 2000).

32. Jocelyn White and Mark H Townsend, editorial, "Transgender Medicine: Issues and Definitions," *Journal of the Gay and Lesbian Medical Association* 2, no. 1 (1998): 3.

33. Namaste, *Invisible Lives*, 168.

34. Public Health Service Task Force on Women's Health Issues, "Women's Health," 73–106.

35. Deborah Bowen, Diane Powers, and Heather Greenlee, "Lesbian Health Research: Perspectives from a Research Team," in *The Lesbian Health Book*, ed. White and Martínez; Andrea L Solarz, ed., *Lesbian Health: Current Assessment and Directions for the Future* (Washington D.C: National Academy Press, 1999), viii. On the findings from the WHI concerning sexual orientation and women's health, see Barbara G. Valanis et al., "Sexual Orientation and Health: Comparisons in the Women's Health Initiative Sample," *Archives of Family Medicine* 9 (September/October 2000): 843–53.

36. Bowen, Powers, and Greenlee, "Lesbian Health Research"; Pat Dunn, interviewed by author; Haynes, interview. On the findings from this study concerning sexual orientation and women's health, see Patricia Case et al., "Sexual Orientation, Health Risk Factors, and

Physical Functioning in the Nurses' Health Study II," *Journal of Women's Health* 13, no. 9 (2004): 1033–47.

37. Peri Jude Radecic and Marj Plumb, "Lesbian Health Issues & Recommendations" (Washington, DC: National Gay and Lesbian Task Force Policy Institute, April 1993), 1, 12, 15.

38. Plumb, "Blueprint for the Future," 366.

39. Haynes, interview; Marj Plumb, "Undercounts and Overstatements: Will the IOM Report on Lesbian Health Improve Research?" *American Journal of Public Health* 91, no. 6 (June 2001): 873.

40. Mastroianni, Faden, and Federman, *Women and Health Research*, vol. 1.

41. Haynes, interview; Solarz, *Lesbian Health*.

42. Solarz, *Lesbian Health*, 6.

43. "Scientific Workshop on Lesbian Health 2000: Steps for Implementing the IOM Report," pamphlet (Washington D.C: Department of Health and Human Services, 2000), 1–3.

44. U.S. Department of Health and Human Services, *Healthy People 2010: Understanding and Improving Health* (Washington, DC: U.S. Government Printing Office, 2000).

45. Martin Rouse, assistant to DHHS Secretary Donna Shalala, made this observation at the Gay Men's Health Summit II, Boulder, CO, July 19–23, 2000 (author's field notes).

46. "LGBT Nixed in Fed Plan," *GLMA Report*, spring 2000, 1; Bob Roehr, "Master Plan for US Health Now Includes Gays," *San Francisco Gay and Lesbian Times*, January 27, 2000, 27; Rhonda Smith, "Healthy Criticism: Activists Complain Report Omits Gays," *Washington Blade*, February 25, 2000, 1, 21, 23.

47. Dunn, interview.

48. Martin Rouse, interviewed by author; Christopher Bates, interviewed by author; Haynes, interview; Dunn, interview.

49. Kathi Wolfe, "Gay Health Off Radar Screen of Bush HHS," *Washington Blade*, October 11, 2002.

50. Ibid.

51. Moreover, the push for greater emphasis on LGBT health research has continued in other venues. For example, the *American Journal of Public Health*, the official publication of the American Public Health Association, published a special issue on LGBT health in June 2001. Mary E. Northridge, editor's note, "Advancing Lesbian, Gay, Bisexual, and Transgender Health," *American Journal of Public Health* 91, no. 6 (June 2001): 855–56; Ilan H. Meyer, "Why Lesbian, Gay, Bisexual, and Transgender Public Health?" *American Journal of Public Health* 91, no. 6 (June 2001): 856–59. That same year, GLMA was granted formal admission by the American Medical Association as an AMA section for specialty societies.

52. NIH, "Behavioral, Social, Mental Health, and Substance Abuse Research with Diverse Populations," NIH program announcement PA-01-096, May 21, 2001.

53. According to one report, Allen was placed at the DHHS on the suggestion of presidential adviser Karl Rove, in order to promote the agenda of the Christian right within the agency. See Doug Ireland, "The Bush Theocracy," *LA Weekly*, January 14–20, 2005. Allen went on to become a key domestic policy adviser to President Bush. In March 2006, Allen was arrested by police in Maryland and charged with theft. John Files, "Former White House Aide Is Arrested on Retail Theft Charges," *New York Times*, March 11, 2006, A28.

54. A separate question is *whether* LGBT health is best promoted via the framework of

the inclusion-and-difference paradigm. I address this important issue in Epstein, "Sexualizing Governance."

55. Dunn, interview; Haynes, interview. On the operationalization of sexual orientation for health research purposes, see Randall L. Sell and Jeffrey Blake Becker, "Sexual Orientation Data Collection and Progress toward Healthy People 2010," *American Journal of Public Health* 91, no. 6 (June 2001): 876–82.

56. Edward O Laumann et al., *The Social Organization of Sexuality: Sexual Practices in the United States* (Chicago: University of Chicago Press, 1994).

57. I discuss the potential risks of such biologizing of sexual identity in the conclusion to this book as well as in Epstein, "Sexualizing Governance."

58. Terry, "Agendas for Lesbian Health," 338.

59. Indeed, part of the explanation for why lesbian health research seemed to take off ahead of (non-HIV-related) gay men's health research may be that, in the popular imagination, gay men are more "sexualized" than lesbians. As Pat Dunn, the former policy director for GLMA, observed: "I have heard political analysis that lesbians are easier to talk about: it's not as politically or socially unacceptable to talk about lesbian health issues, [while the perception is that] gay men's health issues have a lot to do with anal intercourse and that kind of thing." Dunn, interview.

60. Edward O. Laumann, Robert T. Michael, and John H. Gagnon, "A Political History of the National Sex Survey of Adults," *Family Planning Perspectives* 26, no. 1 (January–February 1994): 34–38; Julia A. Ericksen, *Kiss and Tell: Surveying Sex in the Twentieth Century* (Cambridge, MA: Harvard University Press, 1999); Janice M. Irvine, "'The Sociologist as Voyeur': Social Theory and Sexuality Research, 1910–1978," *Qualitative Sociology* 26, no. 4 (winter 2003): 451.

61. Steven Epstein, "The New Attack on Sexuality Research: Morality and the Politics of Knowledge Production," *Sexuality Research and Social Policy* 3, no. 1 (March 2006): 1–12.

62. Alan Fram, "House Rejects Bid to Block Sex Research," *Associated Press*, July 10, 2003.

63. "NIH Questions Researchers on AIDS Grants," *New York Times*, October 28, 2003; Jocelyn Kaiser, "NIH Roiled by Inquiries over Grants Hit List," *Science* 302, no. 5646 (October 31, 2003): 758.

64. Jennifer Block, "Science Gets Sacked," *Nation*, September 1/8, 2003, 5–6; Matt Smith, "Vicious Cycle: Federal Investigators Clear AIDS Prevention Programs of Wrongdoing—and Then Reinvestigate Them," *SF Weekly*, May 7, 2003.

65. Marie Cocco, editorial, "White House Wages Stealth War on Condoms," *Newsday*, November 14, 2002.

66. Gardiner Harris, "Morning-after-Pill Ruling Defies Norm," *New York Times*, May 8, 2004, 13. A subsequent decision to continue postponing licensing led to the angry resignation of Susan Wood, the FDA's assistant commissioner for women's health and director of the FDA's Office of Women's Health. See Harris, "Official Quits on Pill Delay at the F.D.A.," A12.

67. To put it another way, the failure to achieve biopolitical citizenship in this case is linked to the failure to achieve "sexual citizenship." On sexual citizenship for LGBTs, see, for example, Diane Richardson, "Sexuality and Citizenship," *Sociology* 32, no. 1 (February 1998): 83–100; Jeffrey Weeks, "The Sexual Citizen," *Theory, Culture and Society* 15, nos. 3–4 (1998): 35–52.

68. On the effects of "political opportunity structures" on the likelihood of activist

mobilization and success, see Kitschelt, "Political Opportunity Structures and Political Protest"; Doug McAdam, John D. McCarthy, and Mayer N. Zald, eds., *Comparative Perspectives on Social Movements* (Cambridge: Cambridge University Press, 1996); Sidney Tarrow, *Power in Movements: Social Movements and Contentious Politics* (Cambridge: Cambridge University Press, 1998).

69. Women in Congress continued to meet under that name, but they were deprived of the caucus office, its six-member staff, and its $250,000 annual budget. See Primmer, "Women's Health Research," 328.

70. "Women's Health Office Act Passes House Health Committee," *Sexx Matters: Research News from the Society for Women's Health Research*, summer 2002.

71. Kaufman and Connolly, "U.S. Backs Pediatric Tests in Reversal on Drug Safety," *Washington Post*, April 20, 2002, A3. More recently, the Bush administration also has sought to pull the plug on a long-planned Children's Health Study (a longitudinal study of one hundred thousand children), but in June 2006 a House of Representatives spending panel insisted the study remain in place. Jocelyn Kaiser, "NIH Gets Off to a Slow Start," *Science* 312, no. 5780 (June 16, 2006): 1585.

72. Advocates of women's health in Congress have introduced a Women's Health Office Act in the hope of extending the statutory authorization to the remainder of the women's health offices within DHHS agencies, so far without success. Society for Women's Health Research, "Women's Health Office Act Reintroduced in Senate," June 2003, www.womens-health.org/policy/Coalition/hot0603.htm (accessed July 14, 2003).

73. Bowker and Star, *Sorting Things Out*, 14. See also Kingdon, *Agendas, Alternatives, and Public Policies*, 201.

74. Margaret Weir, *Politics and Jobs*, 19. See also chap. 1, n. 56.

75. See http://crchd.nci.nih.gov/.

76. I return to these issue in the conclusion to this book. To some degree, congressional mandates require DHHS agencies to focus on health disparities. For example, in compliance with the Minority Health and Health Disparities Research and Education Act of 2000 (which transformed the NIH's Office of Research on Minority Health into the National Center on Minority Health and Health Disparities), the NIH is obliged to prepare a strategic plan on reducing health disparities; see *Minority Health and Health Disparities Research and Education Act of 2000*, P.L. 106–525, 108th Congress, 2nd session, November 22, 2000; NIH, *Strategic Research Plan and Budget to Reduce and Ultimately Eliminate Health Disparities*, vol. 1 (Bethesda, MD: National Institutes of Health, October 30, 2003), www.ncmhd.nih.gov/our_programs/strategic/pubs/Volume1_031003EDrev.pdf.

77. On how knowledge claims travel, see Latour, *Science in Action*; Steven Shapin, "Here and Everywhere: Sociology of Scientific Knowledge," *Annual Review of Sociology* 21 (1995): 306–8. On the complexities of the transnational extension of scientific materials, claims, and categories, see Lakoff, "Diagnostic Liquidity."

78. Health Canada, "Policy Issue from the Drugs Directorate: Inclusion of Women in Clinical Trials during Drug Development," September 25, 1996, www.hc-sc.gc.ca/dhp-mps/prodpharma/applic-demande/pol/women_femmes_pol_e.html.

79. Health Canada, "Inclusion of Women in Clinical Trials," November 1997, www.hc-sc.gc.ca/dhp-mps/prodpharma/applic-demande/guide-ld/clini/womct_femec_e.html.

80. Health Canada, "Health Canada's Gender-Based Analysis Policy," June 19, 2002, www.hc-sc.gc.ca/hl-vs/women-femmes/gender-sexe/policy-politique_e.html.

81. Health Canada, "About the Bureau of Women's Health and Gender Analysis," Decem-

ber 8, 2003, www.hc-sc.gc.ca/ahc-asc/branch-dirgen/hpb-dgps/pppd-dppp/bwhga-bsfacs/index_e.html.

82. Ruth Merkatz, interviewed by author.

83. Health Canada, "Policy Issue from the Drugs Directorate."

84. Health Canada, "Inclusion of Women in Clinical Trials."

85. Statistics Canada, "Ethnocultural Portrait of Canada," December 1, 2004, www12.statcan.ca/english/census01/products/highlight/Ethnicity/Index.cfm?Lang=E. Other questions on the census are used to identify members of "First Nations."

86. Angela Marrocco and Donna E. Stewart, "We've Come a Long Way, Maybe: Recruitment of Women and Analysis of Results by Sex in Clinical Research," *Journal of Women's Health and Gender-Based Medicine* 10, no. 2 (2001): 176.

87. Paula A. Rochon et al., "Reporting of Gender-Related Information in Clinical Trials of Drug Therapy for Myocardial Infarction," *Canadian Medical Association Journal* 159, no. 4 (August 25, 1998): 323.

88. Rathore and Krumholz, "Race, Ethnic Group, and Clinical Research," 763.

89. National Health and Medical Research Council of Australia, "Women, Clinical Trials Involving," June 2001, www.nhmrc.gov.au/hrecbook/02_ethics/46.htm.

90. For a sophisticated discussion by Dutch scholars of the issue of differences within subject populations, see Nicolien Wieringa et al., eds., *Diversity among Patients in Medical Practice: Challenges and Implications for Clinical Research* (Amsterdam: Universiteit van Amsterdam, 2005).

91. Mary Foulkes, interviewed by author.

92. On French data-collection policies with regard to race and ethnicity, see also De Zwart, "Dilemma of Recognition," 139.

93. Maurizio Bonati et al., "Closing the Gap in Drug Therapy," *Lancet* 353, no. 9164 (May 8, 1999): 1625.

94. European Commission, Enterprise Directorate-General, "Detailed Guidance for the Request for Authorisation of a Clinical Trial on a Medicinal Product for Human Use to the Competent Authorities, Notification of Substantial Amendments and Declaration of the End of the Trial," April 2004, http://eudract.emea.eu.int/docs/Detailed%20guidance%20CTA%20.pdf.

95. Xavier Bosch, "Pediatric Medicine: Europe Follows U.S. in Testing Drugs for Children," *Science* 309, no. 5742 (September 16, 2005): 1799.

96. FDA, "International Conference on Harmonisation; Guideline on Studies in Support of Special Populations: Geriatrics; Availability," *Federal Register* 59, no. 147 (August 2, 1994): 39399.

97. ICH Steering Committee, International Conference on Harmonisation of Technical Requirements for Registration of Pharmaceuticals for Human Use, "Draft ICH Consensus Principle: Principles for Clinical Evaluation of New Antihypertensive Drugs," March 2, 2000, 2.

CONCLUSION

1. On the importance of moving beyond simple notions of social movement "success," see Marco Giugni, "How Social Movements Matter: Past Research, Present Problems, Future Developments," introduction to *How Social Movements Matter*, ed. Giugni, McAdam, and Tilly, esp. xx–xxi.

2. On classification and standardization, see the references in chap. 1, nn. 32 and 50.

3. See chap. 1, nn. 35 and 64.

4. See chap.1, n. 39.

5. Paul Rabinow has described this phenomenon as the creation of "biosociality"; see Rabinow, *Essays on the Anthropology of Reason*, 91–111.

6. See the references in chap. 1, n. 42.

7. Latour, "Give Me a Laboratory."

8. My language here borrows from (but oversimplifies) Howard Winant's summary of the racial formation approach. See Winant, "Race and Race Theory," 182; and see also Omi and Winant, *Racial Formation in the United States.*

9. See my discussion of this concept in chapter 1, as well as the references in chap. 1, n. 13.

10. Frickel and Moore, "Prospects and Challenges."

11. Knorr Cetina, *Epistemic Cultures*, 10.

12. On the epistemic role of organizations, see Vaughan, "Rôle of the Organization."

13. See chap. 1, n. 19.

14. See chap. 1, n. 20.

15. Cathy Tokarsi, "For-Profit Research More Favorable in Drug Trials," Medscape Medical News, August 20, 2003, www.medscape.com/viewarticle/460329.

16. See Cohen, *Overdose*. For a perceptive analysis of the problem of adverse drug reactions, see also O. Corrigan, "Risky Business."

17. See my discussion of this issue in chapter 5.

18. On the distinction between efficacy and effectiveness in clinical trial methodology, see, for example, Piantadosi, *Clinical Trials*, 197–98. In a discussion of the NIH guidelines, Ann Hohmann and Delores Parron suggested in 1996 that the intent was precisely to focus attention on "effectiveness research," as opposed to "efficacy research." What I am proposing here is a move further in that direction. See Hohmann and Parron, "How the New NIH Guidelines," 853.

19. Bird and Rieker, "Gender Matters," 747. The study of the relation between social and biological factors in health has been promoted within the NIH by its Office of Behavioral and Social Sciences Research; see Christine A. Bachrach and Ronald P. Abeles, "Social Science and Health Research: Growth at the National Institutes of Health," *American Journal of Public Health* 94, no. 1 (January 2004): 22–28.

20. Schiebinger, *Has Feminism Changed Science?* 14–15, 118.

21. Shim, "Bio-Power and Racial, Class, and Gender Formation," 191.

22. For an intersectional approach to the study of various kinds of health disparities, see Schulz and Mullings, *Gender, Race, Class, and Health.*

23. Shim, "Race, Class, and Gender across the Science-Lay Divide," 178–82.

24. J. Stevens, "Racial Meanings and Scientific Methods," 1075–76.

25. I discuss some of the specific complications that arise when thinking about sexual identity within the rubric of the inclusion-and-difference paradigm in Epstein, "Sexualizing Governance."

26. Vogel, *Woman Questions*, 127.

27. Katzenstein and Reppy, "Rethinking Military Culture," 4–5.

28. For an excellent overview of debates concerning public participation in biomedical research, see Dresser, *When Science Offers Salvation.*

29. I review these developments and their implications in Epstein, "New Attack on Sexuality Research."

30. Society for Women's Health Research, public statement, "Society for Women's Health Research Statement on NIH Peer Review and Politicization of Research," 2003, www.cossa.org/CPR/SWHR.pdf.

31. In thinking about this debate over public participation, I am also influenced by Alan Irwin, *Citizen Science: A Study of People, Expertise and Sustainable Development* (London: Routledge, 1995); H. M. Collins and Robert Evans, "The Third Wave of Science Studies: Studies of Expertise and Experience," *Social Studies of Science* 32, no. 2 (April 2002): 235–96; Mark Elam and Margareta Bertilsson, "Consuming, Engaging and Confronting Science: The Emerging Dimensions of Scientific Citizenship," *European Journal of Social Theory* 6, no. 2 (2003): 233–51; Bruno Latour, "Why Has Critique Run out of Steam? From Matters of Fact to Matters of Concern," *Critical Inquiry* 30 (winter 2004): 225–48; Abby J. Kinchy and Daniel Lee Kleinman, "Democratizing Science, Democratizing Values," *Dissent* 52, no. 3 (summer 2005): 54–62.

32. Epstein, "New Attack on Sexuality Research." See also Epstein, *Impure Science*, 337–46.

33. Wylie has argued that this project requires extracting the "promising core" of feminist standpoint theory from its contested history and recasting it in nonessentialist terms. Wylie, "Why Standpoint Matters," 26–27. See also Haraway, *Simians, Cyborgs, and Women*, chap. 9.

34. Weisman, *Women's Health Care*, 88. I discuss the broader theme of cooptation of health movements in Epstein, "Patient Groups and Health Movements."

35. I discuss these concerns in more detail in Epstein, "Sexualizing Governance."

36. Wendy Brown, *States of Injury: Power and Freedom in Late Modernity* (Princeton, NJ: Princeton University Press, 1995), 196.

37. Morone, *Democratic Wish*, 1.

38. In recent years, critics have questioned not only identity politics, but the very utility of the analytical category of identity. For example, Rogers Brubaker and Frederick Cooper have proposed, in an insightful article that, unfortunately, may throw the baby out with the bathwater, that it is time to move "beyond identity." Brubaker and Cooper, "Beyond 'Identity.' " As Craig Calhoun has noted in a response, none of the authors' proposed substitute terms are adequate to the task. Craig Calhoun, "The Variability of Belonging: A Reply to Rogers Brubaker," *Ethnicities* 3, no. 4 (December 2003): 561. For a valuable discussion of how to retain the concept of identity though not in its "originary and unreconstructed form," see Stuart Hall, "Who Needs 'Identity'?" in *Questions of Cultural Identity*, ed. Stuart Hall and Paul DuGay (London: Sage, 1996), 1. On identity and difference, see also John Rajchman, ed., *The Identity in Question* (New York: Routledge, 1995); Kathryn Woodward, ed., *Identity and Difference* (London: Sage, 1997).

39. I. Young, *Justice and the Politics of Difference*, 11.

40. I. Young, "Polity and Group Difference," 264–65.

41. Ibid., 281–82. See also the references in chap. 3, n. 54.

42. Kymlicka, *Multicultural Citizenship*. A complex question here concerns the adequacy of a "rights-based" formulation to address issues of social justice and citizenship; see Gerald Doppelt, "Liberalism, Multiculturalism, and the Politics of Identity," *Applied Ethics* (1999): 149–62, esp. 150.

43. Eckenwiler, "Pursuing Reform in Clinical Research." For another example of the application of Young's framework to the case of the inclusion of women, see DeBruin, "Justice and the Inclusion of Women."

44. Skrentny, *Minority Rights Revolution*.

45. De Zwart, "Dilemma of Recognition," 138–39. De Zwart also described a third option, "replacement," in which government programs intended ultimately to benefit specific groups are framed using more inclusive categories—as in William Julius Wilson's call for broadly universal federal programs as the best means of helping the urban "underclass" (140).

46. De Zwart, "Dilemma of Recognition," 138–39. Whether or not De Zwart intended the Freudian resonances, the term *denial* seems appropriate to describe this latter strategy— especially in light of events in November 2005, when socially disenfranchised French citizens of Arab and African descent rioted and torched cars in Paris and throughout the country.

47. Fraser, "From Redistribution to Recognition?" On the politics of recognition, see also Charles Taylor, "The Politics of Recognition," in *Multiculturalism*, ed. Amy Gutmann, 25–73 (Princeton, NJ: Princeton University Press, 1994).

48. L. A Kauffman, "The Anti-Politics of Identity," *Socialist Review* 20 (January–March 1990): 68; Wendy Brown, "Wounded Attachments: Late Modern Oppositional Political Forms," in *The Identity in Question*, ed. Rajchman, 221. Here, of course, Brown is not using "therapeutic" in the clinical medical sense, but rather to refer to ideas of psychic healing.

49. Bernstein, "Celebration and Suppression," esp. 535.

50. Fraser, "From Redistribution to Recognition?"

51. Iris Marion Young, "Unruly Categories: A Critique of Nancy Fraser's Dual Systems Theory—Comment," *New Left Review*, no. 222 (March/April 1997): 147–60.

52. Todd Gitlin, *The Twilight of Common Dreams: Why America Is Wracked by Culture Wars* (New York: Metropolitan Books, 1995).

53. Crenshaw, "Mapping the Margins," esp. 93.

54. Haraway, *Modest_Witness@Second_Millenium*, 265.

55. Bernstein, "Celebration and Suppression"; Paul Lichterman, "Talking Identity in the Public Sphere: Broad Visions and Small Spaces in Sexual Identity Politics," *Theory and Society* 28, no. 1 (1999): 101–41; Bernstein, "Identity Politics."

56. Craig Calhoun, *Critical Social Theory: Culture, History and the Challenge of Difference* (Oxford: Blackwell, 1995), 219.

57. For an example, see Simon LeVay, *The Sexual Brain* (Cambridge, MA: MIT Press, 1993).

58. V. Taylor, *Rock-a-by Baby*, 168.

59. Tavris, *Mismeasure of Woman*, 169. For a defense of women's strategic use of biological essentialism in a particular context, see Linda M. Blum, *At the Breast: Ideologies of Breastfeeding and Motherhood in the Contemporary United States* (Boston: Beacon Press, 1999), 7.

60. Howard Winant, "Postmodern Racial Politics in the United States: Difference and Inequality," *Socialist Review* 20, no. 1 (January–March 1990): 121–47; Skrentny, *Ironies of Affirmative Action*, 225–31.

61. See the discussion in chapter 2, as well as Sander L. Gilman, *Difference and Pathology: Stereotypes of Sexuality, Race and Madness* (Ithaca, NY: Cornell University Press, 1985); Jennifer Terry and Jacqueline Urla, eds., *Deviant Bodies: Critical Perspectives on Difference in Science and Popular Culture* (Bloomington: Indiana University Press, 1995); Waldby, *AIDS and the Body Politic*; Scarce, *Smearing the Queer*; Terry, *American Obsession*.

62. Waites, "Fixity of Sexual Identities in the Public Sphere," 555.

63. Ian Hacking has referred to this phenomenon as "the looping effect of human kinds." See Hacking, *Social Construction of What?* 34.

64. Foucault, *History of Sexuality*, 1:101.

65. I. Young, *Justice and the Politics of Difference*, 156–91; Lichterman, "Talking Identity in the Public Sphere," 101–41; Chantal Mouffe, *The Return of the Political* (London: Verso, 1993), 84; Stuart Hall, "Conclusion: The Multi-Cultural Question," in *Un/Settled Multiculturalisms: Diasporas, Entanglements, 'Transruptions,'* ed. Barnor Hesse (London: Zed, 2000), 235; Steven Seidman, *Difference Troubles: Queering Social Theory and Sexual Politics* (Cambridge: Cambridge University Press, 1997).

66. Gayatri Chakravorty Spivak, "Subaltern Studies: Deconstructing Historiography," in *The Spivak Reader: Selected Works of Gayatri Chakravorty Spivak*, 2nd ed., ed. Donna Landry and Gerald MacLean (New York: London, 1996), 203–35.

67. S. Lee, Mountain, and Koenig, "Meanings of 'Race' in the New Genomics," 69. The authors make this point with reference to race, but I have broadened the argument by substituting *difference*.

68. Paul Krugman, "Little Black Lies," *New York Times*, January 28, 2005, A21.

69. In 1900, the gap in life expectancy between whites and blacks (males and females combined) born in that year in the United States was 14.6 years. By 1950, the gap had been reduced substantially but still stood at 8.3 years. As of 2002 (the last year for which data were available in 2006), the gap stood at 5.4 years. These data are from the 2004 version of the National Center for Health Statistics's annual report, *Health, United States* (www.cdc.gov/nchs/data/hus/hus04.pdf; for the most up-to-date figures, see www.cdc.gov/nchs/hus.htm).

70. For an insightful discussion of the distinction between "differences" and "disparities" in health, see Jonathan Kahn, "From Disparity to Difference." For a somewhat different analysis of this distinction, see Saif S. Rathore and Harlan M. Krumholz, "Differences, Disparities, and Biases: Clarifying Racial Variations in Health Care Use," *Annals of Internal Medicine* 141, no. 8 (October 19, 2004): 635–38.

71. See the NCMHD's Web site, www.ncmhd.nih.gov/, for more information on their activities.

72. Nancy Krieger, "Stormy Weather: Race, Gene Expression, and the Science of Health Disparities," *American Journal of Public Health* 95, no. 12 (December 2005): 2155–60.

73. For an excellent recent summary, see LaVeist, *Minority Populations and Health*. See also Geiger, "Health Disparities."

74. Smedley, Stith, and Nelson, *Unequal Treatment*, 5.

75. Jonathan Skinner et al., "Racial, Ethnic, and Geographic Disparities in Rates of Knee Arthroplasty among Medicare Patients," *New England Journal of Medicine* 349, no. 14 (October 2, 2003): 1350–59.

76. Risa Lavizzo-Mourey and James R. Knickman, "Racial Disparities—the Need for Research and Action," *New England Journal of Medicine* 349, no. 14 (October 2, 2003): 1379.

77. Richard M. Campanelli, editorial, "Addressing Racial and Ethnic Health Disparities," *American Journal of Public Health* 93, no. 10 (October 2003): 1624.

78. David Firestone, "Frist Points to Racial Inequities in Health Care," *New York Times*, January 9, 2003, A19. Frist had just replaced Senator Trent Lott as minority leader after the latter made comments that were widely seen as insensitive to African Americans.

79. The Minority Health and Health Disparities Research and Education Act of 2000

(which created the NIH's National Center on Minority Health and Health Disparities) required the DHHS's Agency for Healthcare Research and Quality to "annually submit to the Congress a report regarding prevailing disparities in health care delivery as it relates to racial factors and socioeconomic factors in priority populations," beginning in fiscal year 2003. *Minority Health and Health Disparities Research and Education Act of 2000*, P.L. 106-525, 108th Congress, 2nd session, November 22, 2000.

80. Committee on Government Reform—Minority Staff Special Investigations Division, U.S. House of Representatives, "A Case Study in Politics and Science: Changes to the National Healthcare Disparities Report" (Washington, DC: January 2004), 1. See also Jocelyn Kaiser, "Democrats Blast a Sunny-Side Look at U.S. Health Disparities," *Science* 303, no. 5657 (January 23, 2004): 451. The story of the leak by a DHHS employee is from M. Gregg Bloche, "Health Care Disparities—Science, Politics, and Race," *New England Journal of Medicine* 350, no. 15 (April 8, 2004): 1568–70.

81. Robert Pear, "Taking Spin out of Report That Made Bad into Good," *New York Times*, February 22, 2004, A12.

82. Ibid.

83. Bloche, "Health Care Disparities," 1568.

84. Quoted in Robert Steinbrook, "Disparities in Health Care—from Politics to Policy," *New England Journal of Medicine* 350, no. 15 (April 8, 2004): 1488.

85. For one review of studies of these latter questions, see David Benjamin Oppenheimer and Marjorie M. Shultz, "Gender and Race Bias in Medical Treatment," *Journal of Gender-Specific Medicine* 2, no. 4 (July 1999).

86. Denise Grady, "Little Access to Pain Drugs in Some Areas," *New York Times*, April 6, 2000; John O'Neil, "Disparities in Drug Availability," *New York Times*, May 11, 2004, D6.

87. Shostak, "Environmental Justice and Genomics."

88. Nancy Krieger, "Does Racism Harm Health? Did Child Abuse Exist before 1962? On Explicit Questions, Critical Science, and Current Controversies: An Ecosocial Perspective," *American Journal of Public Health* 93, no. 2 (February 2003): 194–99.

89. David R. Williams and Chiquita Collins, "Racial Residential Segregation: A Fundamental Cause of Racial Disparities in Health," *Public Health Reports* 116 (September–October 2001): 404–16.

90. Baird, "New NIH and FDA Medical Research Policies," 542.

91. Watanabe, "Amid Criticism, NCI Tries to Boost," 1, 4–5.

92. An important question in this regard concerns the extent to which disparities described as racial or ethnic are more correctly characterized as class-based. Researchers increasingly have demonstrated that race and class are independent as well as intersecting determinants of health and health disparities. As Smedley, Stith, and Nelson observe in the National Academy Press report, racial and ethnic "disparities are associated with socioeconomic differences and tend to diminish significantly, and in a few cases, disappear altogether when socioeconomic factors are controlled. The majority of studies, however, find that racial and ethnic disparities remain even after adjustment for socioeconomic differences and other healthcare access—related factors." Smedley, Stith, and Nelson, *Unequal Treatment*, 5.

93. *Minority Health and Health Disparities Research and Education Act of 2000*.

94. Bird and Rieker, "Gender Matters," 745–55; Krieger, "Embodying Inequality"; Duster, "Buried Alive"; Fausto-Sterling, "Bare Bones of Sex: Part 1"; Ossorio and Duster,

"Race and Genetics"; Simon J. Williams, "Medical Sociology and the Biological Body: Where Are We Now and Where Do We Go from Here?" *Health* 10, no. 1 (2006): 5–30.

95. C. Roberts, "Biological Sex?" 1–2.

96. Duster, "Buried Alive," 273. In the United States, conservative opponents to affirmative action have taken precisely this tack on a number of occasions, for example in an unsuccessful ballot initiative in California in 2003 that would have protected "racial privacy" by preventing the state of California from collecting or publishing any information related to the race or ethnicity of its citizens.

97. R. R. Chapman and J. R. Berggren, "Radical Contextualization: Contributions to an Anthropology of Racial/Ethnic Health Disparities," *Health* 9, no. 2 (April 2005): 147.

98. Yet another part of the answer (as reformers have suggested all along) involves increasing the number of *researchers* drawn from communities that suffer from health inequalities; see Amri Johnson, "Where Are the Black Scientists?" *Scientist* 19, no. 21 (November 7, 2005).

99. Heath, Rapp, and Taussig, "Genetic Citizenship," 157 (authors' original emphasis removed). I am adapting the authors' argument, which is about the related concept of "genetic citizenship."

pharmaceutical companies (*continued*)
information, 123; required to provide
pediatric information, 61; and sex-based
biology, 241; supporting inclusion,
54, 84, 279; supporting the SWHR,
84, 247; transnational dimensions,
152–54, 197–201, 276, 356n74; use of
unnecessarily high doses, 286
pharmaceutical drugs: efficacy versus
effectiveness, 286, 389n18; "gendering
of," 180; generic, 222–23; prominence of
United States in industry, 7; "racializing
of," 180; testing (*see* clinical research);
therapeutic index, 234. *See also specific
drugs*
Pharmaceutical Manufacturers Association, 84
Pharmaceutical Research and Manufacter-
ers of America (PhRMA), 106, 178–79,
223
pharmacodynamics, 237, 249
Pharmacogenetic Research Network, 226
pharmacogenetics, 374n106. *See also*
pharmacogenomics
pharmacogenomics, 138, 333n78; and racial
profiling, 225–27; and sex profiling, 252
pharmacokinetics, 237, 249
PHS 398 (grant application form), 130
physicians: as intermediaries between
patients and medical researchers, 195;
prescribing "off label," 224
Physicians' Health Study, 78, 100–101, 108,
143–44, 239, 290, 340n22, 378n29
Piantadosi, Steven, 104, 106, 114, 164
Pill, the, 40
Pinn, Vivian, as director of Office of
Research on Women's Health, 81, 174,
265; president of the National Medical
Association, 70–71, 81; role in relation
to Congress, 112; role in monitoring
inclusion, 150, 156, 165, 169, 172; on
women's health movement, 247
platform, 317n2, 325n58
Plumb, Marj, 265
policy: feedback, 25, 117, 273; legacies, 25,
117, 148, 273, 334n5; paradigm, 17, 318n3
political correctness, 9, 102–9 passim, 114,
207, 216, 235, 297, 315n22

political opportunity structures, 277,
386n68
politics of identity. *See* identity politics
politics of recognition, 293, 391n47
Polletta, Francesca, 58, 342n64
Pollitt, Katha, 245
populations: health disparity, 300;
homogenous or heterogeneous, 49–50;
medically distinguishable, 1; and niche
standardization, 135; priority, 124, 126;
special, 75, 95, 126, 173, 258–273 passim;
target, 261. *See also* clinical research,
with vulnerable or captive populations
Porter, Theodore, 350n54
Post-Fordism, 178
postpartum depression, 294
poverty, global, 199
Powell, Walter, 117
power, 284; in researcher-subject
relationship, 193–202
practices, 140, 281
pregnancy, 64, 261–63; registries, 262
Prescott, Heather Munro, 41
Primmer, Leslie, 77, 79, 81
principle of specificity, 36, 45–46
Proctor, Robert, 72, 329n35
prostate cancer, 229–30, 250
proxy: race used as (*see* racial profiling);
sex used as (*see* sex profiling)
Prozac, 179
Public Health Service (PHS), 42–43, 74
Public Health Service Task Force on
Women's Health Issues, 75, 119, 272
public participation. *See* participation, of
laypeople in scientific debate
Puerto Rico, 41

QT interval, 233, 249
Quetelet, Adolphe, 45
Quintiles, 198
quotas, 9, 109
quotas frame, 101–103

Rabinow, Paul, 21
race: approach to studying, 27–28; as
biological, 10, 204, 206–207, 228–29,
287 (*see also* differences, as biological);
census bureau definition, 148–49;

sex/gender, as hybrid term, 29, 254–55, 350n64

sex profiling, 11, 180, 281; lack of debate concerning, 234, 376n6; problems with, 248–55; relation to racial profiling, 204–205, 234–36, 255–56, 281; stereotyping, 248

sexual identity, 327n70, 386n57

sexuality, 270–71, 291, 327n70, 386n59; research on, 271

sexual orientation, 16; as biological, 270, 294; operationalizing of, 267, 269, 386n55; partial incorporation within paradigm, 263–71, 291

Shafir, Gershon, 321n26

Shalala, Donna, 87, 121, 265, 267

Shapin, Steven, 367n66

Sherman, Sherry, 57

Shim, Janet, 158, 164, 287, 381n88

Shostak, Sara, 299

sickle-cell anemia, 38, 212, 370n37

Simon, Viviana, 234, 252

Sims, J. Marion, 40

single nucleotide polymorphisms (SNPs), 212, 370n32

Skrentny, John David, 88, 147, 259–60, 316n27, 335n21, 350n47, 351n6

slavery, 36, 40, 194, 330n43, 370n22

Smart Mom Act, 262

Smith-Doerr, Laurel, 359n68

smoking, 140, 208–209, 369n19

Smoller, Sylvia, 110

Snow, David, 58

Snowe, Olympia, 76–84 passim, 167

social class, 39, 92, 143–44, 287, 300, 353n33

social justice, 11, 18, 44, 73, 90, 92, 102, 143, 146, 262, 282, 297

social movements, 20, 333n1; adopting similar critiques, 54; as classifiers, 91; and domain expansion, 259; "mediators," 88, 342n64; and medicalization of identity, 294; and organizations, 284; organizing around identities, 283; and political opportunity structures, 386n68; possessing fuzzy boundaries with the state, 88, 283; promoting inclusion, 54–58; sex-based biology as,

240. *See also* activism; framing; health advocacy; interpenetration; reform; *and specific movements*

social sciences, 192

social worlds, 12, 317n41

Society for the Advancement of Women's Health Research. *See* Society for Women's Health Research

Society for Clinical Trials, 106

Society for Women's Health Research (SWHR), 54, 141; defends autonomy of science, 289–90; founding of, 76; and medical school curricula, 176; promotes sex-based biology, 240–43, 251; and publication of subgroup analyses, 168–69; and study of sex differences, 234, 238, 240, 287; supported by pharmaceutical industry, 84, 247

socioeconomic status. *See* social class

solidarity, 294

Sosa, Aníbal, 196

Specialized Centers of Research on Sex and Gender Factors Affecting Women's Health, 242

special populations. *See* populations, special

standard human, 12, 30, 41, 47, 50, 66–68, 81, 87; and Fordism, 178; framing the critique of, 53–73; and pharmacogenomics, 226; replacement of, 135–54, 234; resistance to, 25, 91, 127, 231, 277; "typological" versus "statistical" conceptions of, 68, 338n58

standardization, 24–25; 127–28, 282–83, 350n52, 350n55; attitudes toward, 67–68; in European Union, 276; in medicine, 8, 45–50; of pharmaceutical drug development, 152, 276; of patients, 46–47; procedural, 111, 128–33; in science, 33, 324n50; by the state, 136. *See also* niche standardization

standpoint epistemologies, 316n36

Star, Susan Leigh, 22, 24, 91, 128, 172, 251, 324n49, 346n55, 350n52

Starr, Paul, 22

state, the: approach to studying, 20; bureaucratization of, 128, 291; influence of outside forces on, 127; infrastructural

CPSIA information can be obtained
at www.ICGtesting.com
Printed in the USA
FSHW011250100521
81314FS